The New Science of Medicine & Management

Jon A. Chilingerian • S. Abbas Shobeiri
Mark A. Talamini
Editors

The New Science of Medicine & Management

A Comprehensive, Case-Based Guide for Clinical Leaders

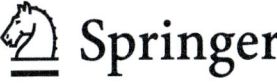

Editors
Jon A. Chilingerian
Heller School
Brandeis University
Newton, MA, USA

S. Abbas Shobeiri
INOVA Health System
Division Chief of Gynecology
Falls Church, VA, USA

Mark A. Talamini
Northwell Health
Senior Vice President and Executive Director Northwell Health Physician Partners
Great Neck, NY, USA

ISBN 978-3-031-26509-9   ISBN 978-3-031-26510-5   (eBook)
https://doi.org/10.1007/978-3-031-26510-5

© Springer Nature Switzerland AG 2023

This work is subject to copyright. All rights are reserved by the Publisher, whether the whole or part of the material is concerned, specifically the rights of translation, reprinting, reuse of illustrations, recitation, broadcasting, reproduction on microfilms or in any other physical way, and transmission or information storage and retrieval, electronic adaptation, computer software, or by similar or dissimilar methodology now known or hereafter developed.

The use of general descriptive names, registered names, trademarks, service marks, etc. in this publication does not imply, even in the absence of a specific statement, that such names are exempt from the relevant protective laws and regulations and therefore free for general use.

The publisher, the authors, and the editors are safe to assume that the advice and information in this book are believed to be true and accurate at the date of publication. Neither the publisher nor the authors or the editors give a warranty, expressed or implied, with respect to the material contained herein or for any errors or omissions that may have been made. The publisher remains neutral with regard to jurisdictional claims in published maps and institutional affiliations.

This Springer imprint is published by the registered company Springer Nature Switzerland AG
The registered company address is: Gewerbestrasse 11, 6330 Cham, Switzerland

This book is dedicated to the memory of Professor Jon Chilingerian and his surviving wife, Dianne, and children. Jon, better known as Professor Fantastico by his students, was a force of nature. He led innovation at the frontiers of health care and management with unmatched passion and insight. Central to jon's impact was his clear moral compass, teaching, and training his students that the business of medicine is nothing if it does not solve for the health and care of people, above simply a profit motive.

Heller Social Impact MBA was launched with Jon's leadership in 1998. Stuart Altman had brought Jon to the Heller School and was a wonderful colleague and dear friend. In 2016 Jon led the launch of the Executive MBA (EMBA) for physicians. The EMBA program has graduated over 200 physician leaders advancing the frontiers of health care in the United States and worldwide. Jon was a national leader in working with medical societies to advance professional development for physicians, including work with the American College of Surgeons, the

Thoracic Surgery Foundation for Research and Education, the European Health Leader's Program, and the Advanced Health Policy and Leadership Academy in partnership with the Hanley Center in Maine. Jon brought practical expertise to his studies, building on his service before graduate school as Assistant Health Commissioner for the City of Boston. In addition to his continued work advancing practice, Jon served as a leader among scholars, including being past-chair of the Health Care Management Division of the Academy of Management, the 2010 recipient of the Myron Fottler Exceptional Service Award for the Academy of Management, and the 2016 recipient of the Dr. Royce Laycock Recognition of Excellence Award, American College of Surgeons, Association for Surgical Education. Jon was awarded the Heller Teaching Excellence Award based on enthusiastic votes by EMBA students.

As a scholar, Jon coauthored International Health Care Management in 2005 and The Lessons and the Legacy of the Pew Health Policy Program, published in 1997. He published scholarly papers and review essays in journals such as Annals of Operational Research, Medical Care, European Journal of Operational Research, Health Services Research, Health Care Management Review, Medical Care Research and Review, Inquiry, Health Services Management Research, and the Journal of Health Politics, Policy, and Law. He pioneered using Data Envelopment Analysis in health care, advancing quality, productivity, and technical change in orthopedic, cardiac, and breast cancer surgeries. Jon brought Heller the Agency for Healthcare Research and Quality (AHRQ) predoctoral fellowships. This work has greatly impacted the direction of health services and policy research nationally and internationally.

As book co-editors and on behalf of the book chapter authors, we were fortunate to work closely with Jon on compiling this book. We feel honored to be part of his long-lasting legacy.

Foreword I

It is a pleasure to write a forward for this wonderful compilation of projects that advance the new science of medicine and management. The essays that appear in this manuscript were written by senior physicians who were students in Brandeis University's Executive MBA physician program (EMBA). It also includes an introductory article by the Executive Director of the program and the principal editor of the manuscript, Professor Jon Chilingerian.

This book is the outcome of the students' 18 team consulting projects. Each of the projects was problem-driven and had a purpose—to improve medical care by creating "value." The discovery and interpretation of the problems, the methods, conclusions, and lessons came solely from the students. I believe the findings from their work are significant and come at a crucial point in the development of clinical leaders in medical care. They also highlight the new and emerging science of medicine and management.

As these essays demonstrate, it is possible to generate value for patients in terms of excellent clinical outcomes and improved patient experience, value for caregivers and staff, value for health care organization, and to do so while improving the efficiency of how health care services are provided.

The importance of fostering more efficiency and value in the way we organize and implement the delivery of health care has never been greater. While the US health care system has been able to provide high-quality health care to most of its population, it has done so by spending large amounts of money in an inefficient system. The United States spends about twice as much per capita as the average industrialized country; however, on many measures of health, Americans do not measure up to those in other countries [1].

This era of big spending may be coming to an end, as government at both the national and state levels are limiting what they will pay for care, and the populations that they provide coverage for are increasing. If we do not improve the efficiency of our delivery system, these lower spending rates could lead to less access to care and/or lower quality of the care provided.

When the Medicare and Medicaid programs were enacted to help pay for the care of our aged and low-income populations, they were required to pay rates to hospitals and physicians that were similar to what was paid by private insurance. Within a few years, legislation was passed that allowed states to develop new Medicaid payment systems for the care of their low-income populations which, in many cases, were significantly less than private rates. Medicare, however, continued to pay rates that were close to what hospitals and physicians received from private carriers. This is no longer the case. As late as 2002, Medicare payments to hospitals were close to the average cost of treating a Medicare patient, and for many hospitals Medicare payments generated a positive operating margin. However, by 2021, Medicare payments were significantly less than private rates and the average hospital witnessed negative margins of more than 11%. Even big teaching hospitals, which receive extra funding for training new physicians, showed significant negative margins [2].

Fortunately for hospitals, they have been able to maintain positive overall margins by receiving significantly higher payments from private patients, which average over 80% higher than Medicare rates [3]. Currently, there is little incentive to provide care efficiently at lower costs. How much longer will private insurers be able to pay these private rates is open to debate. This will become even more difficult in the coming decade as most of the growth in patient care will come from the growth in the populations covered by Medicare and Medicaid, not private insurance [4]. This is why the need to develop a more efficient health care system is so important.

The editors have structured the book into four components: the value of good physician management, the importance of good physician leadership, the use of technical innovation to improve value and patient experiences, and the importance of improving clinical efficiency to lower costs. The 20 chapters offer the reader an excellent road map on how to plan for the future of a health care system that can produce high-quality care with lower rates of spending than we have seen in the past.

These are lessons we must learn.

References
1. OECD, Health at a Glance, OECD November 9, 2021.
2. Medpac, March 2020 Report to Congress, Pg. 90.
3. Op. Cit., Pg. 82.
4. CMS, National Health Expenditure Projections, January 2020.

The Heller School for Social Policy and Management   Stuart H. Altman
Brandeis University
Waltham, MA, USA

Foreword II

This book on the science of medicine and management is written largely by physician leaders. Each chapter is devoted to medical practitioners dedicated to developing solutions to the many challenges facing the health care system. I have had the privilege of working with Dr Chilingerian in his capacity as one of the country's leading experts in physician leadership for over a decade. In a time where health care transformation is occurring at warp speed and physician leadership is paramount to influencing the best possible outcomes in health care and the economy, his knowledge and expertise is unprecedented.

This book represents a commitment to ensuring there is a strong pipeline of physicians who are prepared to lead in this transformation. The cases underscore the value of physician leadership and is the reason the Physicians Foundation is so committed to helping train physicians to lead.

Dr Chilingerian has spent the majority of his career teaching physicians about leadership and managing health care organizations. His compassion toward his students is unparalleled, and he truly motivates physicians to take on leadership responsibility and more "ownership" on how the health care system evolves. His boundless energy and enthusiasm, combined with his expertise and commitment to academic rigor, breeds success.

The Physicians Foundation is thinking strategically about how it can help shape the future of health care policy and management and by implementing bottom-up initiatives and innovations that refocus daily actions and behaviors. To effectuate that change requires a cadre of physician leaders, catalysts, and cocreators. The foundation believes that the missing link has been the deep engagement of physicians leading change. Today, physician leaders understand the importance of creating value not only for patients and communities, but also for the well-being of caregivers and staff.

A critical step in health reform is giving physicians the permission as well as the education and training to rethink their clinical services and processes of patient care. We want healthy and sick patients to obtain better quality, better experiences, and lower costs. Rather than waiting for administration to initiate a project, physicians have to take the lead and work with administration to fix simple as well as more complex problems because it is just the right thing to do for their patients, their colleagues and staff, and the medical care organizations in which they practice medicine.

The Physicians Foundation is a mission-driven organization with four pillars:

- Pillar 1: The Social Drivers of Health
- Pillar 2: Physician Wellness
- Pillar 3: Physicians' Perspectives of the Delivery of Health Care
- Pillar 4: Physician Leadership and Change

These pillars are our vision, what we aspire to do to help improve the health care system. This book fits with our belief that physicians can play a key role in creating high-value care. In order to do that, we need to scale the number of well-trained MDs who know what to do to help their medical practices and organizations perform. No doubt this book contains many examples of physician leadership and is invaluable to anyone who has a leadership role in health care.

The Physicians Foundation Robert W. Seligson
Raleigh, NC, USA

Preface

Countries around the world entrust the health and wellness of their population to autonomous public and private caregivers,[1] medical care organizations, and systems. If these caregivers and organizations perform poorly, there will be significant social impacts. Medicine's purpose is to care for patients and keep communities healthy, and its vision is to create value.

Today "value" means the simultaneous pursuit of improving patient outcomes and experiences, lowering long-term costs, and taking responsibility for the wellness of the caregiver workforce. Value is not about quality or technical outcomes alone, any more than it is about prices and costs alone, although both of these are constraining factors. Further, if value requires satisfying human needs and wants, success in achieving value may always present a moving target.

This book describes what physician leaders need to know and do to fix problems that can erode value in the complex health care environments in which they practice medicine. Hospital readmissions, inefficiency, poor care coordination, and costly but unnecessary services that do not improve health weaken value. Improving patient outcomes, safety, affordability, and employee well-being restore value.

When value is restored and maintained, clinical leaders succeed. Success requires leaders with fortitude—that is, the ability to tolerate managing the change of difficult, complex processes and to persevere when situations become unpleasant without giving way.

Taken as a whole, the book offers a grand tour of what the three editors call the blossoming new science of medicine and management—the concepts, methodologies, techniques, and tools that create value for patients, populations, caregivers and staff, and the health care organizations.

Every chapter in this book is about physician-led change. There are nearly 200 physician-led EMBA physician projects that could have been included. This book chronicles 18 of those physician-led projects. The book is based on the collective efforts and experiences of its 33 authors and coauthors, 28 of whom are physicians,

---

[1] When we use the word "caregiver," we are referring to all of the clinical professionals who care for patients, including physicians, nurses, other clinical practitioners and staff who have direct contact with patients and their families.

and 19 of whom have an MD and MBA degrees.[2] Their willingness and ability to work hard and to record their first-hand, lived experiences as physician leaders made this book possible.

These physician authors were action researchers[3] directly involved in the planned change. They take a problem-driven and data-driven approach, putting the concepts, tools, techniques, and skills of the science of medicine and management into practice. The essential contribution of each chapter is in the lessons learned for the physicians and now also for the readers.

Nearly every chapter describes a physician-led project, and after the introductory chapter, the book is divided into four parts.

Chapter 1 Introduction to the New Science of Medicine and Management
Part I: The Well-Managed Health Care Organization: Building Implementation into Strategic Thinking
Part II. Physicians Leading and Implementing Change: Improving Operating Strategy and Changing Culture While Overcoming Organizational Inertia
Part III: Value Creation in Health Care I: Improving Technical Outcomes and Patient Experience
Part IV: Value Creation in Health Care II: Improving Clinical Efficiency and Lowering Costs

Chapter 1 is an introduction written by the lead editor. To title of this book, *The New Science of Medicine and Management*, required some explanation and a little background. The aim, scope, and purpose of medicine and management as a discipline are discussed. Medical care organizations increasingly depend on the leadership of every physician every day, challenging assumptions, practice behaviors, and systems of authority. While there are many new and complicated tasks ahead, perhaps the most critical task is integrating medicine and management into a discipline to guide clinical leaders and the future of health care.

---

[2] Each year about 30 physicians enroll in a 16-month executive MBA program for physicians at Brandeis University. The program attracts eminent physicians from all over the United States as well as internationally. The curriculum meets all the requirements to obtain an MBA accredited by AACSB and one of the requirements is to undertake an executive team consulting project. The project's five stated objectives were:

1. Develop a change management initiative that is at the nexus of medicine and management science
2. Build a cross-functional collaborative team committed to the goals of your leadership challenge
3. Practice applying concepts and knowledge acquired during the Brandeis EMBA program (see Appendix A)
4. Gain insight and direction by using your colleagues as sounding boards, sources of feedback, information, and advice
5. Be a high-impact clinical leader with a proven track record of effectiveness by implementing a successful change

[3] Virtually every chapter is an action-research project except Chaps. 1, 2, 10, and 11, which are case studies. The authors of the other 16 chapters create an organizational change and study the process.

Part I

Part I describes two cases of a well-managed health care organization. Chapter 2 (Chilingerian, Reinhorn, and Sbayi) describes and analyzes the case of Shouldice Hospital, an 89-bed hospital specializing in abdominal wall hernias and recurrent hernias. This hospital not only offers a high-quality hernia repair with a lifetime guarantee, outstanding patient experience, and caregiver satisfaction but also efficient, low-cost services for patients and payers. Shouldice exemplifies a well-managed organization and how the new science of medicine and management works in practice.

Chapter 3 (Nuki) reports on an underperforming rural hospital struggling financially to survive and the actions taken for the turnaround. The first responsibility of its clinical leaders is to improve quality and patient satisfaction while generating enough revenue to cover current and future costs. Rather than slashing prices, the physicians focus on improving decision-making efficiency, reducing patients who leave the emergency room without being seen, and implementing better management practices. The physicians also address cultural and relational issues needed to improve overall performance. The case reveals how a poorly managed hospital destroys value for patients, caregivers, and staff, resulting in financial loss and even a potential for bankruptcy.

Part II

Part II chronicles physicians leading and implementing clinical and managerial change. The breadth of clinical problems addressed includes on-time surgical starts and operating room turnover; early extubation in perioperative management following congenital heart surgery; postoperative feeding protocols for surgical patients with hypertrophic pyloric stenosis, and what newly appointed chief medical officers do during their first 3–4 months.

Chapters 4 and 5 take on the challenge of improving operating room (OR) performance while teaching lessons on changing surgical cultures. Chapter 4 (Tomashev, Alsheik, and Shobeiri) describes the complex metrics that must be managed in the OR: protocol compliance, canceled cases, average room readiness times, delayed first case starts, average room induction/extubation, and turnover times. They apply lean principles and root cause analysis to identify inefficiencies in patient flow and demonstrate the importance of creating cross-functional teams and relational mapping.

Chapter 5 (Chen) tackles the performance of the operating room and on-time starts with the realization that it required changing the surgical culture and the authoritative political system. Because surgery is busy and generating revenue, there was a strong need to motivate people to want to change current practices to create more value.

The change management team analyzed the organizational structure using the relational coordination theory. They identified the current state as a "shame and blame" culture, with infrequent communication and weak interactions among the caregivers and staff. They crafted the desired state to be a surgical culture with shared values, mutual respect for caregivers and staff, more frequent communications, and increased trust. They describe how they embedded these new values and proposed new solutions.

Utilizing relational mapping, observation, and interviews revealed that the "administration" had tasked nurses with enforcing surgeon compliance. That meant nurses were caught in the middle, and it affected nursing morale.

Physicians were not responding to nurse requests; the team realized that surgeons needed "social proof." The principle of social proof hypothesized that if another "trusted" surgeon organized frequent huddles and requested that they follow new practices, most surgeons would be more likely to respond. The project team experimented with a new boundary-spanning role—called "physician of the day" (POD). With the POD communicating with other physicians and changing the surgical culture and relationships among stakeholders on-time starts increased coordination and patient flow improved.

The sixth chapter (Polimenakos) implemented early extubation protocols and fast-track strategies to improve patient outcomes for pediatric heart surgery. They applied time-driven activity-based costing to present the cost and value advantages. It turned out that the logic of the change was necessary but not sufficient.

They did not start with an explanation of the rationale of early extubation. In contrast, they engaged the team to explore the problem and discover what might improve pediatric heart surgery outcomes while reducing costs. To anchor the change into the care program, they relied on collaborative team building and fair process leadership.

Chapter 7 (Fischer) underscores how minimizing the variability of a postoperative feeding regimen by standardization can improve patient experiences, enhance patient recovery, shorten hospital stays, and lower costs. Prior to this project, clinical pathways were randomly set according to the habits and practices of each attending surgeon. By going into the frontlines of clinical service, the clinical leaders and team learned that nurses were not "empowered" to move patients along the prescribed pathway. The attending surgeon insisted on using their "favorite" feeding program, blocking the nurses on any given day. The multi-disciplinary change team developed an intervention, and the experiment was successful.

Chapter 8 (Tracy) reflects on what a physician needs to know and do during the first 3–4 months when appointed chief medical officer (CMO) at a major medical center. The Dean wanted a redesign of care programs to provide better patient access to primary and specialty care. The chapter describes a fair process model of leadership that starts by engaging relevant stakeholders, exploring problems and brainstorming new ideas, discussing and explaining the rationale for solutions, and setting expectations for results. At the end of the 3–4 months, the newly appointed CMO could (1) build commitment to future goals and (2) establish working relationships with key stakeholders as future allies.

Part III

Part III is about value creation to improve technical outcomes and patient experiences. Some serious patient safety challenges are being addressed in these seven chapters: reducing catheter-associated urinary tract infections, prolonged intubation, surgical site infections, perioperative myocardial events, informed consent in procedural sedations, and care for neonates with congenital heart disease. This section also describes how community-based primary care can help the United States deal with the public health opioid crisis, and team-based care can create value in primary care. The last two chapters deal with creating a complex cranial surgical center and a robotic program in a safety net academic hospital.

Chapter 9 (Talamini and Tassiopoulos) describes the roll-out of standardized NSQIP measures of risk-adjusted outcomes in a surgery department. They were using a data-driven "learning from outliers" analysis. Four areas were identified as having "unimpressive" patient results. To improve outcomes, they built a multi-specialty team with key stakeholders, including a surgeon champion, NSQIP nurses, information technology (IT) specialists, and quality management staff, reporting to a four-person executive team. Although they developed strategies, tactics, and new protocols in each of the four areas. After the first year, there was no improvement; however, critical lessons were learned.

One of the powerful insights in this chapter was that risk-adjusted NSQIP measures are not evaluating surgeon performance. They evaluate a surgical system consisting of people, care processes, behavioral norms, and hidden internal problems such as poor coordination and/or weak incentives. They also learned that the change initiative needed to be more inclusive—engaging more surgeons, as well as anesthesiologists, nurses (from the OR, recovery rooms, and floors), and people from IT. Another insight was recognizing that risk-adjusted measures are suitable for identifying problems but not for clinical and managerial control. The data was clinically accurate but not timely—the data arrived 6–12 months later. They had to develop a dashboard to track results in real-time.

Chapter 10 (Larson and Agarwal-Harding) is focused on the challenge of opioid addiction. The authors assessed the research on strong community-based networks as a clearinghouse for resources and action. These networks showed great promise to reduce death rates as they focus on the community ecosystems that can some of the social determinants of health, such as malnutrition, housing, transportation, and better access to Buprenorphine, a medication for heroin addicts.

Chapter 11 (Larson) makes a compelling case that highlights evidence on how team-based primary care can add value to patients, caregivers, and organizations. Team-based models that adopt and assimilate (1) co-location workstations, (2) pre-visit planning, (3) morning huddles, and (4) four-stage office visits can increase and boost patient engagement and workforce morale. If the implementation is effective, the model can enhance patient flow and improve patient outcomes. Most importantly, team-based primary care can increase the time a physician spends with patients and help to close the gaps in primary care.

Chapter 12 (Schears and Bellolio) confronts the challenge of educating physicians about serious adverse events following procedural sedation. After diagnosing the problem, they surfaced a need to improve the informed consent procedure. They studied the literature and developed an intervention to evaluate caregiver knowledge, training on patient safety, and a post-test. Using a Delphi method, they created a visual aid to supplement the physician-patient informed consent conversation.

Chapter 13 (Pelletier) explores the factors that can help parents choose a care program (surgeon and hospital) for neonates diagnosed with congenital heart disease. The team learned that payer contracts (15%) were less important than physician referrals (73%) and the parent's choice (89%). Upon reflection, valuable lessons were learned about teams, coordination, and the importance of leadership style.

The last two chapters of Part III discuss how to obtain center of excellence (COE) status for surgical programs. Chapter 14 (Kandregula, Demand, Ingraffia, Trosclair, and Guthikonda) discusses how to employ a value innovation process to become the premier intracranial surgery center in Louisiana. The "blue ocean" case identifies what to eliminate and reduce to raise and create value for patients, caregivers, staff, and the institution. Creating value (better decision-making, outcomes, convenience, relationship with caregivers, and overall patient experience) requires a multidisciplinary center. Creating a COE required a new organizational design. Oncology, Neurology, Radiology, and Endocrinology needed to move into one center around a core team from (1) ENT, (2) Interventional Neuroradiology, and (3) Oral Maxillofacial Surgery.

Chapter 15 (Johnson and Danner) also describes the process for becoming a center of excellence (COE) for a robotic surgery program at a safety net hospital. The case for developing the program for patients of lower socioeconomic status is clear—reducing disparities, fewer complications, shorter lengths of stay, decreased narcotics use, and better patient experience. Earning that designation also affects the institution's operating efficiency, finances, and long-term costs. How do you build support for this vital program?

Along the way, there were unexpected challenges—loss of executive support, concerns from surgeons and managers that the costs would be prohibitive, and loss of other supporters. This social impact case reveals the importance of adaptive leadership, drawing on the concepts and tools of medicine and management.

Part IV

The final section, Part IV, focuses on value creation aimed at clinical and managerial efficiency to lower patient care costs. These chapters take on what the Japanese call "Muda," or waste. The chapter teaches us how to fix clinical programs that are costly, error-prone, and lead to the low morale of all stakeholders. The clinical focus is on anatomic and physiologic testing to assess vascular pathologies, primary care testing; improving cholecystectomy, abdominal hernias, varicocelectomy, and artificial urinary sphincters; pediatric surgical cancellations; and radiographs of pediatric wrist and forearm fractures.

Chapter 16 (Lipsitz) discusses the implications of justifying, adopting, and assimilating an advanced data management and imaging system in a non-invasive vascular lab. The investment of $1.1 million is a "big ask." The question is, *what economic value does this innovation give the vascular lab?* The project employed time-driven activity-based costing, cash flow, and net present value.

The project is instructive as an analytic demonstration of fixed and variable cash outflows, revenue projections, and a net present value calculation. What is revealed, however, is a concept of productivity that can be defined as equipping the vascular lab with human and material resources with new value-adding capacity. Making the lab more productive requires creating an excess of benefits for patients and lab employees that exceeds the cost of this innovation. Other vital lessons are leveraging relationships and using relational coordination and boundary spanners to manage the key stakeholders.

Chapter 17 (Savarise and Kragen) assesses four common ambulatory procedures at two ambulatory surgical centers and one central hospital to identify best practices. Controlling for case mix (ASA scores of 3 or less and BMI of less than 50), the team found that three of four procedures had a shorter net average operating room time, lower costs and better patient satisfaction in the two ambulatory centers than the main hospital. Although the cost study revealed that shifting these cases to ambulatory centers would increase efficiency, lower costs, and improve patient experience, there was significant resistance. The chapter explains how the clinical leaders overcame the resistance by negotiating and building coalitions and solid political support.

Chapter 18 (Ariyabuddhiphongs and Kragen) is about reducing low-value care in population health. Though engaging physicians is essential to managing variations in practice behavior, so is the selection of the problem. They selected four lab tests (Vitamin D, cholesterol, thyroid-stimulating hormone, and chemistry that was costing $3 million annually. Building a small team, they (1) combed the literature, (2) developed clinical guidelines for testing, (3) studied lab utilization behavior, and (4) identified the top 25 physician utilizers for each of the four tests.

They created an intervention where one group received monthly meeting reminders and performance reminders, and two groups received less intense follow-ups. The group with the most intense intervention reduced lab testing by 10 and 19% for two tests. The project learned that setting goals, giving feedback on utilization, and gently holding people accountable at monthly meetings can change physician practice behavior and improve population health.

Chapter 19 (Singh, Beijnen, and Taghinia) focuses on an overlooked inefficiency—late surgical cancellations. It is a well-known fact that the operating room is a high fixed-cost resource in the health care system. When they studied more than 10,000 surgeries, more than 440 (4%) were canceled less than 24 h before the surgery. They learned that 75% of preventable and possibly preventable could be attributed to the patient (often due to an illness) and 12% to the surgical team. They developed excellent recommendations that have a strong social impact on the cost of care.

Chapter 20 (Cruz) is the last in the book. His team studied one of the most prevalent emergency evaluations—pediatric forearm and wrist fractures. The team he led organized an excellent process improvement project to improve performance. They apply lean methods with a flow analysis and cost analysis to understand the impact of eliminating post-reduction radiographs on value. Utilizing mini-C-arm imaging and uploading images to the health record reduced unnecessary testing inefficiencies and improved cost control.

The author ends with two central ideas. First, with pressure to demonstrate value, minimizing those "unnecessary services" is low-hanging fruit for physicians. Second, clinical leaders can learn from experience by taking action, observing results, explaining what happened and why, and adapting future actions. His last sentence states:

> These projects can serve as examples on how to effect process change within health care organizations particularly within the context of the Plan-Do-Study-Act paradigm.

That quote reminds us that the Plan-Do-Study-Act paradigm applies the scientific method to every action-research project. Improvement is a continuous and relentless pursuit. And the quote hints at the importance of rapid experimentation and physicians becoming faster learners. We conclude this preface with a few summary comments.

Summary

Most of these projects discovered that acquiring new technology or adopting a clinical innovation or a care process improvement was not the most difficult part. The real challenge was in assimilating and anchoring the innovation or improvement in the culture, setting measurable strategic goals, and holding people accountable for the creation of real value. Many projects encountered the problem of obtaining the engagement and endorsement of the senior clinicians or changing the habits of clinicians who were resistors or part of a "buddy network." Another common problem was a medical culture of individualism and an autonomous department silos. These physicians could find a solution by drawing on relational coordination theory. Many of the projects identified and mapped vital stakeholder relations. This tool helped them to uncover hidden issues such as (1) disrespect for other caregivers and staff, (2) weak interpersonal communications with group dynamics, and (3) goal conflicts. These issues can block process improvement decision-making, collaboration, and working together as a team.

Each chapter has told a story, a contextual narrative, describing how physician leaders defined a shared clinical vision and tried to implement medical ideas that often challenged assumptions, practice behaviors, and systems of authority. The cases in this book are all about leading change and creating value in health care by improving outcomes, patient experience, and efficiency. They are contextual analyses based on the events, the people, and their experiences. Cases are an excellent way to teach physicians how to diagnose and reframe problems as opportunities, apply analytic concepts, and use a specific management technique or tool to find a solution.

We believe the cases have been reported accurately through the interpretive lens of the authors. And yet there is always the potential that the cases may be underanalyzed. There are and will be many new ways to reinterpret these case studies as we continue to learn about medicine and management as a discipline.

We hope that this book will help prepare present-day and future physicians for the practice of medicine and management. The health of every individual and society increasingly depends on physicians becoming the instruments of strategic direction, decision-making, and a higher order and people-centered leadership that enables health care organizations to perform in accordance with a more modern definitions of value that include innovation and cost efficiency while also protecting medicine's most important human and social values.

Newton, MA, USA Jon A. Chilingerian
Falls Church, VA, USA S. Abbās Shobeiri
Great Neck, NY, USA Mark A. Talamini

Acknowledgments

This book was a partnership and a truly collaborative effort. The original contributions of the 33 authors and coauthors of the 19 chapters became the basis for this book. We thank each of the 28 physician authors and 5 non-physician authors for their hard work and their patience.

We graciously thank Dr Stuart Altman, PhD, Sol C. Chaikin Professor of National Health Policy and former Dean of The Heller School for Social Policy and Management and Mr. Robert W. Seligson, MBA MA, the Chief Executive Officer of the Physicians Foundation. Dr Altman has dedicated his career to advancing federal and state health policy and helping medical care organizations. Mr. Seligson has dedicated his career to advancing health care innovation and promoting physician leadership. We were honored that they wrote the foreword to this book.

We owe a huge debt of gratitude to the EMBA Physician Program at the Heller School and all its faculty and staff. More importantly, eight individuals had a great influence on this project. Our sincere gratitude goes to two professors, Dr Sally Ourieff, MD, and Carole Carlson, M.CityPl., MBA who taught the Executive Team Consulting Projects, offering their questions and comments. Eighteen of these projects became Chaps. 3–20.

We thank Priya Agarwal-Harding, Corrie Holliday-Stocking, and Ben Kragen, three Brandeis University PhD. students. They used their health care expertise to read, edit, and critique several chapters. A heartfelt thanks to our wonderful EMBA team, Annalisa Valadez and Amy Dimattia. Both read, edited, and critiqued chapters and Amy provided much of the logistical support.

We are especially indebted to our colleague, Annalisa Valadez, who was our project manager. She contributed much to the development of this book—turning drafts into manuscripts, managing the entire editing process, organizing editor meetings, sending messages to the authors, and managing the deadlines.

We want to take very special notice of one more individual, Stephanie Frost, our Springer development editor. Stephanie performed yeoman's work editing and formatting the entire manuscript. This project was delayed owing to our 30 physician authors and editors being in the throes of COVID-19. Stephanie was beyond patient and for the three editors a source of continuous encouragement and inspiration. She is always so positive, optimistic, energetic, and competent.

Authoring manuscripts and editing a book takes time away from families. On behalf of the 33 authors, we acknowledge their families' support and forbearance. And to our spouses, Dianne Chilingerian, Eileen West, and Carol Talamini, we thank you.

To all our aforementioned colleagues—GRATITUDE.

Contents

1	**Introduction to the New Science of Medicine**........................ Jon A. Chilingerian	1

Part I The Well-Managed Health Care Organization: Building Implementation into Strategic Thinking

2	**Shouldice Hospital from Interviews and Observations: The Well Managed Organization**.. Jon A. Chilingerian, Michael Reinhorn, and Samer Sbayi	23
3	**Improving Leadership and Business Structures in a Rural Emergency Department**.. Guy Nuki	95

Part II Physicians Leading and Implementing Change: Improving Operating Strategy and Changing Culture While Overcoming Organizational Inertia

4	**Improving the Operating Room Efficiency through Communication and Lean Principles**........................... 111 Roni Tomashev, Jonia Alshiek, and S. Abbās Shobeiri	
5	**Implementing Change in Surgical Culture**........................ 135 Mike K. Chen	
6	**Fast Track Approach Following Heart Surgery in Infancy and Early Childhood: Implementation Strategy with Outcome and Cost Analysis**................................... 145 Anastasios C. Polimenakos	
7	**Decreasing Variance in Care: Implementation of Protocolized Postoperative Feeding as a Proxy for Discharge**.................. 163 Anne C. Fischer	

8	Institutional and Professional Transition: The Foundations of Business Management in the First 100 Days of a Chief Medical Officer 183
	Thomas F. Tracy

Part III   Value Creation in Health Care I: Improving Technical Outcomes and Patient Experience

9	National Surgical Quality Improvement Program (NSQIP) Improvements: A Case Study................................. 199
	Mark A. Talamini and Apostolos Tassiopoulos
10	Addressing America's Opioid Crisis through Community-Based Primary Care 211
	Heidi M. Larson and Priya Agarwal-Harding
11	Team-Based Care: A Foundation for Success in Value-Based Payment Models 225
	Heidi M. Larson
12	Impacting Risk Communication: Educating Providers to Improve Informed Consent Conversations in Procedural Sedation 237
	Raquel M. Schears and Fernanda Bellolio
13	Factors Influential in Seeking Care for Neonates with Congenital Heart Disease.................................... 251
	Glenn J. Pelletier
14	Creation of the LSU Health Shreveport Complex Cranial Surgical Center of Excellence: Needs Served, Process to Obtain, and Lessons Learned 261
	Sandeep Kandregula, Audrey Demand, Patrick Ingraffia, Krystle Trosclair, and Bharat Guthikonda
15	Obtaining Center of Excellence Accreditation of a Robotic Program in a Safety Net Academic Hospital 273
	Shaneeta M. Johnson and Omar K. Danner

Part IV   Value Creation in Health Care II: Improving Clinical Efficiency and Lowering Costs

16	Vascular Diagnostic Laboratory Improvements Through Effective Data Management................................... 293
	Evan C. Lipsitz
17	Use of Operations Management Tools to Improve Efficiency for Ambulatory Surgery Procedures........................... 317
	Mark Savarise and Ben Kragen

18	**Physician Engagement in Population Health: A Case Study in Project Selection and Practice Variation** 331
	Kim D. Ariyabuddhiphongs and Ben Kragen
19	**Late Surgical Cancellations in a Pediatric Surgical Practice** 343
	Vivek Singh, Usha E. A. Beijnen, and Amir H. Taghinia
20	**Routine Post-reduction Radiographs After Closed Reduction of Pediatric Wrist and Forearm Fractures Is Unnecessary: Effecting Process Change and Eliminating Waste in the Pediatric Emergency Department** 351
	Aristides I. Cruz Jr

Index 363

List of Contributors

Priya Agarwal-Harding, MA The Heller School for Social Policy and Management, Brandeis University, Waltham, MA, USA

Jonia Alshiek INOVA Women's Hospital, Falls Church, VA, USA

Department of Obstetrics and Gynecology, Holy Family Hospital, Nazareth, Israel

Stuart H. Altman The Heller School for Social Policy and Management, Brandeis University, Waltham, MA, USA

Kim D. Ariyabuddhiphongs Beth Israel Lahey Health Performance Network, Westwood, MA, USA

Usha E. A. Beijnen Department of Plastic and Oral Surgery, Boston Children's Hospital, Boston, MA, USA

Fernanda Bellolio Department of Emergency Medicine, Mayo Clinic, Rochester, MN, USA

Mike K. Chen Department of Surgery, Children's of Alabama Hospital, Heersink UAB School of Medicine, Birmingham, AL, USA

Jon A. Chilingerian (Deceased) Health Care Management, EMBA Physician and MD-MBA Programs, Institute for Health Systems, Heller School for Social Policy and Management, Brandeis University, Waltham, MA, USA

Public Health and Community Medicine, Tufts University School of Medicine, Boston, MA, USA

Aristides I. Cruz Jr Department of Orthopaedic Surgery, Hasbro Children's Hospital, Warren Alpert Medical School, Brown University, Providence, RI, USA

Omar K. Danner Department of Surgery, Morehouse School of Medicine/Grady Memorial Hospital, Atlanta, GA, USA

Audrey Demand Department of Neurosurgery, LSU Health, Shreveport, LA, USA

Anne C. Fischer Palm Beach Children's Hospital, West Palm Beach, FL, USA

Tenet Healthcare Corporation, Dallas, TX, USA

Charles E. Schmidt College of Medicine, Florida Atlantic University, Boca Raton, FL, USA

Bharat Guthikonda Department of Neurosurgery, LSU Health, Shreveport, LA, USA

Patrick Ingraffia Department of Neurosurgery, LSU Health, Shreveport, LA, USA

Shaneeta M. Johnson Department of Surgery, Satcher Health Leadership Institute, Morehouse School of Medicine, Atlanta, GA, USA

Sandeep Kandregula Department of Neurosurgery, LSU Health, Shreveport, LA, USA

Ben Kragen Heller School for Social Policy and Management, Brandeis University, Waltham, MA, USA

Heidi M. Larson Cape Elizabeth, ME, USA

The Heller School for Social Policy and Management, Brandeis University, Waltham, USA

Evan C. Lipsitz Division of Vascular and Endovascular Surgery, Department of Cardiothoracic and Vascular Surgery, Montefiore Medical Center and the Albert Einstein College of Medicine, Bronx, NY, USA

Guy Nuki BlueWater Health, Brunswick, ME, USA

Glenn J. Pelletier Nemours A. I. duPont Hospital for Children, Nemours Cardiac Center, Wilmington, DE, USA

Anastasios C. Polimenakos Pediatric Cardiothoracic Surgery, Medical College of Georgia, Children's Hospital of Georgia, Augusta, GA, USA

Michael Reinhorn Boston Hernia, Wellesley, MA, USA

Mark Savarise Department of Surgery, University of Utah South Jordan Health Center, South Jordan, UT, USA

Samer Sbayi Surgery Department, Emergency General Surgery, Stony Brook University Hospital, Stony Brook, NY, USA

Raquel M. Schears Department of Emergency Medicine, University of Central Florida, Orlando, FL, USA

Robert W. Seligson The Physicians Foundation, Raleigh, NC, USA

S. Abbās Shobeiri Professor of Medical Education, The University of Virginia, Charlottesville, VA, USA

Faculty of Bioengineering, George Mason University, Fairfax, VA, USA

Women Service Line, NOVA Health System, Falls Church, VA, USA

Vivek Singh Department of Plastic and Oral Surgery, Boston Children's Hospital, Boston, MA, USA

Amir H. Taghinia Department of Plastic and Oral Surgery, Boston Children's Hospital, Boston, MA, USA

Mark A. Talamini Northwell Health Physician Partners, Manhasset, NY, USA

Northwell Health, Manhasset, NY, USA

Zucker School of Medicine at Hofstra/Northwell, Manhasset, NY, USA

Apostolos Tassiopoulos Division of Vascular and Endovascular Surgery, Department of Surgery, Stony Brook University Hospital, Stony Brook, NY, USA

Roni Tomashev INOVA Women's Hospital, Falls Church, VA, USA

Assaf Harofe Medical Center, Zrifin, Israel

Department of Obstetrics and Gynecology, Tel Aviv Faculty of Medicine, Shamir Medical Center, Be'er Yakov, Zriffin, Israel

Thomas F. Tracy The American Pediatric Surgical Association, East Dundee, IL, USA

Adjunct Professor of Surgery and Pediatrics, Brown University, Providence, RI, USA

Krystle Trosclair Department of Neurosurgery, LSU Health, Shreveport, LA, USA

Introduction to the New Science of Medicine

Jon A. Chilingerian

In 2001, the Institute of Medicine's (IOM's) Committee on the Quality of Health Care in America threw down the gauntlet. They had been charged with developing a strategy to improve health care quality by 2008. The opening sentences of their book on the "quality chasm" stated:

The American health care delivery system is in need of fundamental change. Many patients, doctors, nurses, and health care leaders are concerned that the care delivered is not, essentially, the care we should receive…The frustration levels of both patients and clinicians have probably never been higher. Yet the problems remain. Health care today harms too frequently and routinely fails to deliver its potential benefits [1, p 1].

That was more than 20 years ago, so where are we today? In 2018, Dr. Zeke Emanuel, a leading expert on US health care, wrote about the continuing underperformance:

On even the most basic measures of health system quality—life expectancy, maternal, infant and youth mortality, immunization rates, asthma survival, heart attack survival, control of diabetes, and mental health—the United States falls well below other developed countries. There are endless complaints about impersonal care, hospital-acquired infections, rushed office visits, excessive admissions to the ICU, and too many high-tech interventions at the end of life [2].

Jon A. Chilingerian was deceased at the time of publication

J. A. Chilingerian (✉)
Health Care Management, EMBA Physician and MD-MBA Programs, Institute for Health Systems, Heller School for Social Policy and Management, Brandeis University, Waltham, MA, USA
e-mail: chilinge@brandeis.edu

Public Health and Community Medicine, Tufts University School of Medicine, Boston, MA, USA

More recently, two physicians wrote:
As physicians, we know that we often spend our days doing the wrong work for our patients [3, p. 2452].

Despite these assessments, people live longer and are healthier today than previous generations were. Premature infants survive, new molecules can attack hard-to-treat cancers, 90% of children with leukemia have an excellent chance of cure, and remote patient monitoring of vitals and advanced telemedicine have improved outcomes and access.

Medicine's purpose is to care for patients and to keep communities healthy. Technically, medicine's mission is investigating and diagnosing, offering therapies, and managing recovery and follow-up. In fulfilling that purpose and technical mission, medicine has been successful. What has failed in the descriptions above is the management of medical care through human and social organizations. Management succeeds when it designs and implements work processes, structures, and a culture of deep engagement that enable patients, caregivers,[1] and staff to jointly achieve clinical objectives and outcomes [4].

Why has management failed? There are at least three reasons why health care management has failed to address the IOM's quality challenges. One reason is that health care managers have been unable to obtain deep physician engagement. A second reason is that although physicians are high achievers, improving the quality of care represents an unclear goal. Quality is multi-dimensional and ill-defined, which makes it hard to measure and difficult to assess. A third reason is that until recently, physician leaders were not trained in management as a discipline and a practice. Each one of these reasons will be addressed in the coming pages.

Difficulty Involving Physicians in Health Care Performance Improvements

Experience has shown that physicians contribute significantly when participating in quality improvement and other changes [5]. However, one recurring theme is the difficulty of involving physicians in performance improvements [6]. National surveys reveal that 3 out of 5 physicians working in health care are feeling disengaged [7].

Why has it been challenging to involve physicians? It is unlikely that the reason is that they are too busy or too skeptical. Physicians do care about quality and their patients' experience. It is also unlikely that physicians are less involved because it is uncompensated work [Berwick 1990]. That may have been true 20 years ago, but in 2022 74% of US physicians are hospital, system or corporate employees and are well compensated [8].

The answer may lie partly in the science of persuasion and the limited influence nonclinical leaders have on physicians. The psychology of persuasion has taught us

---

[1] When I use the word "caregiver," I am referring to all of the clinical professionals who care for patients, including physicians, nurses, other clinical practitioners and staff who have direct contact with patients and their families.

that people follow the lead of others with similar professional backgrounds, work roles, or identities [9]. When physicians take a leadership role in a process improvement, this offers "social proof," making the call to action credible to the other physicians. As one physician said:

I would trust a physician vs. a non-physician in an administrator position in probably 90% of cases [10].

It has been well documented that physician leadership is a critical success factor in quality, patient experience, and overall performance improvement [5, 10, 11]. The health management literature documents the importance of a deep bench of physician leaders who enlist, communicate with, and coach other physicians [12–16]. However, it is not the title "chair" or "chief" that makes a clinical leader; it is whether the physician leaders have shown they are competent, truthful, dependable and take actions that demonstrate they understand physician interests. However, trust in clinical leaders can erode quickly. An excerpt from a physician interview exemplifies that point:

The half-life of clinical credibility is about 6 months [after becoming an administrator] [10].

So, part of the problem is the need to train and educate physicians to take on leadership roles in quality and other performance improvement projects. Next, we address the second reasons why we have made little progress in improving quality.

Quality as Ambiguous Versus the Value Revolution in Health Care

Throughout the 70 s, 80 s, and 90 s, attempts to contain rising health costs failed. From 2000 to today, the focus shifted to quality and patient-centered care with marginal progress in improving patient outcomes and experiences. For caregivers and especially physicians, organizational life became more difficult. Pressure to increase revenues and reimbursable physician activity (measured by arcane relative value unit activity) has meant shorter patient visits, spending less time with more patients, or delivering more physician services to patients. Structured observations of how physicians allocate their time reveal that 50% of a physician's time can be spent on electronic health deskwork, and clinical documentation is often done on nights and weekends [17].

One of the most important variables affecting health care today is changing societal expectations about the value of health services in relation to its "costs." Patients want excellent end results and a service process that has more benefits with regard to the sacrifices they make to obtain any health service. Caregivers want a supportive workplace and a strong people proposition that enables high-quality care. Third-party payors want to reduce or eliminate unnecessary services that do not improve health but increase per-unit costs/prices.

The good news is that these are not conflicting goals from a value perspective. We see the beginning of a value revolution in health care that is creating a more robust motivating environment for overall performance improvement.

After five decades of muddling along with vague and unclear cost and quality goals, we now have a purpose and a beacon for action—it is called "high-value health care" [2]. High-value care is a vision for the future that aims to create value for patients (excellent technical outcomes and patient experience), caregivers, staff, and the health care organization.[2] This is sometimes referred to as the quadruple performance problem.

The Importance of Training Physicians in Management

Obtaining high-value health care requires using the right concepts and tools, which brings us to the third reason the quality movement failed—most physicians have not been trained in management as a discipline and a practice. Principles and practices that bridge medicine and management have not been part of the mindset of caregivers. That requires equipping caregivers with the right concepts, tools, skills, and attitudes concerning the actual performance of patient care. To be more specific, every physician needs to understand how to manage and improve what already exists in their clinical work. How to redirect people and resources from processes or areas showing poor results to achieving more productive results.

Physicians need a deep understanding of how mission, goals, and strategy can be managed. They need the knowledge and skills to team with others to redesign care processes and cultures to achieve better clinical outcomes and to ensure that clinical activities are productive for patients.

Physicians also need leadership training. Every physician should be able to lead and collaborate with caregivers and staff to keep their clinical practice performing today and build commitment to a new vision that develops a capacity to perform, grow, and change for the future.

This book starts with the proposition that there is a new science of medicine and management. The discipline is not taught in medical school or most business schools. But we can see that it is much needed in medical care and clinical practice.

Given that proposition, we begin with three assertions:

1. The clinical side of complex professional medical organizations such as hospitals has traditionally been led by highly skilled, highly experienced medical practitioners trained in the underlying biomedical disciplines and applied medical sciences.
2. There is research evidence that managers with clinical backgrounds can run better healthcare organizations, and a growing number of physician-led multispecialty groups are outperforming organizations run by lay managers.
3. Physicians and other caregivers should have some training in the new science of medicine and management; however, the transition from clinician to clinical manager and leader is challenging and requires training in the new science of medicine and management.

---

[2] As a ratio, value is (1) the perceived clinical benefits in relation to (2) foregone opportunities and sacrifices made to obtain the clinical service, including time, inconvenience, costs, and prices of care.

The Science of Medicine and Management[3]

Health care organizations are among the most complex social organizations. The growth of knowledge in the biomedical sciences has led to differentiation and specialization—a proliferation of sub-specialties—and patient care has become increasingly fractionated and customized. As new medical disciplines and subspecialties develop, care coordination and accountability for outcomes become more difficult challenges [1].

In the past, complex health care organizations like hospitals have been organized into two fragmented and distinct domains: one where patient care and clinical services are delivered; and one where management is practiced. In the past, these domains have conflicting goals and problematic communication. In the future, these domains will need to share common goals, develop trusting relationships, and have a great deal of activity and interaction to achieve high-value care.

Many hospitals have established cooperative, not hierarchal, relations with physicians out of respect for physician expertise and the need for decision-making autonomy. This has remained the case even after growing numbers of physicians have become employed. Because patient care in hospitals involves temporary multiperson workgroups, each performing a sequence of highly interactive micro care processes, there is poor communication and coordination and, ultimately, only the illusion of control. These problems are at the intersection of medicine and management.

Given health care complexity and clinical frustration, the day-to-day operational problems of the biomedical sciences and the management sciences have been blossoming into what can be called a new science of medicine and management [18].[4] Other industries have followed similar pathways owing to chance and necessity.

For example, after the second industrial revolution (1870–1914), factories and manufacturing plants had unique problems that required the application of the engineering sciences to the design of human work and production systems. At the turn of the twentieth century, James Gunn recommended a new profession, curriculum, and discipline called industrial engineering to deal with the problems and performance of manufacturing plants, such as how to combine complex production technology and people systems or how to achieve an optimal product workflow. When colleges began to teach students the science of (1) applied mathematics, (2) factory economics, (3) applied motion studies, and the like, a new discipline of industrial engineering emerged.

---

[3] Later in this introduction it is acknowledged that neither medicine nor management are sciences. Although medicine and management are informed by and make use of basic and applied sciences and social sciences, physicians do not practice biochemistry and managers do not practice political science or sociology [4]. Medicine and management are two distinct disciplines that if combined can teach evidence-guided paradigms and competing paradigms that help medical practitioners, among other things, to frame, diagnose and solve problems in medical care performance.

[4] Likewise, when biology and chemistry became biochemistry, that integration resulted in a far more powerful science.

Over many decades, industrial techniques and factory models have been proposed to solve health care problems. Some health care experts have pointed out fundamental differences between manufacturing and health care. Recently, an article appeared in a clinical journal that stated, "...a hospital is not a factory but a complex adaptive system..." [19]. Similar arguments have been made in the past. Unlike manufacturing plants with a single managerial hierarchy with control over professionals, hospitals are more decentralized, almost loosely coupled organizations with temporary teams forming and dissolving around patients [20].

The word "science" overstates the more important fact about the nature of medicine and management as disciplines. As others have observed [4, 21], medicine draws from an enormous curriculum of basic and applied sciences such as biochemistry, physics, physiology, and anatomy. Management draws on a much smaller base of knowledge from the social and behavioral sciences such as economics, applied mathematics, political science, psychology, social psychology, and anthropology [4, 21]. But neither medicine nor management is a "true" science. Although they draw on knowledge, evidence, and systematic studies of the underlying and applied sciences, both are practices based on the practitioners' skills, experience, and mindsets.

There has always been tension between medical practices based on scientific evidence and clinical trials and medical practices based on experience [22]. On the one hand, when medicine wants to study the efficacy of a surgical procedure or a drug, randomized controlled trials (RCT) are the scientific way to aim for truth. That is evidenced-based medicine. On the other hand, if medicine wants to study the efficacy of teams in health care, qualitative methodologies are often superior to RCT. Why?

Consider, for example, cardiac resuscitation teams (CRTs), a medical practice that improves in-hospital cardiac arrest survival rates. Hospitals that adopt CRTs can have a wide range of survival rates due to implementation quality. Unlike adopting an evidence-based surgical procedure or drug, CRTs in hospitals require not only understanding the key features of the practice (protocols and procedures, role of people, technology, etc.) but also how to integrate them into an existing care process and a complex adaptive social and cultural system.

The reason some resuscitation teams are more effective than others might include factors like leadership styles, relationships among team members, the stability of team membership, cross-specialization group dynamics, clarity of roles and responsibilities, commitment to goals, and systems of accountability [23]. This will be addressed in a later section.

There is another feature of both medicine and management that makes science difficult, the existence of uncertainty. In some situations, judgments are based on incomplete or ambiguous information about diagnosis, objectives, alternatives, risks, trade-offs, and the complete set of consequences. Not everything is known.

Atul Gwande talks about medicine as a practice that draws on the medical sciences, but owing to decision-making under conditions of high residual uncertainty, the application of an evidence-based science can be equivocal:

> Every day, surgeons are faced with uncertainties. Information is inadequate; the science is ambiguous; one's knowledge and abilities are never perfect. Even with the simplest operation, it cannot be taken for granted that a patient will come through better off—or even alive. [24 p. 15].

So, Gwande calls medicine "an imperfect science" [24].

Likewise, managing uncertainty is a significant problem for management. As Dorner has observed about decision-making and human judgment with incomplete information:

> When someone simply walks away from difficult problems or "solves" them by delegating to others …when someone solves the problem she can solve rather than the one she ought to solve, when someone is reluctant to reflect on his actions, it is hard not to see in such behavior a refusal to recognize one's impotence and helplessness… [25, pp, 25-26].

As in medicine, management is training for uncertainty. How to maintain self-confidence when there is no easy answer to a problem. An ability to take responsibility for the outcomes of high-risk decisions when there is a lack of scientific knowledge or incomplete information. Like medicine, management draws on the certainty and security of scientific knowledge and evidence. As a practice, managers must develop skills and experience to make choices while inspiring confidence.

Managers in any industry need basic or generic skills such as strategic thinking, allocating resources, engaging in difficult conversations, making decisions with limited information, entrepreneurial or innovative thinking, and the like. Health care organizations have unique problems, such as highly autonomous professionals and experts, incentives and policies that distort motivation, and protocols that are adopted but never fully assimilated into practice. The complexity and uniqueness of health organizations support the idea that health care organizations need an organized body of knowledge at the intersection of medicine and management that can be taught and practiced.[5]

We have described the division of labor and the emergence of two domains in medical care organizations. On the one hand, medical decision-making and clinical work have been performed by highly skilled physicians and other caregivers trained and licensed to practice medicine but have no serious training in management. On the other hand, managerial work has been performed by highly skilled people trained in management science, many lacking serious training and experience in the biomedical sciences. This model can work well when the managerial and clinical domains share goals, trust each other, and share a lot of activity and interactions.

Would we, however, observe much better results if these two jobs were combined into one professional discipline? Physicians who practice clinical medicine and have studied management? Clinical leaders who can attract, recruit and lead top

---

[5] Although the science of medicine and management is nascent, health care organizations and clinical leaders have been advancing foundational ideas for more than a century. During a 1911 congressional hearing, Fredrick Winslow Taylor was asked for an organization that practiced "scientific management." He replied, "the Mayo Clinic." [4 , p. 168]. Mayo was and still is a physician-led organization.

physicians and be the instrument of strategic direction and innovative operations. Physicians who can redesign care processes and care programs that achieve higher levels of performance.

This leads us to our first assertion.

The Clinical Side of Medical Organizations Are Led by Medical Practitioners Trained in the Bio-Medical Sciences

There has been an ongoing debate about whether technical experts trained in the underlying science should lead technical organizations or merely advise professionals prepared to be general managers.[6] Health care organizations have a unique organizational configuration called a "professional bureaucracy" with highly trained and specialized knowledge workers [26]. These highly trained people (physicians, nurses, other caregivers, and support staff) deliver high-quality patient services, conduct all tasks related to patient care, and innovate. So, the critical part of any health care organization is the operating core that performs all the clinical work [26].

The complexity of hospitals requires that decision-making be decentralized to the caregivers with some hierarchal top-down control for support staff who provide indirect services. In the past, the prime coordinating mechanism was standardizing skills from prior professional training, licensing, continuing education, and following practice norms. Coordination and motivation have always been problematic [1].

The operating core in complex biomedical science organizations, such as academic medical centers, acute general hospitals, or specialty hospitals, have traditionally been led by professionals trained only in the underlying disciplines and applied medical sciences, i.e., physicians, nurses, and other licensed caregivers. In some medical centers, as many as 80 semi-autonomous surgeons might report to one chair of surgery with other vice chairs.

This decentralized structure works well when two conditions hold. When it can be presumed that the environment is stable and caregivers work together regularly as a team. Second, it works well when the individual attending physicians assigned to a patient earn the privilege of having the autonomy to make clinical decisions for their patients because they achieve desired outcomes, and their practices are consistent with the most current professional knowledge.

Today, health care environments are more turbulent than stable and societal expectations about care and value have intensified. Value, as stated in the preface, is a moving target and best care practices diffuse slowly. And in most physician departments, practice styles, utilization behaviors, and patient outcomes vary. If performance matters, physician practice behavior should be monitored, evaluated, and benchmarked by clinical leaders. That means replacing wholesale physician

---

[6] Consider, for example, who ought to run a technocratic organization like Google? One answer is the people trained in the basic underlying science, such as programmers and software engineers who will be seen as competent by the other professionals with that identity.

autonomy with a new medical culture, where there are conversations about practice styles and next practices. And each physician takes more responsibility for resource utilization and outcomes. That is a bittersweet pill for any professional, but the alternatives are far worse.

Consider the range of problems medical care organizations confront every day such as (1) central line bloodstream infections, (2) surgical site infections, (3) prolonged ventilation, (4) reducing readmission rates for congestive heart failure and chronic obstructive pulmonary disease, (5) procedural sedation in the emergency rooms, (6) early extubation protocols, (7) in-hospital cardiac arrest, and on and on. Only physicians, as medical practitioners, have the knowledge, experience, and qualifications to understand and solve these problems.

A chair or chief cannot possibly lead and hold dozens or hundreds of physicians accountable for the range of problems just mentioned without a deep bench of clinical leaders who understand management concepts, practices, and techniques and are supported by robust information systems. While caregivers have led the clinical side, there is a growing need to develop more physician leaders who can improve performance.

The next question is how many physician leaders are needed to improve performance?[7] Whatever the correct answer is to that question, the people who and willing and able to lead should be trusted physician leaders—seen by the rank-and-file caregivers and staff as (1) competent, (2) reliable, (3) honest and truthful, and (4) have the best interests of others in mind [10].

We have argued that owing to their medical training, physicians are uniquely qualified to manage medical care operations. We stop short of claiming physicians "should" lead medical care organizations. Now we will explore our second assertion—What do we know about the effect of physician leadership on performance?

Impact of Physician Leadership on Health Care Performance

Based on years of research, our second assertion is that physician leadership can significantly affect healthcare delivery outcomes and efficiency in hospitals [27–30]. The most recent data suggests that physician-led hospitals seem to outperform hospitals led by non-physicians. Studies of hospitals with physician CEOs have better clinical performance versus CEOs with non-clinical backgrounds, though there is less evidence about financial performance [29, 31, 32].

One observational study in 2022 that compared 250 physician-led versus non-physician-led acute care facilities found better access to care, evidence of more

---

[7] Imagine you want to make a quality improvement in a medical department with 55 FTE caregivers who are known to each other and are socially connected. What is the minimum number of people you should engage to be trained and to lead the quality change? A heuristic used to determine how many professionals you need to train and engage to have a performance impact was to take the square root of the total number of people whose behavior you want to change; so, if n = 55 people, that answer is 7 or 8 people. Advances in network theory suggest a simpler formula, multiply the number of people by @20%--55 * 20% = 11.

affordable care, and better patient experiences (NDP Analytics). The direct involvement of frontline physicians in healthcare management improves overall organizational performance.[8]

Historically the most effective healthcare organizations are the multispecialty, physician-led groups. These organizations nurture and integrate physician leaders who are prepared to bring management science closer to clinical operations and medical decisionmaking. The Mayo Clinic studied more than 2500 physicians and found that frontline physician leader affected physicians' satisfaction and their well-being—11% of the variation in burnout and 47% of the variation in physician satisfaction with their organization were associated with higher leadership rating of the physicians who supervise them [17]. Guided by this evidence, health organizations may be better off with more clinical leaders. This brings us to our third and final assertion in the next section.

The Difficult Transition from Clinical Staff Member to Clinical Manager

Our third assertion is that transitioning from being a clinical expert to becoming a manager and from manager to leader can be difficult [30, 33–35]. Many studies have reported that many clinicians feel they did not receive any management training, so they were not prepared to manage [30, 33, 35]. These studies report that doctors often feel they were "thrown into a management position."

The newly appointed physician managers also feel they are intuitive managers because they are trained as physicians to be action-oriented—ready to use their expertise to fix problems as they present. Being action-oriented and task-oriented can work. However, physicians who use their expertise to fix problems are guided by an arbitrary list of emergent complaints [25]. They may end up with an inescapable 7 am to 11 pm workload. Or they invest their time and attention in less important, nice-to-do issues and miss the enormously critical strategic opportunities.

Clinicians who become managers discover that to be effective as a manager requires learning how to get work done through people. Physician leaders must have the patience to listen to concerns, establish priorities and build commitment to measurable goals. They learn that decision-making has political, social, and cultural tensions. And they must learn how to empower other physicians to solve their own problems by coaching and monitoring, not by fixing problems themself.

Managerial work requires fewer transactional tasks and more relational activity. Up to 85–90% of a health care leader's time can be spent in verbal communication. Physicians learn they need relational skills such as team building, as well as

---

[8] One research study in 2010 on 1200 hospitals found that hospitals with more clinically trained managers outperform all the others [27]. No surprise. They hypothesized that clinical managers obtain higher levels of street-level credibility, competence, and authoritative clinical expertise are difficult to achieve for nonclinical managers. This is what behavioral scientists call "social proof." [9]

budgeting, and other financial skills. They must understand patient flow and management of medical care as efficient and high-quality service. Not every self-taught physician can make that transition.

Nevertheless, many medical care organizations have been successful because their physicians have been solving problems that apply the ideas and principles of the science of medicine and management. The following section discusses examples from the frontiers of medicine and management.

The Early Frontiers of Medicine and Management

The following four studies highlight valuable lessons that have led us to an emerging discipline of medicine and management. In the past, the clinical literature and managerial literature have been separated. While that has been changing, the next study would never have been read by clinical leaders. Why? It was buried in one of the premier management journals, *Management Science*.

Organizational Learning and the Case of Minimally Invasive Cardiac Surgery

In the early years of minimally invasive cardiac surgery (MICS), a study followed 16 hospitals among the first to adopt the technique following FDA approval [36]. The research team was composed of one physician and two management scientists. The purpose was to study organizational learning. The measure used to demonstrate organizational learning was the reduction in the procedure time to perform the MICS. They studied variations in procedure time among the 16 sites with cumulative experience [36].

They found that the net average procedure time was reduced with more case experience.[9] Though every hospital team had the same three-day training, some teams learned faster than others, displaying different learning rates across hospitals. Two outlier hospitals stood out—a fast-learning team at hospital M and a slow-learning team at hospital R.

Hospital M had a slower start, the net adjusted procedure time for the first case was 500 min, but by case 50, they had the shortest procedure time, an average of 132 min versus 220 min for the rest of the sample. The 88-min advantage translated into a savings of $2250 per case, enabling the Surgical team to perform more daily procedures. Hospital R was one of the slowest learners, taking more than 2.5 h longer than hospital M. What made the difference? The physician investigator conducted some interviews, and here is what he found.

The cardiac surgeon at Hospital M was a more junior and less-experienced cardiac surgeon. However, he played a critical leadership role in creating a stable process and a stable team culture. For example, he handpicked his own MICS team

---
[9] The rest of this section is based on the MICS study [36].

based on the prior history of people he knew and could work well together. He insisted that the surgical team have a stable membership and, as a team, be willing and able to take responsibility for outcomes.

After the three-day training, the team began to have frequent face-to-face meetings. Seeing a need for effective communication, the perfusionist, operating room nurse, and anesthesiologist met to agree on standard terminology and learn how to communicate. During those meetings, they shared information about each other's backgrounds, roles, and responsibilities and how they would communicate during the surgery.

While the team was meeting, the cardiac surgeon realized that to keep a dedicated team, he needed referrals. He organized weekly meetings with the cardiology department to introduce the MICS technology. Those meetings built trust with referring cardiologists and resulted in a steady flow of future cardiac patients with sufficient volume to guarantee that the team could stay together.

The cardiac surgeon scheduled six cases in the first week, allowing enough process stability so the team could learn how to make incremental improvements to the procedure. The cardiac surgeon insisted that the team stay together for the first 15 cases without changing membership. The team met before each of the first 10 cases and after the first 20 cases to debrief. The perfusionist went to the ICU each day to check on the patient. The cardiac surgeon met with cardiology each week to discuss each case. The team analyzed process and outcome data, which they presented at national surgical congresses. These practices differed distinctly from hospital R, with less organizational learning and a much higher average procedure time.

At Hospital R, the team was selected randomly based on willingness and availability and because they worked well together. Only three of the four team members who attended the training showed up for the first MICS case. The first six cases had different team members each time. As one nurse said, there were no stable teams; different people were assigned to the team on any given day. The cardiac surgeon did not have team meetings before or after the surgery. Finally, there was no data collection on outcomes and weak clinical leadership [36].

Lesson

When health organizations adopt a new clinical technique, team stability, cohesiveness, leadership behavior, and management practices matter. Organizational learning is critical if health care organizations want to assimilate new technology and obtain better performance. While there is extensive literature on hospital performance in relation to volume, the clinical literature assumes that the learning is uniform—i.e., medical care organizations have similar resources and capabilities to learn. However, organizational sciences teach us there is a difference between natural experience owing to volume and different rates of organizational learning owing to medical and managerial practices.

Explaining Variations in Risk-Standardized Mortality

A three-year (2005–2008) study of 30-day risk-standardized mortality rates for acute myocardial infarction (AMI) found a wide range of rates from a low of 11% to a high of 25% [37]. Controlling for socio-economic factors, when they tried to understand the factors that were associated with lower 30-day mortality, only three hospital variables were associated with lower mortality (1) higher volume, (2) urban settings, and (3) teaching status). Those factors could only explain 17% of the variation in mortality. The researchers were stumped, and some members of the research teams conducted a follow-up study [11].

This time they ranked the top 5% of hospitals with the lowest 30-day risk-stratified mortality rates and the bottom 5% with the highest mortality rates [11].[10] They conducted face-to-face interviews with physicians, nurses, and staff at both hospitals. They discovered that these hospitals had followed the same technical protocols and care practices. The difference between the best and worst 5% was clinical leadership, accountability systems, and a more or less inclusive culture.

Staff at high-performing hospitals described physician leaders as passionate about getting the best outcomes, embedding those values in the culture, and inspiring people. Nurses and pharmacists were highly engaged with clear roles, responsibilities, and systems for holding people accountable for poor performance. When adverse events occurred, the problem-solving approach was data-driven and backed up by root cause analysis.

Staff at low-performing hospitals cited weak physician leadership, nurses feeling unvalued, irregular team meetings, inadequate IT, a general lack of respect, clinical leaders with a 'me-me-me' mentality, and minimal use of management tools such as root-cause analysis.

Lesson

What differentiated the top and bottom 5% was not clinical expertise alone but clinical teams and medical practices supported by management: better leadership, a more inclusive and performance-driven culture, and effective use of data and other management practices. While clinical medicine would assume professional expertise, technical protocols, and care processes (such as rapid response teams, drug reconciliation, and use of hospitalists) explain why lower mortality rates, they turned out to be a necessary but not a sufficient condition.

---

[10] The rest of this section is based on the follow-up study [11].

For most medical care practitioners, culture is an opaque spirit or climate inside an organization. In the science of medicine and management, culture is no mystery but a critical part of informal organizational structure.[11] Culture can not only be decoded and analyzed, but clinical leaders can also embed new values and beliefs to change cultures [38].

In the following example, the researchers the discipline of medicine and management to solve a clinical mystery. Why do some hospitals have lower mortality rates following an in-hospital cardiac arrest?

In-Hospital Cardiac Arrest

Each year, in the US, it has been estimated that 290,000 patients experience an in-hospital cardiac arrest (IHCA), with three-fold variations in risk-standardized patient survival among hospitals [39, 40]. Despite the widespread adoption and implementation of clinical practices such as standardized protocols for chest compressions and ventilation, defibrillation, and resuscitation training, the survival rates are poor.

One study of risk-standardized survival rates following IHCA distinguished the top-performing hospitals from the rest. The critical factor was how they organized and managed the resuscitation teams [23]. They found four practices that top-performing hospitals with higher patient survival rates adopted:

- they established dedicated resuscitation teams with clear roles and responsibilities and effective leadership
- every hospital had a similar team composition (physicians and respiratory therapists); the top performers were more inclusive, adding additional staff from the pharmacy and security and clergy members.
- given the diversity of the team, the leaders and team members practiced multidisciplinary communication and mutual respect.
- Finally, the training, which included mock codes, was well-organized and taken seriously [23].

Lesson

None of these practices used by the top-performing hospitals were difficult or costly. They merely confirm some of the findings from the previous examples. Medical

---

[11] According to Schein, culture is a pattern of deep unconscious assumptions that groups discover and learn when trying to cope with and solve external and internal problems [17, 38]. When a solution to a problem is successful, the group adopts a way to understand, frame, and make sense of the external environment. At the same time, the group discovers a successful and "valid" way to work together when interacting, communicating, and making decisions. So, given that definition of culture based on the group's past experience solving problems together, physicians practice in health organizations with unique cultures.

care organizations with dedicated teams, better team communication, and effective physician leadership outperform the others. This is another example of a slowly emerging discipline that integrates medicine and management to improve performance. The fourth example concerns the importance of building implementation into improvement-oriented strategic thinking.

Adoption of LEAN Management Is Not Implementation

In the health care management literature, there are examples of the importance of building implementation into technology adoption. A recent study of 1222 hospitals found that "simply" adopting a LEAN management system as a targeted intervention was not associated with better performance [41]. Merely adopting a performance improvement method does not guarantee that it is working to improve performance.

In that same study,[12] they found that hospitals able to assimilate LEAN effectively into a more significant number of organizational units had a much better overall performance. For example, hospitals with more widespread execution of LEAN had (1) lower adjusted inpatient expense per admission, (2) lower 30-day unplanned readmission rates, (3) less low-value care, and (4) higher patient experience scores. Adopting LEAN throughout the organization means bringing teams of people together to solve waste and low-value problems by observing process and value streams, standardizing, using root cause problem-solving, and employing other lean methods.

Lesson

Extraordinary medical advances in the biomedical sciences, emerging technologies, and novel clinical treatments continue to race ahead. Organizations that can identify the value of these advances to achieve their clinical goals can identify new technology opportunities. However, the ability to adopt new medical knowledge or avant-garde clinical treatments to achieve higher levels of clinical performance is only the beginning.

Once adopted, health care organizations must assimilate that knowledge into their organizational cultures, develop the requisite human skills and experience, and turn that knowledge into outputs that result in better patient care. Developing the capability to adopt, assimilate and perform better is called "absorptive capacity" [42]. Adoption with poor implementation can be a function of cognitive inertia, truculent caregiver resistance, resource munificence, and the capacity of professionals and service workers to take on one more initiative.

The following example is how the science of medicine and management was used at Intermountain Healthcare to deliver better quality, lower costs, and high value to patients, caregivers, supporting staff, and the Intermountain organization.

---

[12] This section focuses on the study of the adoption of LEAN [41].

Managing for Medical Results at Intermountain Healthcare: Putting Medicine and Management Science to Work

Between the 1990s and into the millennium, Intermountain Healthcare (IHC) may be one of the best longitudinal illustrations of the benefits of merging the sciences of medicine and management [43]. IHC began by focusing on six diagnoses and procedures, i.e., prostatectomy, cholecystectomy, total hip replacement, coronary artery bypass graft, pneumonia, and implanting pacemakers. They then tracked all the clinical inputs and outcomes for these procedures.

IHC physician leaders learned that 80% of the patients within these six diagnoses and procedures had the same admission severity and complexity and were discharged without complications and satisfactory outcomes. However, there were significant variations in physician utilization behaviors, and these leaders also discovered that utilization costs per case were two times higher for the least efficient physicians.

Combining the two disciplines of medicine and management, leaders focused on process improvements that would result in the best clinical outcomes at the lowest necessary costs. Over the next decade, they launched 100 successful cost-quality improvements—and nearly every improvement project was physician-led. For example, physicians could reduce costs for a total hip replacement by one-third without sacrificing quality outcomes or patient satisfaction. During that time, they also redesigned their leadership structure to create physician-nurse dyads that convened monthly to review costs, quality, and other outcomes. These are just a few examples of the potential of the new science of medicine and management.

A Few More Lessons about Medicine and Management

This section illustrated four illustrations of the practice of medicine and management. Those examples are a small part of a hidden literature that describes the rudiments of knowledge—an evolving set of ideas, some observational research studies and experiments, and many case-based findings, Knowledge, however, cannot accumulate scientifically because it is often bounded by contextual and organizational factors such as organization culture, personalities, weak systems of accountability, imbalance of power, group dynamics, and other situational variables. There are three points in summary.

First, adopting an innovative idea or a successful practice from another organization without knowing the organizational factors that helped it become a success is like an experiment that is difficult to repeat. The critical resources and capabilities associated with success may not be available in other health care systems. With an incomplete recipe, success and failure can fluctuate.

Second, in each of the four cases, effective clinical leadership is one key ingredient for success. Leadership matters to effectuate an innovative, value-driven health care system [2]. Our most effective health care systems identify physician leaders who can bring management discipline closer to clinical operations and medical decision-making [12, 43, 44]. These physician leaders are the instruments of direction, decision, fairness, and justice. They define a shared clinical vision and implement medical reforms that challenge assumptions, current practices, and systems of authority.

Finally, being an effective clinical leader requires a combination of two leadership characteristics. The thoughtful and reflective clinical leader who can use the right analytic concepts and tools to diagnose problems and situations and build relationships and commitments. And the action-oriented risk-taking clinical leader who can make a series of timely adaptive responses when dealing with the inevitable uncertainty, novelty, and time pressure in a given organizational context.

The Way Forward

Physicians in health care organizations are often not motivated to improve care processes because of the push of a crisis situation or the pull of a value-adding opportunity. These forces tend to motivate extrinsically, with seeming benefit in the short term, but these momentary positive outcomes are quickly extinguished in light of overall value to medical care organizations.

When not under pressure, physicians are intrinsically motivated to put their patients first. By and large, physicians are people-centered and empathic. Their gratification lies in relieving the suffering of their patients, and patient experience matters. They want to understand best practices and learn how to lead teams better. Finally, they want to work in organizations that aim for a culture of continuous improvement with no tradeoff between quality and efficiency. In short, physicians are motivated to bring value to their work.

Zeke Emanuel says that while the Affordable Care Act is a necessary policy change, it is insufficient to improve health care delivery. Getting to the next level requires:

> …physicians, hospitals, and other providers to comprehensively rethink the processes of care delivery—from the simple, like scheduling office visits and rooming patients, to the more complex, like rolling out standardized care protocols, implementing effective chronic care coordination, and integrating behavioral health services into routine office flows. [2, p. 5].

That statement is a call to action. The way to fix health care is not by policy initiatives alone but by continuously having physicians and other caregivers redesign and work to improve care processes and programs. When value is created or restored, clinical leaders succeed.

This book was written by physician leaders answering that call to action by initiating team-based, clinical implementation management projects. The projects focused on new initiatives to change operating strategy and culture, obtain better patient outcomes and experiences, improve internal morale, or raise clinical efficiency and lower costs.

Each chapter described a case study on a physician-led clinical implementation management initiative. In each case, the project team had to confront and adjust to surprises, both desirable and undesirable. The lessons learned in each chapter are invaluable and provide insight as to how and why these initiatives worked or did not work as planned.

These cases provide an excellent opportunity for physicians, health administrators, and medical practitioners to learn about the science of medicine and management as a discipline, and a foundation to support their ongoing efforts to develop physician-led teams. Investing in future physician leaders who can close the gap between the very top performers offering high-value care and the majority will reap benefits for patients, caregivers, hospitals, and the health care delivery system overall.

References

1. Committee on Quality Health Care in America, Institute of Medicine. Crossing the quality chasm: a new health system for the 21st century. Washington, D.C.: National Academy Press; 2001.
2. Emanuel EJ. Prescription for the future: the twelve transformational practices of highly effective medical organizations. New York: Public Affairs; 2018.
3. Sinsky CA, Panzer J. The solution shop and the production line–the case for a frameshift for physician practices. N Engl J Med. 2022;386(26):2452–3. https://doi.org/10.1056/NEJMp2202511. Epub 2022 Jun 25
4. Drucker P. The Frontiers of management. New York: Harper and Row; 1986.
5. Berwick DM, Godfrey AB, Roessner J. Curing health care: new strategies for improvement. San Francisco: Jossey-Bass; 1990.
6. Mahbooba Z, Chera B, Evarts L. Engaging physicians in quality improvement in a hospital setting: a scoping review. Am J Med Qual. 2021;36(5):328–36. https://doi.org/10.1097/01.JMQ.0000735456.03039.2e.
7. James TA. Engaging physicians to Lead change in health care. Trends in medicine. Harvard Medical School 2020. https://postgraduateeducation.hms.harvard.edu/trends-medicine/engaging-physicians-lead-change-health-care. Downloaded August 1, 2022.
8. Gooch, K. Becker's hospital review. 2022. https://www.beckershospitalreview.com/hospital-physician-relationships/74-of-physicians-are-hospital-or-corporate-employees-with-pandemic-fueling-increase.html
9. Cialdini CR. Influence, new and expanded: the psychology of persuasion. New York: First Harper Business; 2021.
10. Chilingerian JA. Exploring trusted relationships among physicians, organizational practices, and the influence of both on hospital citizenship behavior. Unpublished working paper. Waltham, MA: Heller School for Social Policy and Management, Brandeis University; 2022.
11. Curry LA, Spatz E, Cherlin E, Thompson JW, Berg D, Ting HH, et al. What distinguishes top-performing hospitals in acute myocardial infarction mortality rates? A qualitative study Ann Intern Med. 2011;154(6):384–90. https://doi.org/10.7326/0003-4819-154-6-201103150-00003.
12. Cosgrove T. The Cleveland Clinic way: lessons in excellence from one of the world's leading healthcare organizations. New York: McGraw-Hill; 2014.
13. Kralewski JE, de Vries A, Dowd B, Potthoff S. The development of integrated service networks in Minnesota. Health Care Manag Rev. 1995 Fall;20(4):42–56.

14. Coddington DC, Chapman CR, Pokoski KM. Making integrated care work: case studies. Englewood, CO: Medical Group Management Association, Center for Research; 1996.
15. Shortell SM, Gillies RR, Anderson DA, Erickson KM, Mitchell JB. Remaking health care in America. Hosp Health Netw. 1996;70(6):43. -4, 46, 48
16. Gillies RR, Zuckerman HS, Burns LR, Shortell SM, Alexander JA, Budetti PP, Waters TM. Physician-system relationships: stumbling blocks and promising practices. Med Care. 2001 Jul;39(7 Suppl 1):I92–106.
17. Shanafelt TD, Gorringe G, Menaker R, Storz KA, Reeves D, Buskirk SJ, et al. Impact of organizational leadership on physician burnout and satisfaction. Mayo Clin Proc. 2015;90(4):432–40. https://doi.org/10.1016/j.mayocp.2015.01.012. Epub 2015 Mar 18
18. Chilingerian JA. Teaching surgeons how to Lead. In: Köhler T, Schwartz B, editors. Surgeons as educators. Cham: Springer; 2018. https://doi.org/10.1007/978-3-319-64728-9_20.
19. Mahajan A, Islam SD, Schwartz MJ, Cannesson M. A hospital is not just a factory, but a complex adaptive system-implications for perioperative care. Anesth Analg. 2017 Jul;125(1):333–41. https://doi.org/10.1213/ANE.0000000000002144.
20. Chilingerian JA, Sherman HD. Managing physician efficiency and effectiveness in providing hospital services. Health Serv Manag Res. 1990;3(1):3–15. https://doi.org/10.1177/095148489000300101.
21. Schein E. Professional education: some new directions. New York: McGraw Hill; 1972.
22. Berwick DM. The science of improvement. JAMA. 2008;299(10):1182–4. https://doi.org/10.1001/jama.299.10.1182.
23. Nallamothu BK, Guetterman TC, Harrod M, Kellenberg JE, Lehrich JL, Kronick SL, Krein SL, Iwashyna TJ, Saint S, Chan PS. How do resuscitation teams at top-performing hospitals for in-hospital cardiac arrest succeed? A Qualitative Study Circulation. 2018;138(2):154–63. https://doi.org/10.1161/CIRCULATIONAHA.118.033674.
24. Gawande A. Complications: a surgeon's notes on an imperfect science. New York: Picador; 2002.
25. Dorner D. The logic of failure. Reading: Perseus Books; 1996.
26. Mintzberg H. Managing the myths of health care: bridging the separations between care, cure, control and community. Oakland: Berrett-Koehler; 2017.
27. Dorgan S, Layton D, Bloom N, Homkes R, Sadun R, van Reenan J. Management in Healthcare: why good practice really matters. Technical Report: Joint with McKinsey & Co and Centre for Economic Performance at the London School of Economics; 2010.
28. Sarto F, Veronesi G. Clinical leadership and hospital performance: assessing the evidence base. BMC Health Serv Res. 2016;16(169) https://doi.org/10.1186/s12913-016-1395-5.
29. Tasi MC, Keswani A, Bozic KJ. Does physician leadership affect hospital quality, operational efficiency, and financial performance? Health Care Manag Rev. 2019;44(3):256–62. https://doi.org/10.1097/HMR.0000000000000173.
30. Sullivan EE, Stephenson AL, Hoffman AR. Engaging physicians in leadership: motivations, challenges, and identity based considerations. J Healthc Manage. 2022;67(4):254 65. https://doi.org/10.1097/JHM-D-21-00224.
31. Goodall AH. Physician-leaders and hospital performance: is there an association? Soc Sci Med. 2011;73(4):535–9. https://doi.org/10.1016/j.socscimed.2011.06.025. Epub 2011 Jul 6
32. Kaiser F, Schmid A, Schlüchtermann J. Physician-leaders and hospital performance revisited. Soc Sci Med. 2020;5(249):112831. https://doi.org/10.1016/j.socscimed.2020.112831. Epub ahead of print
33. Spehar I, Frich JC, Kjekshus LE. Clinicians' experiences of becoming a clinical manager: a qualitative study. BMC Health Serv Res. 2012 Nov 22;12:421. https://doi.org/10.1186/1472-6963-12-421.
34. Leicher B, Collins SK. The transition from clinical staff member to manager. Radiol Manage. 2016;38(2):14–9. quiz 20

35. Thompson AM, Henwood SM. From the clinical to the managerial domain: the lived experience of role transition from radiographer to radiology manager in south-East Queensland. J Med Radiat Sci. 2016;63(2):89–95. https://doi.org/10.1002/jmrs.169. Epub 2016 Mar 19
36. Pisano GP, Bohmer RMJ, Edmondson AC. Organizational differences in rates of learning: evidence from the adoption of minimally invasive cardiac surgery. Manag Sci. 2001;47(6):752–68.
37. Bradley EH, Herrin J, Curry L, Cherlin EJ, Wang Y, Webster TR, et al. Variation in hospital mortality rates for patients with acute myocardial infarction. Am J Cardiol. 2010;106(8):1108–12. https://doi.org/10.1016/j.amjcard.2010.06.014.
38. Schein EH. Organizational culture and leadership. Hoboken, NJ: Wiley; 2017.
39. Andersen LW, Holmberg MJ, Berg KM, Donnino MW, Granfeldt A. In-hospital cardiac arrest: a review. JAMA. 2019;321(12):1200–10. https://doi.org/10.1001/jama.2019.1696.
40. Bradley EH. Learning from diversity. Circulation. 2018;138(2):164–5. https://doi.org/10.1161/CIRCULATIONAHA.118.035370.
41. Shortell SM, Blodgett JC, Rundall TG, Henke RM, Reponen E. Lean management and hospital performance: adoption vs. Implementation. Jt Comm J Qual Patient Saf. 2021;47(5):296–305. https://doi.org/10.1016/j.jcjq.2021.01.010. Epub 2021 Feb 5
42. Miles JA. Management and organization theory. San Francisco: Jossey Nass; 2012.
43. James BC, Savitz LA. How intermountain trimmed health care costs through robust quality improvement efforts. Health Aff. 2011;30(6) https://doi.org/10.1377/hlthaff.2011.0358.
44. Vilendrer S, Amano A, Asch SM, Brown-Johnson C, Lu AC, Maggio P. Engaging frontline physicians in value improvement: a qualitative evaluation of physician-directed reinvestment. J Healthc Leadersh. 2022 Apr 8;14:31–45. https://doi.org/10.2147/JHL.S335763.

Part I

The Well-Managed Health Care Organization: Building Implementation into Strategic Thinking

Shouldice Hospital from Interviews and Observations: The Well Managed Organization

2

Jon A. Chilingerian, Michael Reinhorn, and Samer Sbayi

Key Learning Points
- Working as a focused clinic, Shouldice not only cares deeply about their patients, but they also partner with their patients, and they set clinical targets and establish performance standards that are well-defined, measured, and clearly understood

---

We are grateful to the Shouldice Family, especially Dr. E.B. Shouldice, Dr. Robert Bendavid, and Managing Director, Mr. John Hughes, for their generosity and hospitality. This research would not have been possible without their transparency and willingness to spend time with us. Our most heartfelt gratitude goes to John Hughes, whom we had the pleasure to interview. He was a source of many important stories and pieces of information. He not only shared his knowledge of the facts and key enterprise processes, but he also read a draft of the entire manuscript.

We would also like to pay our respects to two thought leaders in the field of hernia surgery who during our interviews and encounters shared their deep knowledge of the evolution of hernia surgery at Shouldice. The first is Dr. Bendavid, who passed away, in September 2019. Finally, we were sad to hear that Dr. E.B. Shouldice passed away in April 2022. He was a humanistic clinical leader, a talented and caring surgeon, and a role model for all of us.

Jon A. Chilingerian was deceased at the time of publication

J. A. Chilingerian (✉)
Health Care Management, EMBA Physician and MD-MBA Programs, Institute for Health Systems, Heller School for Social Policy and Management, Brandeis University, Waltham, MA, USA
e-mail: chilinge@brandeis.edu

Public Health and Community Medicine, Tufts University School of Medicine, Boston, MA, USA

M. Reinhorn
Boston Hernia, Wellesley, MA, USA

S. Sbayi
Surgery Department, Emergency General Surgery, Stony Brook University Hospital, Stony Brook, NY, USA

- The care program and surgical workflow have been scientifically studied with performance standards and protocols that achieve excellent end results.
- A health care organization's culture is the de facto competitive strategy, enabling a collective purpose, and a strong identity as a working team that can partner with patients.
- Health care organizations need a strong people proposition that offers employees challenging goals, continuous learning, and an opportunity to achieve while doing productive work.
- Fair process leadership builds implementation into their strategic thinking; consequently, there is a system of accountability, with no extra layers of management.

Introduction: The Well-Managed Health Care Organization

In November 2016, Dr. Michael Alexander, chief of staff and chief medical officer for Shouldice Hospital, performed his 30,000th hernia surgery. His picture was posted on social media and there were multiple responses. Following is a sample post:

> Almost two years after my surgery, I am so grateful to Dr. Alexander, both for his exceptional surgical skill that ended my mesh nightmare, and for his kind and thorough treatment of me afterward, answering so many questions and allaying my fears about healing (which had not gone so well on my prior two mesh surgeries). I cannot recommend Shouldice highly enough. Shouldice offers a lifetime guarantee for their nonmesh surgical procedure and a success rate of 99% [1].

Dr. Alexander is an example of a hyperspecialized physician. Shouldice Hospital, a focused clinic founded in 1945, specializes in the surgical repair of abdominal wall hernias and recurrent hernias.[1] Shouldice has performed 415,000 hernia surgeries and consistently produced excellent outcomes for more than 75 years.

Shouldice Hospital in Ontario, Canada is an 89-bed hospital with five operating theaters. The hospital offers not only efficient and low-cost services for patients and payers, but also high-quality hernia repair with a lifetime guarantee[2] and outstanding patient and caregiver satisfaction.

Dr. Edward Earl Shouldice started Shouldice Hospital in Canada in 1945, at a time when a traditional hernia surgery meant weeks in the hospital, a painful patient experience, poor outcomes, and months of slow recuperation. He did not try to compete with the general hospitals that performed herniorrhaphy, but instead created a unique surgery and care program, organizational culture and operating strategy that emphasized:

---

[1] When an organ, tissue, or intestine finds a weakness in the abdominal wall and pushes through a tear in the muscle or tissue covering this area, it is diagnosed as a hernia. Often it is obvious to the patient because there is a noticeable bulge of soft tissue. Hernia rupture can become a serious health issue, such as causing an intestinal obstruction. Hernias can occur in the abdomen, belly button, upper thigh, and miscellaneous areas, and they most commonly occur in males. It is estimated that 75% occur in the inner groin, called inguinal hernias.

[2] Although Shouldice fixes hernia failures from other non-Shouldice surgeons five days a week, they estimate that they redo only 50 of their own surgical failures each year.

- superior surgical technical outcomes
- low risk, with respect to patient safety
- high volumes and strict standardization
- low prices/costs
- austerity and simplicity
- surgical and patient productivity with less time in pain
- convenient access with healthy amenities
- homelike and fun ambiance
- memorable and supportive relationships with surgeons, nurses, staff, and patients
- environmentally friendly location

Within a few decades, Shouldice Hospital redefined acute health care services for primary and recurrent abdominal wall hernias. Unlike traditional hospitals offering hundreds of service lines and continuous expansions, Shouldice focused on a *single service line*: primary and recurrent inguinal hernias (85%) and other groin and ventral wall hernia procedures. Shouldice's strategic formulation and execution of services achieved cost efficiency with a stable revenue stream, a strong value proposition for patients, and a strong employee proposition for caregivers and nonclinical staff.

Patient value, as it is used here, means:

> Offering the highest quality to patients at a lower price, and at a reasonable cost to the organization.

Quality of care has both objective components, e.g., outcomes and end results, as well as subjective and emotional components, e.g., patient experience and patient satisfaction. Quality is best understood as a multidimensional construct, operationalized by five variables (1) technical outcomes; (2) overall patient experience and satisfaction; (3) decision-making efficiency; (4) relationships with caregivers and staff; and (5) convenience and amenities [2].

Regarding costs, laparoscopic and mesh repairs have substantially higher variable costs for supplies and materials than pure tissue repairs [3]. The variable operating room costs per non-mesh primary hernia surgery at Shouldice until 2020 were less than $30.[3] Today, owing to Covid19 (PPEs, IV costs and new regulations) they are less than $130. In fact, the price for the entire Shouldice hospital and surgical service (surgeon, nursing, food, laundry and linen) with a three-day to four-day stay is less than the price of a laparoscopic outpatient procedure in the US and Canada.[4] The Shouldice price is about $2950 versus an average outpatient price of $7750 USD in the US. Historically, the cost of a Shouldice hernia surgery to the provincial health system in Canada is also significantly less than that funded through public

---

[3] Throughout this paper monetary references with a dollar sign ($) will be in Canadian dollars and cents. Otherwise, it will be noted as $ US dollars.

[4] That would include the round-trip airfare from major cities in the US to Toronto, Canada.

hospitals and outpatient centers.[5] For example, in Ontario, the average general hospital's surgical cost per comparable hernia surgery case was $1639, compared to $1072 for Shouldice, which excludes the surgeon's fees, the semi-private room and out-of-province fees. The average payment to hospitals and surgeons in Toronto for a comparable hernia procedure may be approximately $4000 versus $2950 for Shouldice.[6]

Shouldice Hospital redefined hospital patient experience with its rave reviews from former patients. For many decades, Shouldice brought a sample of patient cohorts back together for an annual reunion, because patients had expressed a need to see the friends they had made and the surgeons and caregivers they had encountered during their in-patient stay at the hospital.[7]

The Shouldice hernia repair almost never uses general anesthesia; in well over 95% of primary inguinal cases, operations are performed under local infiltration and a light sedative [3, 4].[8] Avoiding general anesthesia significantly reduces the risk of harm to patients. Moreover, Shouldice surgeons are carefully selected and trained based on their prior experience over a 2–4 month period before they are allowed to operate. Where a typical general surgeon may perform 50 hernia repairs a year, each Shouldice surgeon performs on average more than 600 per year. Additionally, the surgery is not done on an outpatient basis. Each patient stays in the hospital for a minimum of three to four days.

What makes some of the clinical work challenging and rewarding for Shouldice surgeons is repairing hernias that other surgeons have been unable to repair permanently. Throughout the day, surgeons operate on patients with a hernia recurrence. These patients may have already had one or two hernia procedures, but the hernia returned because it was not properly repaired. Performing a procedure over old scar tissue is tricky work for any surgeon. Nevertheless, these are the cases that motivate Shouldice surgeons because they provide clinical evidence of the superiority of the Shouldice technique with its specialized incision, suturing, and early ambulation procedures. Shouldice surgeons can guarantee their patients that they are the most experienced hernia surgeons in the world.

---

[5] In Canada hernia surgery is covered under provincial health care plans, as required under the Canada Health Act. There are no co-pays or deductibles, so prices to patients are not relevant. Physicians are paid on a fee-for-service basis by the Ontario Health Insurance Plan (OHIP) and the hospitals are paid a global budget rate.

[6] One of the authors called a Toronto ambulatory care center and received a quote in writing that a laparoscopic hernia procedure was estimated to cost between $6500 and $9000.

[7] In 1947 Dr. E.E. Shouldice was asked by a few patients to organize a "soiree" for himself and his patients. The patients wanted 2 things (1) to renew friendships with other patients; and (2) to stay close with the hospital. This became an annual event and Shouldice patients were encouraged to come back every year to have their hernias checked by surgeons who were in attendance as well. It was a huge event in the ballroom at the Royal York Hotel. During our visit in 2016, the managing director told us, "A few years ago, we stopped the patient reunion. It had to end—it just got too big. The demand was four thousand people every year and growing. We could not accommodate the demand, and it turned into a negative."

[8] General anesthesia is used for large ventral and recurrent hernias.

Shouldice offers not only a hernia repair technique but also a well-designed service proposition that has clinical value for patients. The care process includes a stay in a pleasant and relaxed environment, continuity of relationships, low prices and high quality. The physician-patient interaction differs from most surgical encounters. When patients are admitted to this hospital, the first person they see is their surgeon who confirms their diagnosis, explains the procedure, and tells them what to expect.

Once selected for Shouldice, patients are educated to become partners and coproducers in every aspect of the care process, which builds both trust and self-confidence. For example, they are encouraged to walk into the operating room. They are awake and can talk with the surgeons during the surgery, and they are invited to get off the operating table and walk, with the help of the surgeon and assistant surgeon, to a waiting wheelchair where they are taken to their room. The postoperative room.[9] Early ambulation is part of self-confidence building and the recovery process, with patients being fully ambulatory after 4 h.

Recovery is completely programmed, but more like at a resort or on a cruise than in the military. Each day it starts with getting patients out of bed, taking their medications, walking down a flight of stairs to eat breakfast in the dining hall, and going to exercise classes with rest periods in between. The patients' day continues with a nice lunch in the dining room followed by more exercise and interactive recreation. Later in the day patients have dinner, more recreational activity, snacks, and then lights out [5]. To encourage mobility and interaction, there are no televisions or telephones in the rooms. Meals must be eaten in a dining room after the first day post-op, and patients must take themselves to the toilets. The facility has stairs with low risers, putting greens, exercise cycles, walking paths, and other activities aimed at fostering a speedy recovery. Upon discharge, patients are invited to return for annual hernia checks and to join the Shouldice patient network.

Patients, providers, and staff are fully engaged, understand their roles and responsibilities, and share a supportive and caring attitude and mindset. Through mutual interaction, learning and understanding, they are committed to the mission and goals of the clinical care process and adopt a Shouldice identity. The nurses know that their job is not to perform menial tasks, but to educate patients, help them to exercise, and relieve physicians of simple, nonclinical tasks.

These are powerful lessons in the repositioning of the primary clinical activities and the role of management in the formulation of care practices into a care process. The science of medicine and management aims to create value for patients and value for caregivers, staff, and the health care organization—what has been called the quadruple performance problem (see Fig. 2.1). The Shouldice story is about a well-managed health care organization, and in many ways, it is an exemplar case of the new science of medicine and management.

In this chapter, we present the case of Shouldice Hospital, a complex health care organization that for decades has created value for patients, caregivers, staff and the organization. Our purpose is to account as for the success of Shouldice as a modern

---

[9] General anesthesia patients recover in the PACU.

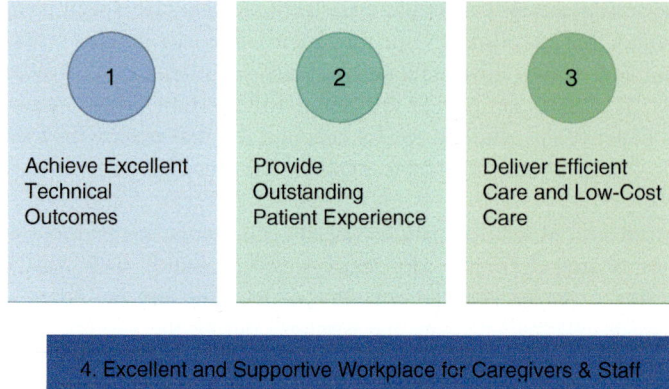

Fig. 2.1 The New Quadruple Performance Problem. Health care organizations are being asked to achieve (1) excellent technical outcomes, (2) outstanding patient experiences, (3) team well-being, and (4) cost-efficient care. For most health care organizations achieving even two out of four is a very difficult management task

well-managed health care organization, especially compared with the apparent satisfactory or malperformance of many general hospitals in recent years. The case study will illustrate how the new science of medicine and management works in practice.

All three authors shared an interest in understanding Shouldice as a health care organization. For decades, the hospital outperformed other hospitals and outpatient facilities doing hernia suture procedures. Thus, the authors decided to do a literature review and organize a visit to Shouldice in 2016, with follow-up interviews and worked together to write this chapter.

Two of the coauthors were highly experienced hernia surgeons. The third author was a professor of health care management.[10] One of the hernia surgeons was recruited, trained, and gainfully employed as a Shouldice staff surgeon for nearly 2 years. As an insider performing Shouldice surgeries, he was able to render very detailed explanations about the repair technique as well as his own journey to Shouldice, his learning curve, and personal development at the clinic. He could talk in detail about the care process, the management practices, the Shouldice culture, the people at the clinic and the administrators.

The other hernia surgeon was in private practice working in a US hospital and had performed several thousand hernia procedures. He spent 2.5 days visiting the clinic. During that time, he toured the facility, conducted many formal and informal research interviews, and keenly observed several surgeries using non-participant

---

[10] The research for this chapter began in the late 1980s when the health care management professor and lead author started a longitudinal study of Shouldice hospital. He conducted follow up interviews in the 1990s and more research in the early 2000s. Over several years he combed the literature on Shouldice, conducted on-site and off-site interviews with key Shouldice informants, and analyzed and taught about Shouldice as a health care organization.

observation. The professor later visited a second time and spent 2 days at the clinic, conducted many formal and informal interviews, and toured the facility. More interviews were conducted in the Summer of 2022. In the next section, we will discuss what we learned from the literature and from our interviews and observations.

Literature Review

We began with a literature review. First, we looked at dozens of studies on the history of hernia surgery, clinical studies of different surgical methods, and comparative studies of performance. Second, we collected dozens of documents concerning Shouldice Hospital—clinical studies, management case studies, reports, newspaper and magazine articles.

We identified three broad streams in the literature (1) the evolutionary history of hernia surgery; (2) studies comparing the Shouldice methods with other techniques; and (3) the literature on focused factories and well-managed organizations. (Each stream will be discussed and drawn together in this chapter.)

The First Stream: The Evolution of Hernia Surgery & the Search for an Optimal Hernia Repair

This clinical literature stream documents how the science and practice of hernia repair evolved and progressed [6].[11] With a better understanding of anatomy and physiology, new hernia repair techniques were introduced.

The first remarkable advance was reported by Edoardo Bassini in 1884, when he described a surgical technique that could fix 90% of hernias without recurrence. Bassini cut into the groin, pushed the intestine back through the hole and sewed together the torn tissue [6, 7]. In the years following Bassini, there were many smaller, open surgical advances, and up until the 1950s hernia repairs were closed using suture.

A second clinical breakthrough was the surgical technique introduced by Dr. E.E. Shouldice in 1945. The procedure is an open transinguinal pure tissue repair dissecting the entire groin area to identify weak areas and secondary hernias. The tension-free repair is performed with a laminated closure and under local anesthesia.

Shouldice hypothesized that a surgeon's knowledge of anatomy coupled with large volumes of cases would lead to a mastery that could prevent recurrences. As the transinguinal technique evolved, follow-up studies of hundreds of thousands of Shouldice patients over the better part of a century support the assertion that the end result was a durable, lifetime repair [4, 8].

---

[11] According to Hori and Yasukawa, 2021 [6], Hernia was first described in 1552 BC in Egypt and the diagnosis comes from the Latin word for prolapse. There is a lifetime risk of 17% for men and boys, and only 3% for women and girls. Females have a 4 times higher risk for femoral hernias.

A third notable event happened in 1958, when a new technique using a polypropylene mesh prosthesis was introduced. By the 1990s Dr. Irving L. Lichtenstein announced the discovery of a "tension-free" repair technique using mesh that was done under local anesthesia so that it could be performed on an outpatient basis with outstanding end results. Since then, the technique has continued to evolve with mixed results.

Although the medical community is still searching for the most optimal hernia treatment, 90% of all hernia procedures in the US today use one of the newer mesh techniques, such as Lichtenstein, Stoppa, laparoscopic, Kugel, mesh-plug or robot assisted [8, 9]. Given the large number of techniques, reaching a consensus on which mesh technique is optimal has created an ongoing and vigorous debate. Some studies report no difference in end results, and other studies report that one or another is superior [9–11].

The literature on the evolution of hernia surgery falls into two categories. First, there are hernia studies that focus on clinical breakthroughs in safety and reliability, anatomical discoveries, technological advances, and controversies among surgeons [6]. The second category comprises comparative studies of alternative repair methods, comparing open versus minimally invasive surgery for elements such as recurrence rates, technical difficulty, quick recovery after convalescence, chronic pain, costs, and efficiency [3, 12–18].

Discovering an optimal surgical repair technique is complicated. Each technique has to be evaluated on dimensions such as (1) low risk of complications, (2) replicable outcomes, (3) efficient and low cost, (4) operative time, (5) recovery, and more.[12] These performance attributes would require multivariate analysis controlling for confounding variables and nonclinical factors, such as the practice setting, a surgeon's ability (e.g., knowledge of anatomy, skills and experience, etc.), trust relationships with members of the surgical team, and other variables [19]. This brings us to the challenges faced in the second literature stream.

The Second Stream: Comparing Shouldice with Other Techniques

Over many decades, when comparing the efficacy of the Shouldice repair methodology and technique with other suture repairs, Shouldice had the lowest (1) cost, (2) recurrence rate, and (3) rate of complications. However, replicating results produced by highly trained focused centers like Shouldice versus general settings using the Shouldice repair methodology created mixed results.

In 2009, European hernia guidelines stated that the Shouldice hernia repair is the best nonmesh repair [20]. This is important since, in 2018, the HerniaSurge consensus recommended mesh repair as the new gold standard. However, since some patients refuse mesh, a surgical alternative is needed.

---

[12] When considering issues of social justice, access, and equity, an important consideration is whether a surgical technique is affordable and scalable to lower resource countries.

In 2012, a Cochrane review that compared all prior randomized clinical trials (RCTs) of Shouldice versus open mesh and nonmesh methods found that Shouldice had lower recurrence rates, less chronic pain, and lower rates of hematoma formation, albeit slightly higher infection rates, longer time in the operating room, and longer lengths of stay [21].

Surgical trials are challenging, however, because the results may only reflect the comparative focus of the techniques being studied and not the overall effectiveness of the implementation of the technique. For example, Shouldice hospital is an expert center with highly trained surgeons who have mastered the technique. Other centers may not have surgeons with equivalent skills. Consequently, some RCTs will be of lower quality, and likely lead to ambivalent results. An example of this occurred in 2002 when the *British Journal of Surgery* reported on a randomized trial of two surgical approaches i.e., the newer Lichtenstein mesh technique versus the Shouldice technique. Although there were no significant differences in postoperative complications, pain, and recovery, the researchers concluded that the Lichtenstein repair was easier to learn, took less time (the Shouldice technique took 7 min longer to perform), and there was a slight difference in recurrence rates [13]. But again, this randomized trial may not tell the whole story.

For that RCT, five surgeons were taught both techniques in a typical surgical training program, and surgery was performed under regional or general anesthesia in an ambulatory setting. The clinical objective was a quick repair, less time in the operating room, and same-day outpatient discharge. From a health care management perspective, the clinical trial not only missed what the Shouldice technique is about, the study completely missed critical aspects of the Shouldice methodology, i.e., pre-operative patient conditioning, immediate and early ambulation with an in-patient postoperative stay. Moreover, Shouldice surgeons are not trained in 8 h, and they are not considered qualified until they perform 300 cases. Further, after experiencing 300 cases, surgeons perform another 700 cases to become clinically efficient.

Our review of both literature streams surfaced important findings. First, new hernia techniques and better data do not necessarily invalidate what was already known-new knowledge is added and integrated into the growing science of hernia repair. When several surgical techniques offered excellent results, evidence-based studies do not arrive at ultimate truth, but often generate ongoing controversy, while still aiming for truth.

Second, discovering the best way to perform a hernia repair has been a frustrating odyssey, owing to the lack of standardized work, difficulty controlling for surgical variations, and lack of clear definitions of outcomes such as pain. Different physicians in the same practice settings using the same hernia repair technique can make hundreds of small decisions that modify the guidelines for a given surgical technique [12, 17]. Without standardized work, there can be no improvement in how the surgery was done [22]. Finally, a major challenge of standardizing hernia repairs is getting every general surgeon to agree on an approach. The hernia repair literature exemplifies all the complexities of surgery with respect to (1) patient safety, risk factors, technical outcomes and recurrences; (2) surgical infections; (3) cost efficiency; (4) learning curves; and (5) physician practice styles.

The Third Stream: Focused Factories and Well-Managed Organizations

Shouldice hospital has been labeled a "focused factory" [23, 24] or focused clinic [25]. In 1974, Wickham Skinner introduced the term "focused factory" to define an organization that would outperform a traditional factory manufacturing hundreds of products. Wickham Skinner described a focused factory as an organization concentrating on a "limited, concise, manageable set of products, technologies, volumes, and markets" [26–28]. In 1996, Skinner further described the ideas behind focused factories [27]:

> A factory is focused if its entire set of manufacturing policies, i.e., its structure, is direct toward one manufacturing task. This has nothing to do with size; it has everything to do with the design of the system. Focus is a state of mind and focusing is the management process of designing a coherent structure to accomplish a strategic task… [27, p. 72].

Although specialty hospitals have long been part of the landscape of delivery systems, a new breed of super specialty-hospital and hyper-focused physician is emerging globally. These organizations are like Skinner's notion of focused factories. Since we are not dealing with the manufacture of products, however, perhaps a better term is a *focused clinic*.

The concept of a *focused clinic*, as it is used here, is defined as:

> A health care organization whose preadmission, investigation, therapeutic, postoperative, and follow-up activities are clearly targeted to meet the unmet and holistic needs of a well-defined patient population segment. Focused clinics deliver a narrow range of services to not only meet a patient's medical needs but also patient's psychological, social and economic needs, and the caregivers' and staffs' psychological, social and economic needs as well, without any tradeoffs.

One hypothesis emerging from the literature is that focused clinics are capable of managing and achieving the elusive quadruple performance problem by creating value for (1) patients (2) caregivers and staff and (3) for the health care organization.

Although this third stream of prior work ignores clinical aspects such as the surgical technique or materials, it makes the connection between management practices and performance. Using anecdotal descriptions, case studies, and performance studies, this stream of literature compares general health care organizations with those that focus [24, 29–35].

Some of these studies compare specialty, subspecialty, or physician-owned hospitals to general hospitals. They hypothesize that with focus comes standardization, fewer variations in quality, such as medical errors, and substantially better quality of care. They find that performance improves when the volume of a given diagnosis or procedure increases, along with the experience curve of professionals. So, physicians, clinics, and hospitals hyper-focused on a few specific diagnoses and procedures may outperform general hospitals that offer a wider scope of medical services.

This third stream of work makes two contributions. First, it identifies the importance of the area of specialization, the importance of work standardization and the importance of volume-outcome effects on performance. Second, it identifies a core set of managerial practices that result in productive efficiency, financial stability, talent retention and operational longevity [23, 36–38].

Our chapter analyzing Shouldice Hospital brings the three literature streams together within an organizational case study of one focused hernia clinic. More specifically, we will take the reader inside Shouldice to analyze how they achieve operational excellence as a focused clinic. First, we will briefly explain the methodology used for the case.

Research Methodology

As we began our study, there were three questions we set out to answer. First, what are the important features of Shouldice Hospital as a care program and delivery system? Second, how does Shouldice create value for patients, caregivers, and the organization? And third, if Shouldice does outperform other outpatient, ambulatory surgery centers and traditional hospitals, what are key lessons that other health care organizations can learn? What underlies these questions is a singular mystery: What accounts for the decades of success of Shouldice as a modern complex health care organization?

The study design was a multi-source, multi-method descriptive and explanatory case study with core qualitative components—using archival data analysis, observation, and interviews with key informants. Prior to the site visit, some archival data was collected and analyzed. Next, we made several site visits to Shouldice to conduct an unstructured observational study of the facility. Two of the authors observed the surgery and all the key processes of the care program. One author was a participant observer working as a surgeon at Shouldice, and the other two were nonparticipant observers who conducted joint and separate individual interviews.

In addition to the observational study, dozens of structured and unstructured interviews with key informants were conducted. Both structured and open-ended questions were asked. The informants included patients, nurses, surgeons, senior executives, and nonclinical staff. To understand the patient and staff experience, meals were taken with patients and staff. Anecdotal data were observed and recorded. Interviews with Dr. E. B. Shouldice,[13] and Mr. John Hughes, the Managing Director, and some surgeons were recorded with their permission and transcribed. Interviews with the chief medical officer, surgeons, nurses, financial and other administrative staff, and patients were informal. Handwritten notes were taken.

To analyze the layout and operations, listening tours and rounds were taken. A considerable amount of that interview data was recorded, transcribed, and later analyzed. Finally, more archival data were collected along with additional literature

---

[13] The late Dr. E.E. Shouldice is the father of Dr. E.B. Shouldice, who also passed away in April 2022.

published from 2016–2022 to generate grounded hypotheses and to retest earlier findings based on interviews and observations. All of the facts and data presented were validated with follow-up interviews conducted Summer of 2022.

Next, we will describe our observations, findings and understanding of Shouldice. We will start with the market for hernia repairs, the historical background and evolution of the care program, and finally the key features of the frontstage and backstage of the care program.

The Current Hernia Repair Landscape: How Attractive Is this Service Line?

There may be no better example of a highly competitive surgical market than the market for hernia repair. According to Michael Porter, five supply-side competitive forces determine the attractiveness, intensity, and profitability of an industry [39]. These forces are (1) rivalry among competitors offering the service; (2) the power of buyers; (3) the power of suppliers; (4) the potential threat of new entrants; and (5) the threat of substitutes. Using that analytic framework, we can determine the attractiveness of hernia repair as a service line (more competitive means less attractive).

Regarding the competitive rivalry, general surgeons perform most hernia surgeries, and there are many general surgeons, except in rural areas. Hernias compose 14 to15% of general surgeons' workload [40]. In the US there are more than 25,000 active general surgeons who do hernia repairs [41]. In Canada, there are more than 2200, and 699 in Ontario, alone.[14] On average, general surgeons in the US and Canada perform about 50 inguinal hernias each year. They are a basic and dependable source of their surgical work. Since most of these surgeons (90%) use mesh, the product has become more standardized.

With respect to supplier power, there are many hernia repair device competitors (mesh, fixators, and other consumables) ranging from large global companies to small startups). Globally, the hernia device market is estimated to be $3.5 billion USD [43]. The hernia repair device market is a powerful supplier force because it is dominated by a few mesh large suppliers with name brands. When supplies are controlled by a few large global organizations, and they are more concentrated than the thousands of hospitals and general surgeons purchasing those products, they exercise influence [39]. Since 90% of hernia repairs use mesh, the concentration of suppliers can add substantially to the cost of hernia repair.

The buyer groups include government health authorities, managed care organizations, insurance companies, and self-insured employers. All of them exercise some power in so far as they control patient volumes and set or negotiate prices. In the US there are large powerful payors like Medicare who have an average fixed price for an ambulatory surgery center of $2039 and $3700 for a hospital ambulatory surgical center [44].

---

[14] Each year 270 or more general surgeons apply for residency in Canada [42].

In Ontario, Canada, the provincial health authority dictates a global budget for hospitals and owing to a recent mandate that required hospitals to primarily serve Ontario patients, medical tourism in Ontario was substantially reduced. Porter tells us that powerful buyers can be curbed only if the service can be delivered at a low cost [39].

The potential threat of new entrants is ever present in the market for hernia repair. There are, however, three features of the market for hernia repair that reduce the threat of new entrants. First, strong brand identification can create a barrier to entry. This can happen when patients can choose where to get a hernia repair and if they remain loyal to a delivery system. Second, since it takes time to build a strong reputation, hernia centers that specialize and build a reputation for obtaining superior surgical outcomes owing to well-trained surgeons can counteract and dominate newer entrants to the market. Third, some hernia techniques such as robotic or laparoscopic surgery, require large financial resources that will limit small or independent entrants.

There are several substitutes in the market for hernia repair. One substitute is called "watchful waiting"—that is, when a physician recommends waiting, patients can put off hernia surgery for many years. Another is avoiding a repair and wearing a comfort truss to support the weak areas of the abdomen. The other substitute is the characterization of emergent surgical solutions, e.g., open surgery versus laparoscopic versus robotic, and mesh versus natural tissue repairs. There will always be the potential threat of a newer, quicker, easier, lower-cost alternative to an open repair.

Porter's supply-side model helps us to understand how the five forces play out and shape strategy. Knowledge of these forces enables organizations to find positions where the forces are the weakest, and that requires making a choice between two generic strategies: either a low-cost service strategy; or one that can offer unique benefits—i.e., a differentiation strategy.

In a price-conscious and regulated industry, the price-performance tradeoffs create a competitive drive to search for innovative surgical technologies. The evolution of hernia surgery illustrates how technology-driven entrepreneurial solutions can backfire, however. For example, the introduction of the "innovative" plug and patch hernia repair became widely accepted in some countries because it offered a shorter operative time, lower cost owing to fewer minutes in the operating room, and it was durable. Plug and patch repairs, as it turned out, were a disruptive and problematic substitute. Over time, they became associated with serious complications such as chronic groin pain and even plug migration into a patient's bladder [45].

Value combines innovation with productive efficiency and excellent outcomes. Consequently, the solution is always to perform a hernia repair with excellent technical outcomes and a lower-cost alternative in the long term. In health care, the Porter model does not work because there can be no trade-off between price and quality outcomes. Patients, payors, and providers want high quality, low prices, and some degree of confidence that a surgical solution works in the long run.

Shouldice Hospital followed a different logic from Porter's, one that was both patient and employee-centered. They anchored their service culture and operating strategy on value—aligning a surgical innovation with excellent outcomes and low prices, supported by productive efficiency.

Shouldice discovered a metaphoric "Blue Ocean" [36, 37] from the clinical insights of founder Dr. E.E. Shouldice, who pioneered a pure-tissue surgical technique.[15] He then set a goal of offering a permanent hernia repair with a lifetime guarantee (any recurrences would be corrected free of charge), organized a collaborative team of focused surgeons running successive experiments, and after successful trials over a decade, selected variants of best practices along with a formulation of a well-managed care program. This will be illustrated by our study of Shouldice, presented next.

Shouldice Hospital: Analysis from Interviews and Observations

History: The Early Years of Shouldice

In the 1930s the outcomes for inguinal hernias were poor. Dr. E.E. Shouldice began a quest to improve not only the surgical technique but also the patient experience across the entire care episode—from preoperative to postoperative care. He continuously searched for the best way to permanently repair a groin hernia, using fewer clinical resources, and creating positive patient and caregiver experiences.

His quest began when he was a senior medical officer in Canada during World War II. He had observed that otherwise healthy recruits were being rejected if a hernia was detected. To help those recruits pass their physicals, Dr. E.E. Shouldice developed an innovative technique for a hernia repair that was coupled with immediate ambulation on the day of surgery.

He continued to challenge traditional surgical assumptions, learning the benefits of local versus general anesthesia, the importance of the suture and ligature material to reduce wound infections, and the importance of the surgical technique to detect secondary hernias for a complete and lasting repair [4].

The results in relation to the costs were significant–Dr. E.E. Shouldice's patients had no major complications and shorter lengths of stay in the hospital, returning home 3 to 4 days after the surgery. The goal was not merely tissue repair but identifying weak areas and preventing recurrences and readmissions.[16]

He also wanted to build a hospital culture where each patient was treated as an individual. To do that, the care program had to be integrated and well-coordinated. That would require strong cross-functional relationships among caregivers and

---

[15] A Blue Ocean discovers a new, sustainable untapped market space that brings prices and costs down and, at the same time, bringing quality up, offering a leap in value for patients, caregivers, and for the organization.

[16] The deep dissection enables the surgeon to identify occult (or hidden) hernias often present but difficult to discover by physical exam or advanced medical imaging technology.

staff. The Shouldice care process begins with preadmission preparation and patient conditioning, local anesthesia, comprehensive inguinal dissection and 4-layered reconstruction, and finally innovative postoperative principles. Next, we will talk about how this system evolved from successive approximations.

The Care Program: A Vision that Reconstructed the Boundaries for Hernia Surgery

By definition, a care program consists of the coordinated delivery of all services provided to a group of patients with similar pathology and care patterns, such as abdominal wall hernias. Activity Centers offer clinical (medical, nursing, or other caregiver services) or nonclinical (administrative or technical support) services to a care program. They are the key steps and operational processes to ensure patient flow and a good result. Underlying a hernia repair care program are hypotheses, assumptions, and assertions based on a testable theory of the service.

Dr. E.E. Shouldice's theory challenged how general hospitals operated and performed hernia repairs in the 1950s.[17] Abdominal wall hernias comprise a group of patients with similar pathology and similar care patterns. With a focus on abdominal wall hernias and high volumes, the care process would aspire to be both efficient, effective, and continuously improving. Although each hernia patient is unique, if Dr. E.E. Shouldice could standardize the repair procedure, poor outcomes and other surgical problems could be identified, analyzed, and resolved [4].

In most hospitals, getting surgeons to agree on a standardized approach can be difficult. Nevertheless, without a standard or protocol, there is no baseline for improvement. Long before Toyota Production Systems were invented, Dr. Shouldice understood that if every surgeon used their own tacit knowledge (e.g., unique hernia dissection and repair technique), surgical improvements might never be recognized or quickly transferred to other surgeons. Dr. E.E. Shouldice shifted the focus of the hernia surgeon from the surgical technique to the scientific study of patient flow through a more holistic lens that planned out the operating strategy and the entire total care process as a health system.

While Dr. E.E. Shouldice understood that standardizing protocols could have a very positive impact on patient safety and technical outcomes, he also understood that surgeons value their autonomy, and the freedom to adopt a surgical technique and develop their own practice style. To preserve physician autonomy, the protocols would be developed by Shouldice surgeons because they were in the best position to document advances based on data organized and sorted from the medical records with careful long-term follow-up of end results of patients.

Standards would not be forced on surgeons, rather Dr. E.E. Shouldice would develop a collaborative, team approach that was data driven and evidence based,

---

[17] History reminds us that hospitals in the 1870s was the place people went to die. By the 1950s hospitals had become such complex organizations that they required clinical leadership and competent management.

where many surgeons employed by Shouldice could contribute new knowledge.[18] Once standards were in place, they could evaluate clinical performance, set up controlled experiments and identify the best results in practice. Being data driven and evidenced based, they could codify and update changes to the hernia repair protocol. Every Shouldice surgeon could contribute new ideas, and by showing the evidence, help the team advance the surgical technique.

In the following quotation, Dr. E.B. Shouldice, the son of Dr. E.E. Shouldice,[19] illustrates how the protocols evolved to become the Shouldice methodology and technique [4]:

> E.A. Ryan joined the group in 1950 and introduced excision of the cremasterics to better view the canal floor. It was also at this time that splitting of the canal floor (posterior wall) was initiated, creating better exposure for finding secondary hernias and weaknesses. This enabled a further improvement, the transversalis fascia repair, starting at the pubic bone where direct hernia recurrences most commonly present. These maneuvers were incorporated into the technique by 1953 and the repair became standardized [4, p. 1165].

Other surgeons who joined the Shouldice staff collectively contributed incremental advances, such as splitting the posterior wall to identify secondary hernias and weak areas. Weaknesses and secondary hernias were hypothesized to be the reason for a so-called hernia recurrence, and the Shouldice methodology was developed to reduce and eventually eliminate recurrences. By the early 1950s, there was growing evidence that the repair method and technique was effective and efficient.

Anesthesia and Conscious Sedation

Another innovation was the use of local anesthesia for hernia surgery, in fact Dr. E. E. Shouldice was the first surgeon to use conscious local anesthesia on thousands of patients [48]. There are four reasons why this practice improves technical outcomes, decision-making efficiency, and patient experience.

First, general anesthesia is more difficult for older patients, who experience urinary retention, deep vein thrombosis, along with pulmonary and cardiac complications [46, 47]. A second benefit of conscious sedation via local anesthesia is that it allows the surgeon to communicate with the patient.[20] During the surgery patients are asked to strain or push to help the surgeons locate hidden or occult herniated

---

[18] According to Bendavid [46, 47] building on more than 100 years of evolution, by the 1950s Shouldice surgeons had incorporated all the steps of the Bassini repair that had been developed in 1886.

[19] Following the death of Dr. E.E. Shouldice in 1965, his son, Dr. E.B. Shouldice took charge of the hospital. For nearly 57 years Dr. E.B. Shouldice led the hospital and in April 2022, Dr. E.B. Shouldice passed away. Today Shouldice is led by the Managing Director, Mr. John Hughes, and Dr. Shouldice's three children, who sit on the Board of Shouldice.

[20] Since 2016, this practice has been reduced. Shouldice surgeons started to perform the procedures with local anesthetic and IV sedation, moving away from the oral sedative that takes longer to metabolize and lowering fall rates postoperatively.

tissue. These hernias cannot be detected by physical examination or ultrasound. Because the patient is a co-producer,[21] surgeons can optimize patient involvement and improve surgical outcomes and productive efficiency.

Third, the literature has found that there is less postoperative coughing when no inhalation agents are used. If older patients have cardiac or pulmonary comorbidities, local anesthesia is safer (a comment made by Dr. E.B. Shouldice to the authors).

Finally, Dr. Shouldice read the medical evidence and postulate about early ambulation by Leithauser following every surgery [12]. He embraced the idea and upon completion of each surgery asked the patient to sit up from the operating table, rise, and walk out of the operating room with the help of two surgeons. Immediate ambulation was made possible because of local anesthesia.[22]

Post-Operative Care: Immediate and Continuous Ambulation

Immediate ambulation, including light exercise on the day of the surgery, is fundamental to the care process. According to Bendavid, postoperative mobilization was nothing short of a medical heresy:

> …the patient walked away from the operating table, bed rest was minimal, and all activities were to be resumed as soon as possible without restriction. Only the patient's discomfort was a limiting factor… [12, p. 1888].

While immediate ambulation has physiological benefits (in terms of respiratory and circulation), there is an equally strong emotional and psychological benefit that builds confidence in oneself and in the surgery. When the patient sits up and gets off the table, it sends a message that they are not sick—they are well. They can resume physical activity. Light exercise and activity are resumed over the next two days, as patients are encouraged to walk around the campus, and use the putting green or game room.

In the 1950s, the hospital admitted sick patients with known or unknown medical problems and after investigation and therapy discharges a patient who is cured or much better only after a very long length of stay. Today, many acute hospitals and outpatient clinics admit a sick patient and discharge a patient with different problems such as anxiety about when they will feel better and get their life back. They bring that anxiety home, or they are discharged to a post-operative rehabilitation clinic or skilled nursing facility.

---

[21] Co-production is about fairness and justice. It implies that the patient is an equal partner with the most responsible caregivers in a reciprocal, two-way relationship. Coproduction means the patient, as a partner, is treated with dignity and respect. Both will be honest and truthful when they share information, and the physicians will explain the rationale for any clinical decisions.

[22] This was practiced safely until 2021, but new guidelines stopped this practice. Now, patients are put in their wheelchairs from the operating table, and ambulation is encouraged after four hours. This innovative practice is done in many outpatient facilities.

There are two parts to a care program. One part is more functional (the price, the sacrifices, and opportunity costs in relation to the benefits such as the technical outcomes), and the other is more emotional (such as the amenities, the overall experience, the trust and confidence in the caregivers, support for pre-post-surgical anxiety). The care program at Shouldice offered excellence in both parts. Dr. E.E. Shouldice always insisted that they would discharge a patient two to three days after the surgery: feeling better, believing they are cured, experiencing great service and new friends, and seeing a minimal surgical scar.

Hyper-Focused Clinic and a Very High Volume of Cases

From 1945 to the present, Shouldice has been a high-volume clinic focused exclusively on the repair of abdominal wall hernias. From 1945 to 2002, Shouldice repaired 280,000 hernias [4]. From the 1980s to 2009, the weekly volume or abdominal wall hernia repairs was 150 by 10 FTE surgeons. From 2010 to 2019 (pre-Covid) the weekly average was 132 repairs a week distributed equally among 10 surgeons. Most general surgeons perform about 50 inguinal hernias each year, Shouldice Surgeons over 600 each year, more than 10xs the average hernia surgeon. By 2022, they had performed over 415,000 hernia repairs.

The next section will describe Shouldice as a health care organization and care program. To understand how value is created at Shouldice, we will characterize activities in two parts, things the patient sees and experiences, and things the patient does not know about. It is what Teboul calls the front and back-stage [49].

The Front Stage and the Key Clinical Activities

The frontstage describes how every interaction and every contact with the patient are customized and integrated. It requires customized co-production with caregivers and staff and an integrated series of seamless interactions. The goal is to produce a durable outcome and memorable experiences. As Teboul states, a service must be "right first time":

> Because service is a performance, it can be neither owned nor accumulated but must be consumed at the moment of production [49, p 25].

Patients should not be passive but active participants for two reasons. First, they are an integral part of the care program, helping with diagnosis, guiding the surgeons, and adhering to the notion of ambulation and exercise. Second, their participation is vital for process improvement.

The backstage describes the organization of the care program, and how it supports service excellence and productivity with two key concepts: division of labor and standardization [49]. Backstage components include mission, senior leadership, operational processes (such as patient flow); how work is carried out; the specialized role of the caregivers and staff; the culture and formal structures such as human resources, and the facility.

There are four traditional clinical activity centers that perform (1) admission, (2) investigation, (3) therapy, (4) discharge/recovery, and follow-up. The way these activities are performed creates or nullifies patient value. The next section will not cover all the front and backstage activities but will highlight key features.

An Admission in Two Visits: Pre-Admission and Investigation

One of the critical dimensions of quality is efficient decision-making that results in finding quicker routes to health [2]. To achieve an efficient admission process requires coordination of the clinical and non-clinical activities. To be scheduled for surgery at Shouldice Hospital, a patient can expect a grand total of two visits. The first visit is a pre-admission screening, which can take anywhere from 2 to 4 h. Here is a description of that process by Shouldice Surgeon:

> During that visit, several activities take place such as triage nurse assessment, GP assessment, a surgical consultation medical history, a dietary consultation, followed by lab tests, and a hospital admission date scheduled.

Patients arrive at the Shouldice clinic in one of several ways: referrals by general practitioners; internet searches; or suggestions from trusted friends, colleagues at work, or family members. Patients do not need to make an appointment, nor have a referral, but can come in during the walk-in hours in the morning, where they will be evaluated by a physician. Next, we describe how walk-ins are managed.

Walk-in Patients Walk-ins are seen between 9:30 am and 3:00 pm. They present at times from 8:30 am and are received at the front desk. The patient may be directed to see a physician (general practitioner) if time permits, who will refer them to the surgeon for further evaluation.[23] The patient receives the benefits of co-locating two physicians so they can experience one visit. Other patients who have had a primary care referral will see the surgeon directly.

In either case, the patient fills out the intake sheet that inquires about past medical and surgical history. If they have a hernia, the location is identified along with a list of prescribed medications. The patient will ask to wait in the waiting room on the main floor and will be seen by a triage nurse who will get his/her height, weight, waist size at the belly button, blood pressure, pulse, and temperature.

The patient then is escorted from the waiting room to a seating area in the surgeon's office area in a hallway, where six offices are located. The offices may be

---

[23] At other hospitals, a hernia repair admission could require up to 7 visits. The GP visit and surgeon referral visit would require 2 or more separate visits in most hospital and hernia centers.

Community Hospital	**Shouldice Hospital: Walk-in Clinic**
• Visit 1: Family doctor appointment • Visit 2: Lab tests • Visit 3: Ultrasound and or CT scan (if recommended) • Visit 4: Surgical consultation	• Visit 1 (4-8 hours): Medical questionnaire, lab tests, triage nurse assessment, GP assessment, Surgical Consultation, Dietary consultation, hospital admission date scheduled
• Visit 5: Pre-admission exam & lab tests • Visit 6: Hospital/outpatient admission	• Visit 2 (admission): Hospital admission examination by a surgeon, lab tests, hospital admission

Fig. 2.2 Comparing Admission Process for Hernia Surgery in Ontario. Obtained from informants at Shouldice Hospital, 2016

staffed by one to five surgeons, affecting the timing that a patient may be seen, thus affecting the waiting period.

Patients who randomly walk in can spend anywhere from 30 mins to 4 h before they see the surgeon. They will be advised of the expected time in advance. The patient will be greeted in the hallway by the surgeon and escorted into the examination room. There, a surgical evaluation is conducted, and a focused examination is conducted. The abdominal wall, groins, and genitalia are examined when evaluating a potential hernia repair at Shouldice. Patients are classified into five groups (1) no hernia present; (2) hernia present, not suitable for the surgery; (3) hernia present and the patient is overweight; (4) hernia present and further medical information is required; and (5) hernia present, patient ready to be scheduled.

If they are diagnosed with a hernia and they are not more than 20 lbs. overweight or require further medical follow-up (i.e., by an internist to evaluate comorbidities), they are provided a surgery date for 8–14 weeks in the future.[24] Patients who have not had a recent ECG or blood work are then taken to the lab where this is all performed. The care process is a series of carefully coordinated steps that result in 2 very productive patient visits. When compared with an average of 4 and a maximum of 6 or 7 visits that can be required for a hernia admission at some centers, 2 visits to Shouldice appears to be more efficient, with less time wasted on multiple trips (see Fig. 2.2).

If they are more than 20 lbs. overweight, but less than 40 lbs. overweight, they are provided with a surgery date. Those patients meet with a surgeon and then meet with the dietitian to create a nutrition program that will allow them to lose weight prior to surgery. Patients more than 40 lbs. overweight meet with the dietitian but are not scheduled for surgery till they have lost enough weight to give them a highly successful outcome.

---

[24] The length of the wait time to schedule the surgery depends on the patient's medical condition, as discussed in this section. Before Covid19, the waits ranged from 2–6 weeks. One estimate from the Managing Director (Summer 2022) is that more hospitals in Toronto have a two-year wait for hernia surgeries versus Shouldice's 8–14 weeks.

To further extend patient outreach, the hospital also operates "remote clinics" where surgeons, supported by administrative staff, rent space in external clinics, and examine prospective patients. These are by appointment only, are advertised in advance, and ensure patients have access to Shouldice surgeons from 100's of miles away and are unable to travel to the hospital.

Self-Diagnosis Questionnaire A second way patients are booked for surgery is by filling out the online medical information questionnaire (see Fig. 2.3). This process is reserved for patients that reside greater than 60 miles from the hospital, as the hospital strongly encourages a physical examination for the best diagnosis, to allow

---

SECTION B • *Mark with an "X" the position of each hernia you want repaired*
(Hiatus, Flank and Parastomal Hernias are not repaired at Shouldice Hospital)

❏ EPIGASTRIC Hernias *are above the navel ("belly button")*
❏ UMBILICAL Hernias *are at the navel*
❏ INGUINAL and FEMORAL Hernias *are in the groin area on either side*
❏ INCISIONAL Hernias *bulge through the scar of any other type of surgical operation that has failed to hold*
❏ OTHER Hernias *are through any other muscular weakness*

SECTION C • *Describe ONLY the hernias you want repaired*
❏ **INGUINAL and FEMORAL HERNIAS**

RIGHT GROIN
Is this your first RIGHT groin hernia? ❏ Yes ❏ No   If no, number of previous RIGHT repairs ? ....
Date of last repair *(mm / yy)*..............   Can you reduce *(push back in)* your hernia? ❏ Yes ❏ No
Size of this hernia: ❏ Walnut (or less) ❏ Hen's egg ❏ Grapefruit (or more) ❏ No noticeable bulge

LEFT GROIN
Is this your first LEFT groin hernia? ❏ Yes ❏ No   If no, number of previous LEFT repairs ? ....
Date of last repair *(mm / yy)*..............   Can you reduce *(push back in)* your hernia? ❏ Yes ❏ No
Size of this hernia: ❏ Walnut (or less) ❏ Hen's egg ❏ Grapefruit (or more) ❏ No noticeable bulge

❏ **UMBILICAL, EPIGASTRIC and OTHER HERNIAS**
Is this your first UMBILICAL, EPIGASTRIC / OTHER hernia? ❏ Yes ❏ No   If no, number of repairs ....
Date of last repair *(mm / yy)*..............   Can you reduce *(push back in)* your hernia? ❏ Yes ❏ No
Size of this hernia: ❏ Walnut (or less) ❏ Hen's egg ❏ Grapefruit (or more) ❏ No noticeable bulge

❏ **INCISIONAL HERNIAS** - *What was the original operation for?*
❏ Appendix?   ❏ Gallbladder?   ❏ Stomach?   ❏ Caesarian?   ❏ Hysterectomy?   ❏ Colon?   ❏ Other?
How many repairs have been attempted on this hernia? ....   Date of last repair *(mm / yy)*..............
Size of this hernia: ❏ Walnut (or less) ❏ Hen's egg ❏ Grapefruit (or more) ❏ No noticeable bulge

ADDITIONAL INFORMATION ABOUT YOUR HERNIA
Has the hernia(s) identified above been diagnosed by a medical doctor? ❏ Yes ❏ No (self-diagnosed)
If yes, how: ❏ Physical Examination   ❏ Ultrasound   ❏ Other ....
Are you experiencing chronic pain from the hernia(s) identified above? ❏ Yes ❏ No
Are you experiencing chronic pain from a previous hernia repair? ❏ Yes ❏ No   Where:..............
Have you experienced a wound infection in any previous surgery? ❏ Yes ❏ No
Was mesh used in your other prior hernia surgery? ❏ Yes ❏ No   Which: ....

Fig. 2.3 Excerpt of the Medical Information Questionnaire. Patients can fill out this form to facilitate their admission

for extended patient out-reach (50% of patients come from the greater Toronto area, the other 50% from greater distances). This is a self-diagnosis that is screened by the on-call surgeon the day it arrives.[25] Patients are booked for surgery on the same selection criteria as those attending the walk-in clinic. They are asked to have and bring all the appropriate medical evaluations and workups on admission.

If appropriate, the patient can be scheduled for surgery without an initial consultation.[26] In this self-referral scenario, occasionally patients are told by the surgeon that (1) they do not have a hernia, (2) they do not need hernia surgery now (watchful waiting), or (3) they may be medically unfit. These patients are sent home with appropriate treatment.

Day One: Admission and Investigation Prior to Surgery

Once surgery has been scheduled, the patients arrive between 10:00 AM and 3:00 PM on the day prior to surgery. Patients that were not examined initially by a Shouldice surgeon come in early for examination to validate the information presented on their on-line application, and those having been seen come in later. Prior to arriving and throughout this first day, the goal is patient orientation and education—preparing them mentally and physically for their surgery. Here are some examples of how this pre-conditioning is carried out.

Patient Preconditioning When they first arrive, they are re-evaluated by the surgeon who will operate on them the next day, which is often different than the surgeon they met previously. Since all Shouldice trained surgeons perform the surgery in the same way, the patients are assured of identical outcomes independent of the surgeon performing their procedure. Some patients may need more lab tests.

At 4:00 pm, all patients attend a 30-min orientation with nurses. At that time, all incoming patients hear more details about their surgery and their upcoming 3–4-night hospital stay. Once done they are often brought to the semi-private room where the patients from the day before are often recovering.

It is a critical part of the patient experience to room with someone in a different phase of care so that postop patients can reassure the incoming patients. At Shouldice they believe that patient relationships offer emotional support. For some, lifelong bonds can be formed in these 3–4 days. These bonds and connections to the hospital have been integral in the word-of-mouth referral of the organization.

At 5:30, there is dinner. After dinner the patients can participate with other patients on the guitar or piano or play shuffleboard, and at 9 PM return to the dining hall for memorable events like the evening snack (tea and cookies). See Fig. 2.4 for an example of the schedule.

---

[25] Several physicians said the online application is reviewed within 24–48 h of its submission.

[26] Questionnaire patients who present a complex medical history or require further investigation of their hernia will have a virtual exam is scheduled.

Fig. 2.4 Example of Shouldice Daily Itinerary. The daily schedule is posted throughout the hospital, to guide patients

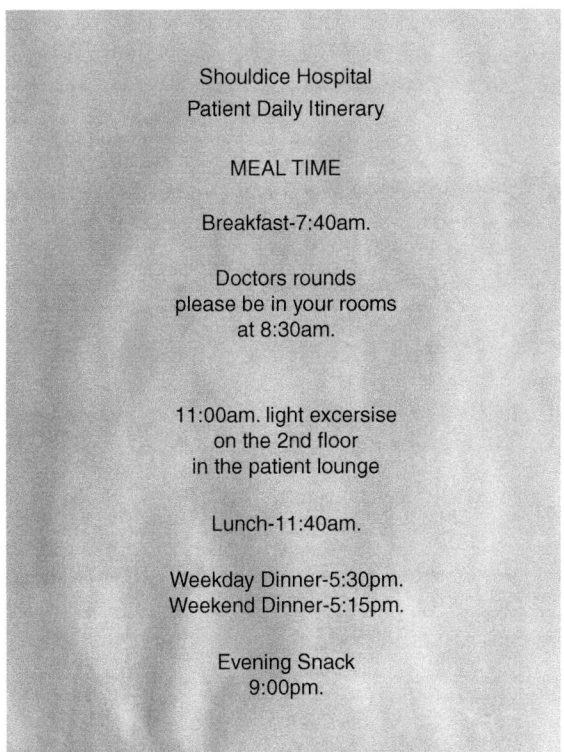

Day Two: Surgery and Therapy

On the day of surgery, the first patients of the day are escorted to the pre-op waiting room while those remaining wait comfortably in their room or patient lounges until approximately 20 min before their scheduled surgery. Few patients require oral sedatives prior to going to the OR as they have been through their orientation and have had the chance to review their upcoming surgical experience with their roommate or others in the lounges who have had surgery—this reduces most of the anxiety.

Patients are always escorted to the Operating Room (OR) by the surgeon and assistant surgeon. In the OR, moderate conscious sedation and local anesthetic are administered as required and there is a great deal of interaction with the patient because they are awake. There are always comforting conversations with the patients, both with their surgeons, but also with the highly trained scrub and circulating nurses.

Once in the OR the patients are situated on the bed and are monitored by the OR circulating nurse. The circulating nurse preps the skin and drapes the surgical site with the surgical nurse tech, while the surgeon and assistant scrub up their hands.

To manage the patient's expectations during the surgery, the nurse and the surgeons are in continual communication with the patient, making the patient comfortable as well as offering information. As one surgeon said:

> ...we ask them to let us know if you have any pain. Throughout the procedure we give the patient information about what to expect: 'there may be some pulling and that is normal. Or we explain what is coming next 'we are going to give you some medications, you feel some burning.

After the surgery is completed, the patient is invited to sit up and link arms with the surgeon and assistant, together they place the patient in the waiting wheelchair and are discharged to their room. General anesthesia patients spend up to 1 h in the recovery room.

Up to 85% of the patients are reported to take only acetaminophen or ibuprofen after surgery. One Shouldice surgeon said:

> I noticed in my hernia practice and in fellowships in US hospitals, nearly every patient needed a script for narcotics. At Shouldice with a local anesthetic, the Shouldice repair, and the 3-night hospital stay, all they require after the surgery are anti-inflammatories (Tylenol, Ibuprofen or Motrin). The same is true when they go home. (Shouldice surgeon)

Patients are received by the floor nurses who check vital signs and monitor their post-operative recovery to ensure ambulation after 4 h. The surgeon also sees the patients to make sure they are recovering well from the surgery and to answer any questions.

Days Three and Four: Post-Surgery Recovery, Follow-Up, and Discharge

Again, Fig. 2.4 is an example of the daily itinerary at Shouldice, illustrating how patient expectations are managed. On day three, patients are instructed to walk down to the dining room for each of the 3 meals of the day plus a 9:00 PM snack. An additional exercise class is also expected during the day and patients are expected to socialize with incoming patients as well as fellow post-op patients.

Patients continue to take acetaminophen or ibuprofen as needed. Many are well enough on the second post-surgical day so they can be discharged after their surgical clips are removed.[27] The rest are discharged on the third post-surgical day. So, patients stay four nights at Shouldice, however, the per diem charge for these 4 postoperative nights in the semi-private room is much less than the cost of a hotel, $305

---

[27] Interviews with two patients on postoperative day 1 revealed that that they only had mild and modest pain when moving, which they were able to do, although at a slow pace. Each one stated that they felt very comfortable going home on the second postoperative day and were planning on returning to a desk job a week after surgery. Both patients were delighted by their choice in Shouldice hospital and team-based care.

each day and it includes all the meals.[28] The quality of the food at Shouldice is not hospital food, it is like dining at a very good restaurant.[29]

Patient Echoes and Frontstage Voices: The Patient Value Proposition

There is enormous literature on mental health and personal anxiety associated with being ill. While the administrative staff is concerned with the overall patient satisfaction, individual patients understand their own experience—based on their perception of the process and how caregivers and staff responded to their needs and their medical condition. Patients not only expect a good technical outcome, but the care process also matters as well.

Over many decades, 98% of Shouldice patients rated their satisfaction with the overall quality of care a 5 and 2% rated it a 4 [5].[30] Here we present excerpts of patients' observations about Shouldice transcribed from video recordings from their website[31]:

> Whatever they did was good. The next day [after the surgery] I had no problem anymore. Staying at Shouldice after the operation was like being on a cruise ship, you're protected. A holiday! (Older male from Canada)

> My first hernia operation [at Shouldice] was a perfect success—no discomfort, I do not have a scar…Staying a few extra days is important. There is always stress and strain at home, you have kids jumping or a dog coming after you…I was very impressed with the staff. They are the highest points of the operation, and the surgery rarely needs to be redone. (Young Male from Canada)

> When I looked into hernia repair in the United States it was in and out…Having to stay here for four days I felt I would be cared for. I researched it and I was hesitating. My sister said there was a place that specializes in hernia, so I contacted them, and I was booked—It is an accommodating experience. When I called them, they called me back, and they always

---

[28] The Ministry pays the per diem when patients stay in a ward. Most Canadians have insurance that covers the semi-private room per diem of $305. Those without insurance pay the per diem rate out-of-pocket.

[29] Two of the Shouldice chefs are certified "Red Seal" Chefs, which means they have advanced culinary skills recognized nationally in Canada. Shouldice patients who go on social media often praise the quality of the dining hall.

[30] Patient satisfaction is rated on a scale from 1 = low to 5 = high

[31] These are not unproblematic, as they are anecdotal information and not scientific. We interviewed a few patients informally and heard only extremely positive comments confirming a more than satisfactory experience. Since we were unable to interview patients in private or interview patients a few months after discharge, we may not have obtained accurate information. We reviewed on-line social media comments and posts (Facebook, Twitter, RateMD) and found it confirmed our impressions. RateMD, a social media cite ranked Shouldice Physicians #1 out of 500. There were, however, some patient complaints about a rusty bathroom sink, a large noticeable scar, 20-year-old furniture, being rejected as a patient owing to co-morbidities, and the like. But far and away most posts extremely positive comments.

responded to me. Why did I wait so long—It has been great. I feel I am part of a big family and not shuffled out the door. (Young female from the United States)

The success ratio for this hospital is amazing…I do believe after surgery you should have enough rest. Staying in the hospital for a few days and having the staff monitor me 24-7 gives me comfort… The staff is professional. Everything flowed the way I was expecting. The staff is friendly, and the food is great. The room is quiet and clean. I absolutely recommend Shouldice. (Young Male from the United States)

I had a mesh repair three years ago that failed. So, I did some research on-line and came across Shouldice. I have a family member who is a surgeon. He heard of Shouldice as world-renowned. Getting his vote of confidence, as an American Surgeon, sold me… For me to go to Canada from California, one of my bigger [concerns] was time and cost of travel plus the surgery cost; it was an easy flight, and they have transportation and hotels set up, it was stress-free. (Younger male from the United States)

If this is an accurate sample of patient experiences, it suggests that Shouldice leaders have succeeded in organizing and creating a care program with a strong patient-centered culture. They have recruited the right people and supported their effort. The next section will describe the backstage at Shouldice and how it supports the frontstage.

The Back Stage at Shouldice

Designing a care program is infused with questions. How do you organize a care program that aims to deliver the world's best surgical outcomes? How do you market and sell patient experience? Can excellent service quality also carry a low-price tag?

Logically, the front stage is supported and operationalized by the backstage. However, the solutions to the problems of the frontstage are different than backstage. There are tensions between: (1) customization and standardization; (2) physician autonomy and service excellence; (3) co-production and no-patient participation; and (4) integration versus specialization. The backstage requires strategic choices, good management practices, and flawless execution. A service vision resolves any frontstage-backstage dichotomies.

Heskett [23] has identified four elements of a strategic service vision[32]:

- targeting both an external and internal segment of the market,
- creating a well-defined service concept that produces results for that segment,
- developing a focused operating strategy by customizing a standard service, managing supply and demand, involving the customer in the service, and controlling quality and costs,

---

[32] Heskett [23] says that a service vision will achieve a superior position by employing three integrating elements: (1) positioning; (2) leveraging value over cost, and (3) integrating the operating strategy with the delivery system. We will use those elements in the discussion section.

- designing a service delivery system with clear roles and responsibilities, motivating job design, facility layout that supports productivity and optimal service flow, and a customer-centered culture.

We use those four elements to describe Shouldice. First, we will describe the external and internal segments.

Targeted Patient Segments

Patient safety and outstanding technical outcomes are central to the mission, and this is not a full-service general hospital with technical backup. So, patient selection criteria are quite strict.

About one-third of the patients who want a Shouldice repair are overweight and require a dietician consult and a diet prior to undergoing the repair. Morbidly obese patients require more anesthesia and longer operative time, making them more appropriate patients for a full-service hospital and mesh repairs.

There is one full-time dietician who can see between 5000 and 10,000 patients each year. The dietician puts the overweight patients on a structured weight loss program. Estimates suggest between 200–300 hernia patients are on an active weight loss program. Many patients will write a comment about how the Shouldice weight loss program helped them to return to a healthier lifestyle and there was no charge for the dietician visit.

Complicated or high-risk patients may not be suitable for open surgery with conscious sedation. For example, patients who are not suitable for this procedure include patients with morbidities or conditions such as malignant hyperthermia, mechanical heart valves, pulmonary embolism, myasthenia gravis, low hemoglobin, ascites, or deep vein thrombosis.

Other hernia patients who are over 70 or who have co-morbidities such as AAA, CVA, liver or kidney disease, diabetes, and cardiac problems, are required to submit a medical report prior to admission. Shouldice has an internist who is brought in to assess all co-morbidities.

Most patients at Shouldice are considered at lower risk for surgery (ASA 1 or ASA 2), and less than 10% of the patients are at higher risk (ASA 3).[33] Since this is not a full-service hospital, complicated or high-risk patients with diseases that pose a constant threat to life cannot be taken care of there. Critics argue that Shouldice is "cream skimming: taking the easy cases and leaving the hard cases for community hospitals. Nothing could be further from the truth.

One study of the distribution of hernia cases found that ASA 1 & 2 comprise 72% of hernia cases, and ASA 3, 28%, and ASA 4, only 5% [50]. That means that Shouldice is taking from 75–85% of the distribution of hernia cases. Figure 2.5

---

[33] The American Society of Anesthesiology (ASA) has for decades developed classification system based on pre-anesthesia medical co-morbidities. It ranges from ASA 1 (normal healthy person) to ASA 4 (a person with severe systemic disease that is a constant threat to life).

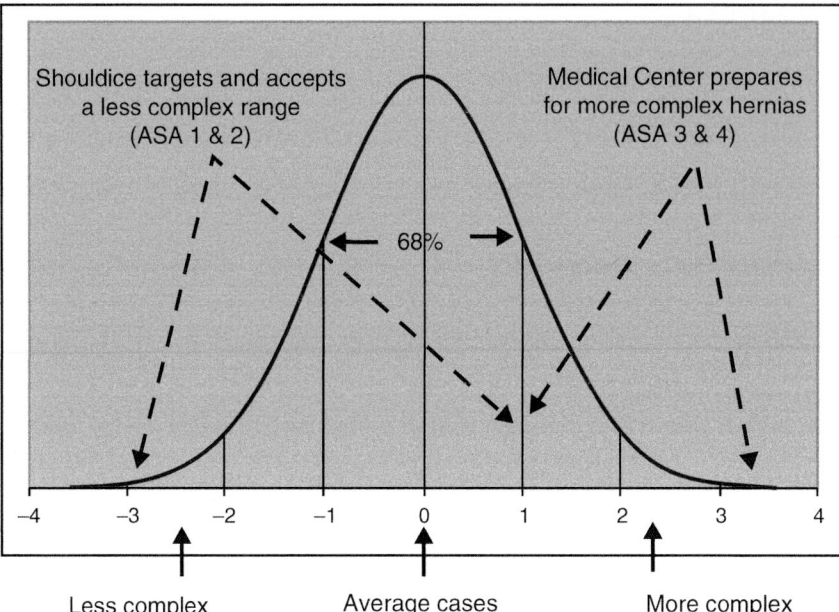

Fig. 2.5 Distribution of the Severity of Hernia Cases from Simple (ASA 1) to More Complex (ASA 4). This chart displays the distribution of the physical status of most hernia patients. It is based on the American Society of Anesthesiology physical status classification system that assesses and describes a patient's pre-anesthesia health status with respect to medical co-morbidities and other factors. For example, ASA I are "normal, healthy," hernia patients. ASA II are hernia patients with mild systemic disease (obesity, mild lung disease, smokers, etc.) ASA III are hernia patients with severe systemic disease, such as poorly controlled diabetes, active hepatitis, end stage renal disease, or history of CVA. ASA IV are hernia patients with a severe systemic disease that is a constant threat to life, such as cardiac ischemia, severe valve dysfunction, shock, sepsis, etc. ASA V is a moribund hernia patient who is not expected to survive the operation. ASA I and II comprise 72% of hernia cases, and ASA III and IV comprise 28%. This illustrates that Shouldice does not take the "easy" abdominal wall hernia cases. They make responsible decisions with respect to patient safety and risk

shows a normal distribution of hernia cases, and Shouldice will take most hernia cases well past the average and towards the more complex cases.

Targeted Physician Segments: Surgeon Recruitment and Training In Canada, the supply of surgeons is less than the demand. To recruit the "right" surgeon, the hospital leadership focuses on the mindset and character of the individual. They must be interested in helping patients and have a strong service attitude. Since attitude cannot be trained, they carefully recruit caregivers.

They also look for physicians with a growth mindset—a willingness to want to be a learner and who want to "learn it all," not physicians who already "know it all." They believe that general practitioners often make excellent hernia surgeons as they often have no qualms about relearning and being retrained to fit the Shouldice way of doing things. They also target general practitioners and non-general surgeons who are willing to be re-trained to learn the "Shouldice Method."[34]

Older, more experienced, physicians are easier to recruit to Shouldice than less experienced surgeons. These older physicians have good handcraft skills, have spent most of their career doing a wide range of surgeries, have spent lots of time in the operating room, and may have leadership experience such as a chief of staff. For the next chapter in their career, they have decided to operate on patients: (1) who are not very sick; (2) who have virtually no chance of mortality or morbidity; (3) who want a great work-life balance, and an opportunity to work in a collaborative and a team-based environment. Their career goals are helping patients and expecting to make "fair" compensation.

New hires are tried out as assistant surgeons for a minimum of 50 cases. After helping to perform 50 cases, they become the primary surgeon with the Chief Surgeon, in the role of assistant, observes them for another 50 or more cases. After this initial training period, a new surgeon will perform 150–200 cases supervised by a rotating group of senior trained Shouldice surgeons. Dr. Shouldice added: "We do not worry about speed. Once you do 1000 cases, the speed picks up."

Trainees become Shouldice surgeons only when both that surgeon in training and the Chief Surgeon agree that the training is completed. Depending on the surgeon's technical background and experience, the training period can last from two to six months.

We have discussed both the patient and physician segments that are targeted. Next, we discuss the Shouldice service concept and how it defines results for patients, caregivers, staff, and leadership.

Shouldice Service Concept

A service concept conveys the way Shouldice wants to be perceived by patients as well as by its caregivers and staff. More importantly, it clarifies the end results and the effort required of both employees and patients. The service concept describes how value will be created for patients and employees in a language that is inspiring and relevant to external and internal stakeholders.

Shouldice's mission is to "deliver the world's best surgical outcomes and patient experience in hernia treatment" with the goal of "exceeding the expectations of our patients by delivering the best surgical outcome and highest quality patient experience" (see Fig. 2.6). Shouldice has a goal of offering a permanent repair with zero defects and a lifetime guarantee. To remain the world leader in hernia surgery, the service concept is not only about a surgical technique that achieves superior results, but it is also about creating a unique patient and employee experience. To realize those aspirations requires an effective operating strategy and service culture with a commitment to solving each patient's problem.

---

[34] General practitioners and surgeons are trained under a structured "GP Change in Scope of Practice Program" supported by Ontario College of Physicians and Surgeons.

Our Mission:	To deliver the world's best surgical outcomes and patient experience in hernia treatment.
Our Vision:	To continue to be the patient's "provider of choice" in hernia treatment and be a global leader in hernia education and research.
Our Core Values:	With an unwavering focus on our patients and commitment to our staff, the following values form the foundation of Shouldice Hospital's operating culture.
Quality/Excellence:	We will exceed the expectations of our patients by delivering the best surgical outcome and highest quality patient experience.
Integrity:	We will adhere to the highest moral principles and standards of professionalism and ethics through our commitment to deal with patients and their families at all times with respect, honesty, confidentiality, transparency, and trust.
Compassion:	We will deliver world-class care to our patients by providing a supportive, sensitive and empathetic environment at all times.

Fig. 2.6 Shouldice Mission, Vision, Values. Downloaded from Shouldice Website 1/8/2022. https://www.shouldice.com/about/#mission

Operating Strategy: Focused on Productive Efficiency and Quality

Shouldice has an operating strategy that is focused on three things: (1) the Shouldice surgical repair and the operating rooms; (2) a team-based, patient-centric motivating environment; and (3) a system of accountability to control quality and cost. The result is very high patient and employee productivity; there is little waste.

The Method and the Operating Rooms: Focused on Quality and Efficiency

There are 5 operating rooms, a central sterilization area, a patient pre/post-operative area, and separate nurses and doctor's lounges. All these spaces are on the same floor and situated close enough that the longest walk between any two rooms takes less than 15 seconds, so no team member walks more than 15 seconds for each step in their job. The proximity of each work area allows for incredible efficiency.

Working as a Team In the Shouldice operating room, there is the surgeon, an assistant surgeon, a circulating nurse, and scrub nurse. Every member of the team is committed to delivering the world's best surgical outcomes and patient experience in hernia treatment. Their goal is "right first time" so the repair lasts a lifetime. They know every step of the surgical method, and they hold themselves mutually accountable. According to Katzenback and Smith that is the definition of a team [51].

Since most of the procedures are the same, each team member and all the equipment have a circular workflow that is uninterrupted and carefully designed. It appears that each person is achieving near efficient "flow" without wasted steps every day on the job, something that is unique to a single hospital that can focus on a smaller set of programs and procedures.

The surgery is performed "nearly" the same way by every surgeon, every time. As one Shouldice surgeon said:

> They have standardized solutions for every part of the surgery. I have rotated with every surgeon at Shouldice. Everything is done the same way—little to no variation. It takes 45 min, and again there is almost no variation. (Shouldice surgeon)[35]

Service Process Flow The surgeon and assistant work so closely together that little conversation occurs between them. Both seemed to be on the same page, with four hands carefully taking care of each patient, always. The surgery is as beautiful to watch as attending a live duet piano performance. In near perfect synchronization, the other teams work together with the surgeon and assistant surgeon to support the OR team. Like a duet, endlessly agile in the twists of individual anatomy and defined by myriad complex shifts of tempo. The surgical nurse in synchronized efficiency started to clean up the tools while the surgeons are closing the incision.

Having standardized the protocols in detail, the surgery takes about 45 min to an hour. If the conscious patient reports some discomfort, they administer more local anesthetic. In all cases, they use intravenous conscious sedation to allow for the relaxed completion of the procedure. Once completed, the patient is placed in a wheelchair that will be used to discharge them directly to their hospital room, where they are asked to stay for the remainder of the day with the required meal service. In the past, many patients went to the dining hall right after surgery,

Immediately after the patient leaves the room, the "scrub" nurse is just behind, heading directly to the central sterilization area where she places the tools in stainless steel buckets and soaked them in antiseptic detergent. The nurse drops off the linens to be laundered in the central laundry that is 15 feet away from the central equipment area. While this is happening the "relief" team is opening all the prearranged and sanitized surgical packs containing all instruments and supplies for the next procedure and the next patient is brought into the room, less than 5 min after the previous patient walked out.[36]

Most hospitals have disposable cloths and gowns. Drapes and gowns at Shouldice are all cloth and recycled and disposable items are avoided whenever possible. The total estimated variable cost of PPE and disposables including anesthesia is less than $130; prior to 2020 and Covid19, the variable costs were less than $30.

All delivery systems have an emergent implicit operating strategy that includes patient flow and clinical procedures, organization, quality & safety, human resources,

---

[35] Owing to Covid19 protocols, baseline surgeries now take about 60 min. Once the pandemic is over, they expect they will return to the 45-min surgical time. Every surgery we observed was less than 45 min.

[36] Prior to Covid in 2020, it was less than 5 min. After 2020 it takes 5–10 min to clean the room and sort out the new instruments for the next case.

accountability, marketing, and financing. In the OR, the 4 team members perform like a quartet and sometimes like a trio or duet. In general, Shouldice operates as a "team of teams." Each team member continually makes a significant contribution to the care process, by doing something for the care of the patient. There is no wasted time, and there are no wasted steps. They rotate on and off teams, so everyone can learn to work together and communicate without much need for verbal interaction. The result is very little variation in the service process and the interarrival rates of the patient and the surgical teams—with few late starts and bottlenecks.

The First Surgery of the Day[37] At the beginning of the day, it feels like a typical operating room with 5 surgeons and 5 assistants prepping for surgery after escorting their patients into the operating room, where the nurse monitors the patient and 'preps' the operative field. Once gowned up, everyone pauses and has a 'time out' to confirm that the surgery is performed on the correct side.

Once the patient is anesthetized, the incision is made with a large blade (#22). Towels are used to protect the skin and the surgery continues. No cautery is used in most cases, so any bleeding vessels are clamped to be tied at a later point. At set times during the case, all clamps are tied with a suture on a reel. Anywhere from 4–10 ties are performed in succession, always with an instrument knot to save on suture.

This appears to be performed for maximal efficiency so that the surgeon doesn't alternate between dissecting and tying knots. Once the external oblique is opened, the first step of the repair is to cut the cremaster fibers and identify the preperitoneal fat or *patent processus vaginalis* (i.e., hernia sac).

Since there is variability in each patient, this step, while performed the same way looked different in each case. Once the indirect portion is complete, the cord is retracted laterally and held back with a retractor while either of the superficial nerves is retracted or dissected out of the way.

The next step is to divide the lateral cremaster fibers along with the genital branch of the genitofemoral nerve. This may be a missing step that is not routinely taught in the US as it opens the view of the transversalis fascia in a way that is almost impossible without this step. An added benefit is that the nerve cannot be entrapped, decreasing postop chronic pain while providing a thick bundle of tissue that can be sutured around the cord laterally, creating a snug, and functional new internal inguinal ring with the proximal cremasteric stump. One Shouldice surgeon described that step as creating a scarf for the cord.

The repair itself was unique in the choice of suture and the number of layers used. It was explained that the numerous layers of continuous steel suture work much like a Chinese finger trap, allowing for flexibility and distribution of pressure minimizing any semblance of tension. The transversalis fascia is always opened, and the peritoneum and preperitoneal fat is dissected off the underside and a

---

[37] These observations about the Shouldice method were made by one of the authors who is a hernia surgeon.

femoral hernia is searched for. The initial suture is tied close to the pubic tubercle, taking care not to suture the periosteum.

The first layer incorporated the inferior edge of transversalis fascia and the underside to the rectus and internal oblique. The lateral most stitch incorporated the cremaster fibers, adjacent to the anterior superior iliac spine, creating the scarf for the new internal ring. The second layer brings the inguinal ligament to the internal oblique muscle, transversus abdominis muscle, transversalis fascia then ends at the pubis incorporating the rectus abdominis muscle and fascia, while taking bites of the pubic periosteum. This layer is very similar to the layer described by Bassini [52]. The 2 remaining layers include a back and forth running layer of more external oblique combined with internal oblique and rectus while taking care to not tighten the deep ring around the spermatic cord but snug enough to avoid a recurrence and continue to take more bites of the pubic periosteum. Finally, the cut distal cremaster is sutured to the external ring that is recreated, to maintain testicular retraction.[38] Dissolvable sutures are used to close the rest of the wound except for the skin which is closed by skin clips (michel clips) which are removed 24 and 48 h after surgery.

Next, the 2–3 nurses in the room get everything ready and start taking care of the next patient, starting the whole cycle again. While the patient is being prepped the surgeon and assistant have time to dictate their previous surgery and even have time for a quick cup of coffee. At this pace often 3–4 hernia repairs are completed before lunch, which the entire team in the room takes between 11:30 AM and 1:00 PM in the staff cafeteria, which is adjoining the patient cafeteria. The room is not utilized for this 30-min chunk each day, but all team members get to socialize in a relaxed environment. Often 2–3 more cases are performed after lunch before 3:30.

Post-Operative Length-of-Stay: 3.2 Days Most hernia surgeries in the US and Canada are outpatient day procedures. When Dr. Shouldice or any Shouldice surgeon is asked why the "long" length of stay, three reasons are offered.

- The first is patient safety—technical complications (bleeding or infection) occur in the first 72 h after surgery. So, surgeons can carefully monitor the patients for 3 nights to make sure the wound has healed well. On the morning of the fourth day, they go to their car and drive themselves home. The clinic may never see these patients again. Re-admissions are rare.
- The second reason for a 3-day stay is to eliminate sewing underneath the skin and using sterile strips across the incision. The body requires 12–14 h for the vasculature to be created underneath the skin. That natural healing becomes the glue and allows Shouldice to use temporary clips to bring the incision together. As the vasculature is being created, half of the clips can be removed the day after surgery, and the rest on the day after that. Patients end up with a very thin scar since subcutaneous sutures are not used.

---

[38] Again, all these observations about the Shouldice method were made by one of the authors who is a hernia surgeon.

- The third reason for three days is the importance of immediate and early ambulation, patient education and emotional support. Encouraging mobility and interaction with patients reduces apprehension, fear and for some, trauma. They admit patients the day before the surgery so the patient can become acquainted with the layout and beautiful surroundings. They can interact with post-operative patients, which increases their self-confidence before the surgery.

Staying several days is critical to the post-operative therapy and the long-term results they obtain. On the first day after the procedure, the patients are coached by nurses to stretch and exercise. Most complications (they estimated 90%) present on the first post-operative day, so if there are post-surgical issues they are observed and dealt with rapidly. They eat with all of the other patients in the dining room—they are not served any meals after post-op day 1 in their rooms. They are encouraged to walk around the hospital grounds, play pool in the patient lounges and attend daily exercise classes.

Most hernia patients enter an outpatient facility of the hospital with a hernia and leave that day with a repair, medicated for pain, but not feeling well, and need to return to check the repair and remove the suture. Shouldice on the other hand allows patients to stay a few more days so they can leave confident and feeling well.

Dr. E.B. Shouldice said:

> The benefits to the patient outweigh the minimal cost of a 3-4 day stay. When you care for a convalescing patient after surgery, it not only builds their motivation and confidence, but they also take less time off from work.

According to Dr. E.B. Shouldice, they return to work, on average, in 7 days. After hernia mesh surgery, patients go home the next day and return to light work between 1 to 2 weeks, however, full recovery can take from 4 to 6 weeks. Complications from mesh will extend recovery in some cases up to 1 year [45].

Creating a Strong Motivating Environment A fundamental question is what motivates a surgeon who is doing hernia surgeries? As one surgeon said:

> If you come to this clinic you have to answer a basic question—are you sure you want to do hernias the rest of your life? (Shouldice surgeon)

When asked what keeps the surgeons and OR staff motivated, the senior leaders gave several answers. First, the surgeon's job has been designed to require a deep understanding of the anatomy and requires technical skills and experience that many general surgeons do not have. Dr. Shouldice said,

> It is a 4-layer repair, where the transversalis fascia is incised from the internal ring laterally to the pubic tubercle medially, and upper and lower flaps are created. These flaps are then overlapped (double-breasted) with two layers of sutures…

While the basic procedure is performed the same way, there is a great deal of variability in each patient's hernia. To an observer, the surgery looks different from case to case. For each surgery, there is one "most responsible surgeon." During each procedure, Shouldice surgeons exercise their autonomy.

Second, surgeons can feel like they are *top-knife* surgeons.[39] One way this is illustrated is by fixing recurrent hernias from other hospitals and surgeons. Owing to their reputation as a hyper-specialized hospital, fixing a recurrent groin hernia from other hospitals soon became a significant part of Shouldice the target patient segment. Going over scar tissue and re-doing other surgeons' hernia work to make a permanent repair made Shouldice surgeons understand that they were practice leaders and world-class hernia surgeons.

Dr. Shouldice said "we are not afraid to take any type of hernia. Some hernias literally hang down to the patient's knees." He also confessed that more than once he came out of the operating room and thought to himself, "that was a masterpiece."

Third, since Shouldice records every case by the surgeon, there is a strong sense of collective responsibility for the surgery and the long-term end result. During every surgery, there is immediate feedback; each team member holds each mutually accountable. Finally, they trust that they are working with a stable and competent surgical assistant and nurse as a team.

Fourth, and most importantly, to keep a team-based culture, the hospital wants to pay every surgeon the same. They are paid a fair wage with a bonus, a paid vacation, a full range of health benefits, reimbursement of all professional and insurance fees, and an allowance for professional development.[40] There are clear workload norms and physicians can exercise some autonomy in deciding when they want to exceed or relax the norms. Surgeons are expected to (1) perform 5–6 surgeries a day, (2) see 12–15 new patients, (3) examine their patients the day before their surgery, operate on them the next day, and visit their patients in their rooms on the day of the surgery. When surgeons exceed those norms, they may obtain a bonus that is, on average, 5%. Finally, surgeons at Shouldice are choosing a lifestyle, they can always finish at 16:30 (4:30 PM) and go home to their families.

For all non-clinical employees, there is a performance-based bonus plan. Each year stretch goals, objectives and performance targets are set for each department such as (1) improving patient satisfaction, (2) staying within the operating budget, or (3) submitting audit information on a timely basis, etc. At an annual meeting the Board discusses the same question—"given each department's contribution to our annual goals and objectives, what do we want to do our employees in that department?" After that discussion, a bonus pool is established without a formula. It is never based on annual profits.

Reviewing the employee records, one finds that annual turnover for surgeons, nurses, and other employees is less than 5%. Most importantly, they retain their "star performers." There is a huge cost to recruit, hire and train new health care

---

[39] Hirschberg and Mattox used the phrase "top knife" playing off the popular film *Top Gun*. The idea was the discipling required to train the very best trauma surgeons—thinking under pressure, adapting to uncertainty and rapidly changing situations [53]. Like the name of the Naval Fighters, you cannot be a Shouldice surgeon without commitment and courage in the face of adversity and being able to cut across any type of hernia and complicated anatomical areas.

[40] In 2022, physician compensation is about $300,000.

employees. In health care, the cost of turnover is the amount of time it takes to get a nurse, a surgeon, or a chef to perform. So, the real cost of turnover is a loss of productivity and/or a decrease in patient satisfaction.

In 2020, during the Covid19 pandemic, all elective surgeries were stopped and Shouldice was ordered to shut down for three months. The Shouldice family and the Board made a conscious decision to keep everyone on the payroll at their current salary.[41] From 2020 to 2022, the hospital had to shut down three times for 7 months. Each time they lost a great deal of money. When they re-opened every employee came back—there were virtually no resignations.[42]

A System and Culture of Patient-Centered Accountability[43]

Going back to the early years, Dr. E.E. Shouldice created a system for knowledge creation and a system for knowledge dissemination that has become part of the culture at Shouldice. They have evolved and become part of the culture at Shouldice. There are 4 processes: (1) one for creating clinical standards and protocols for hernia repair; (2) one for implementing those protocols; (3) another for following the protocol, with rigorous training and closely observing surgeons while being trained; and (4) one for monitoring performance by keeping a track record of end-results for each surgeon and the team holding everyone mutually accountable. The surgeons are under the watchful eye of the assistant and nurses. Here is how it is working.

Quality Control Quality control is very hands-on and performed in several ways. First, if a patient returns with a recurrence, that patient is set up for the follow-up surgery with the original surgeon. Excellent records or score cards are kept for each surgeon, noting OR time as well as those rare recurrences. Additionally, the Chief Surgeon will scrub in and assist frequently during the year to observe the surgeons directly in the OR.

---

[41] The Board not only wanted to support their employees during the pandemic, but they also understood that because of the specific training to work at Shouldice they wanted those well-trained people to come back. They would be hard to replace.

[42] A handful of employees did retire because of their age. After the second shutdown in 2021, they kept everyone on salary, but the second time over the 3 months, they ratcheted from 100% of salary to 90% and then 80%. Again, everyone returned. The last shutdown occurred in January 2022, for one month. This was their third shutdown. Owing to the significant losses in 2020 and 2021, they had no choice but to temporarily lay everyone off. After one month, when they were told they could re-open, every employee returned.

[43] As Dr. Shouldice suggests, for many general surgeons, and hospitals, there are no incentives to keep very accurate track records of successes or hernia recurrence rates, so they are always understated. In addition, he said, "How many patients have a recurrence and choose to live with it? Every day our surgeons are operating on patients who had a repair at another facility, and it failed. So, I did 2 informal studies. I asked these patients 'did you go back and tell your surgeon it failed?' Two-thirds said, 'no' the first study, and one-third said 'no' in the second study. However, 100% said they told their general practitioner."

The senior management team, including the Managing Director, Director of Operations, and Director of Nursing, will make frequent rounds and discuss the surgeons with the surgical scrub nurses who observe every surgeon frequently. They are the first line of alert should a surgeon's technique varies from the fundamental protocol of the surgical repair, or a new surgeon is underperforming and needs further supervision or training.

A relatively new surgeon, who had gone through the training with the Chief Surgeon, did not seem to know his way around the OR. He was a little unfocused, and he spent a longer time in training. Just 2 weeks after he was performing the surgery, one of the assistant surgeons told the senior leadership: "There was no harm to the patient, however, I will not work with that surgeon." He was immediately taken out of OR.

Next, we describe the delivery system.

Well-Designed Service Delivery System

The operating strategy will fail without a service delivery system that integrates and supports the strategy. The important attributes of the delivery system include (1) the formal organizational arrangements and people management; (2) people and job design; (3) extensive training; and (4) a patient-centered facility. We begin with a description of the organization and people.

Organization Structure and People Management

Shouldice is a family-run enterprise managed by a few senior executives.[44] The leaders have created a flat organization with minimal reporting relationships, coordinated by a mission-driven culture and teams of people on the front lines with clear roles and responsibilities. Dr. Shouldice walked through the entire hospital 10 times a day, doing listening tours and having impromptu conversations with all of the physicians and employees right until 3 months before his passing. There are a small handful of top managers and staff, so Dr. Shouldice knew everyone's name.

The hospital is led by the Managing Director, Mr. John Hughes, who told the authors:

> One of the beauties of being in a relatively smaller organization is that you touch everything every day. I will go from finance to human resources…I deal with families, hire a cook or nurse…Every day is a unique challenge.

There is a Director of Operations who oversees the administrative groups, such as maintenance, front office, medical records, IT, research and inpatient services. Working in an executive dyad, the Managing Director and Director of Operations spend a great deal of time on the front lines listening and interacting with employees. They also know everyone's names and if there are any concerns, they take note and act immediately.

---

[44] Shouldice was headed by Dr. E.B. Shouldice, as Chair, until he passed away in April 2022. Today three of Dr. Shouldice's children sit on the Board of Shouldice.

There are 5 service centers (or departments) reporting to the Managing Director and Director of Operations[45]:

1. Medical: Chief Surgeon & Medical Officer, Surgeons (11 FTEs), Assistant Surgeons (8 FTEs), General Practitioners (2 FTEs), Anesthesiologist, (2.5 FTEs), and Clerical Staff.
2. Nursing: Director of Nursing, Manager of Floor nurses and Manager of OR Nurses, Floor Nurses (30 FTEs) and OR and Scrub Nurses (20 FTEs) Personal Support Workers (5) and Lab staff.
3. Administration (Front Office, Finance, Medical Records, IT, HR and Research).
4. In-Patient Services (Housekeeping, Dietary, Dining Room and Laundry).
5. Maintenance (Building and Grounds)

A minimal hierarchy is not a weak structure. On the contrary, when people are "carefully" selected to work together as a collaborative team, and they trust each other, they believe in the mission, and they not only share goals but are committed to accomplishing the goals, they can manage themself.

People and Job Design

Being patient-centric runs to the heart of every job at Shouldice. As an organization, the operating strategy is driven by people: patients, nurses, surgeons, other caregivers, and staff. There is not another single factor more important than the quality of the people. Since the employees deliver services and not technology, selecting and retaining the right people with the right service attitudes cannot be overstated.

Heskett reminds us,

> One person can regard a job in food services as a boring, repetitive task, while another can see the same job as offering an endless variety of opportunities to meet and interact with people [23, p. 123].

Jobs are carefully designed, spelling out tasks, activities as well their broad roles and responsibilities. For example, the duties of an on-call surgeon and surgical assistants are posted on a bulletin board—see Fig. 2.7. That is not special, many organizations have similar job descriptions.

What does distinguish this organization is the way both clinical and non-clinical employees engage in mutually rewarding relationships with patients by sharing knowledge, offering advice, or simple guidance. Everyone's jobs have been enlarged to include listening and talking with patients. Everyone who interacts with patients is educating and counseling patients. The dietician educates and coaches overweight patients on nutrition and eating healthy. Nurses and housekeepers educate and counsel patients about exercise and self-care. Surgeons and assistants counsel patients on the importance of immediate and continual ambulation and light exercise. And postoperative patients counsel newly admitted patients.

---

[45] Everyone reports to the managing director. There are five senior executives and 7 supervisors,

On-Call Surgeon	Week-end On-Call Surgeon
• After finishing in the OR, proceed to the office to see patients and stay until all patients for the day have been seen • Post-op patient rounds are after 4:00 pm and only after all office patients for the day have been seen. Patients are to be examined in their rooms to be sure they are comfortable, the dressing is dry, and intact, and no sign of hematoma. • Do Hx and Px, draw blood on late admissions. • Remain in the hospital until the cardiologist phones. Follow-up on EKG concerns, compare with the previous EKG on the chart...if surgery is canceled record the reason.. • Assess bloodwork results (phone report) • Be on the floor by 6:45 the next morning to attend to any necessary ward work (drawing blood, completing charts) • Be available and reachable by phone and respond to any problems or concerns • On-call hours are from 8 AM to 8 AM (24 hours)	• Ward rounds are to start at 8:30 a.m. and Saturday Office is to start at 10:00 AM • Patients for admission are to be seen after having their EKG work done, their blood drawn and being seen by the admission nurse. The history of the chart is to be reviewed with the patient and any changes in health status or medications recorded. Patients are to be examined (heart, lungs, abdomen, all potential hernia sites, testes, scrotum) and results recorded on the chart. The operative site is to be marked and recorded as marked on the chart. The pre-op orders are to be written following the prepared pre-op Order Sheet taking into account the patient's age and weight • A new complete history and physical are required if the existing history is more than 6 months old or if there is not a previous complete history and physical on the chart • Patients are not to be discharged early on the weekend • Must be available and reachable by phone and respond to any problems or concerns related to Shouldice Hospital Patients. • Hours of on-call from 8:00 A.M. Saturday morning to 8:00 A.M. Monday morning of the first day following a long weekend

Fig. 2.7 Example of On-Call Surgeon's Duties. This is an example of the accountability system supported by setting clear expectations. It also illustrates the standardization of job design even for physicians

To deliver the world's best hernia outcomes and patient experiences, everyone must focus their time and attention on patients. That means treating patients with dignity and respect. By doing that, employees believe they are productive by helping patients find quick routes to health.

Human Resource Investment in Training

Most hospitals assume that once a physician has completed a residency, there is little need for clinical training, aside from some general on-boarding. Shouldice puts newly recruited surgeons through a 2–6-month training program.[46] They take a great deal of time to get new hires comfortable with not only the surgical technique, but also the whole patient journey and experience while at the hospital.

One surgeon spoke about the first week working at Shouldice:

> The first week was shadowing physicians in the clinic, waiting for my malpractice insurance to kick in. They have a simple electronic medical record, where you press buttons and fill in blanks and it is easy to see the patient. I shadowed a surgeon and observed how the physician greets a patient, escorts her or him into an exam room, does a full head-to-toe exam, height, weight,[47] and identifies the hernia. It helped me understand that Shouldice had a patient-centric culture... (Shouldice surgeon)

He explained his experience:

---

[46] New "in scope" surgeons undergo an extensive in-house training program, while surgeons undergoing a "change in scope" are supervised by senior Shouldice surgeons under a program approved by the Ontario College of Physicians and Surgeons of Ontario.

[47] The clinic is invested in the patient having an excellent outcome and being healthy. As described above, to become a Shouldice patient, individuals with hernias must fall into an acceptable weight-for-their-height range (BMI). If they must lose more than 20 pounds, there is a diet that is recommended by the on-site dietician. The physicians and staff support, motivate and encourage the patient to become healthier.

When I started, I observed 100 Shouldice procedures, as every new surgeon must do. Since each surgeon is doing 4-6 a day, you finish your observations quickly. Slowly, they hand over the suture, and the knife and they take you through the four layers. They identified vessels that most general surgeons would never observe... At Shouldice, it is a powerful science driven by surgeons. For males, there is the tube around the spermatic cord called the cremasteric that grows off the internal oblique muscle. That is a tube you slice and open like a banana and peel it off the spermatic cord. The cremasteric must be identified and used in each repair, otherwise, there will be future complications...

Surgeons can take approximately 1000 cases (almost 2 years) to get to a point where the surgery is fast and efficient. Surgeons work approximately 50% of their time in the Shouldice Hospital operating rooms and 50% of their time in the Shouldice Clinic.

This extensive onboarding and training (which occurs for all caregivers and staff) create a work environment that is motivating. The Shouldice approach is unique in its efficacy, every caregiver and staff has knowledge of the results of their effort.

Each surgeon can strive for mastery and to be in an elite set of the best hernia surgeons in the world. Additionally, there is a great work-life balance in that all cases are elective and scheduled with minimal "call coverage"and no emergency work. Surgeons can work predictable hours, with less uncertainty and stress.

A Patient-Centered Facility

There is one building that co-locates two facilities totaling approximately 73,000 sq. ft. a licensed surgical hospital, and a team-based clinic. The hospital is a private, surgical acute care hospital in Thornhill, Ontario, with 5 operating rooms and 10 examination rooms. Shouldice Hospital is restricted to 89-beds under its provincial license and is funded by the provincial government directly from the Ministry of Health. The hospital is not funded by procedure, they get a global budget (see Table 2.1). Consequently, they have to be efficient.

Table 2.1 Shouldice Financial Aspects. These were estimates based on interviews with the Chief Administrative Officer to illustrate the importance of managing costs at Shouldice. The costs and prices are much lower than other facilities even in Canada. Note: price, as it is used here, refers to what the Canadian government "reimburses" Shouldice. There are other sources of revenue from the clinic and other services that are not listed

Ontario Reimbursement to Shouldice	Patient costs: Full Cost Accounting
• $1072 for surgery	• variable OR costs = $130 per patient
• $357 for Surgeon's fee	• fixed costs per patient = $2574–$2774 per patient
• $120 for surgical Assistant's fee	• maintenance of 50-year-old building
• $180 for Anesthetist's fee	1. Replaced boiler, $180,000
• $77 for GP and $92 surgical consult fee	2. Replaced elevator, $265,000
• $34.1 for a post-operative consult on day 1	3. Internal EMR, $400,000
• $34.1 for a post-operative consult on day 2	4. HVAC issues, etc. $200,000
• $60 day of discharge	5. Cosmetic renovation, $1000.000
• $305 each day of stay (average is 3.2 days = $976)	6. New electric beds, $150,000
• Total Hospital and clinic revenue: $2950 per patient	• Total Hospital & Clinic Expenses: $2704–$2904 per patient

Seventy percent of the hospital costs are labor. Shouldice employs 142 FTE employees five managers, seven supervisors, (50 FTE nurses and scrub nurses, 2.5 FTE anesthetists, 1 dietician, and 89 FTE non-clinical staff employees). The only employed physician is the Chief Surgeon/Chief Medical Officer, Dr. Fernando Spencer-Netto, MD., who works for both the Hospital and the Clinic. He performs two roles, he is Chief Medical Officer for the hospital, and he is the Chief Surgeon and the clinical leader for the surgeons. As a player coach, he is part of the group practice actively performing hernia surgeries and training new surgeons.

Shouldice Clinic is a private group practice run by physicians and under the leadership of the Chief Surgeon, Dr. Spencer-Netto. There are 18 FTE physicians in the clinic: 11 FTE surgeons,[48] 2 FTE general practitioner physicians, and 5 FTE surgical assistant physicians. The clinic is funded by the Ontario Hospital Insurance Plan (OHIP). The clinic bills OHIP on a fee- surgical consults, and each hernia surgery (for-service basis and is reimbursed for all physician services such as physical examinations, see Table 2.1).

Over the past few years, the number of FTE employees has been reduced by 10. Since it is not a full-service general hospital, aside from crash carts for rapid response codes, there is no need for advanced technological backup. So capital budget expenditures are minimized.

Most acute hospitals built to handle a high volume of cases look like bureaucratic institutions, with giant parking lots. Shouldice hospital looks more like an estate or a home than a hospital (see Fig. 2.8). The original house was renovated to create a hidden hospital and clinic, designed to reduce anxiety, and promote patient and staff productivity, patient safety, respect, and comfort.[49]

The front door opens to the reception, a large lounge, and a glass solarium with a beautiful view and canteen, a large clinical waiting area and the examination rooms see Figs. 2.9, and 2.10. Going down one flight of stairs there is the dining room, kitchen, housekeeping office and administration. On the hospital side of the first level are the 5 operating rooms, pre-and post-op, laundry and central supplies. On the clinic side of the first level are admissions and discharges, general practitioner clinic and examination rooms and lab. Going up two flights of stairs in the hospital there are more patient rooms, as well as another lounge and exercise room.

There are several ways that the facility was designed to support both the functional care program (patient interaction, exercise and ambulation that stretch muscles) and emotional support—(reducing anxiety, finding antidotes to boredom, and the genuine feeling of enjoying their postoperative stay). First, the facility has multiple levels, and all the stairs and steps were designed with low risers for easier climbs and descents for patients having had groin surgery. Second, the floors and stairs are carpeted everywhere but the OR. Third, showers, televisions, and telephones are in common areas not in the patients' rooms.

The facility has pleasant amenities where patients can have fun. The hospital is located on 23 acres of beautifully landscaped grounds with appropriate inclines to

---

[48] The 11 FTE include the Chief Surgeon.

[49] In 1968 Dr. E.B. Shouldice designed and built a 58,000 square foot addition to the existing estate.

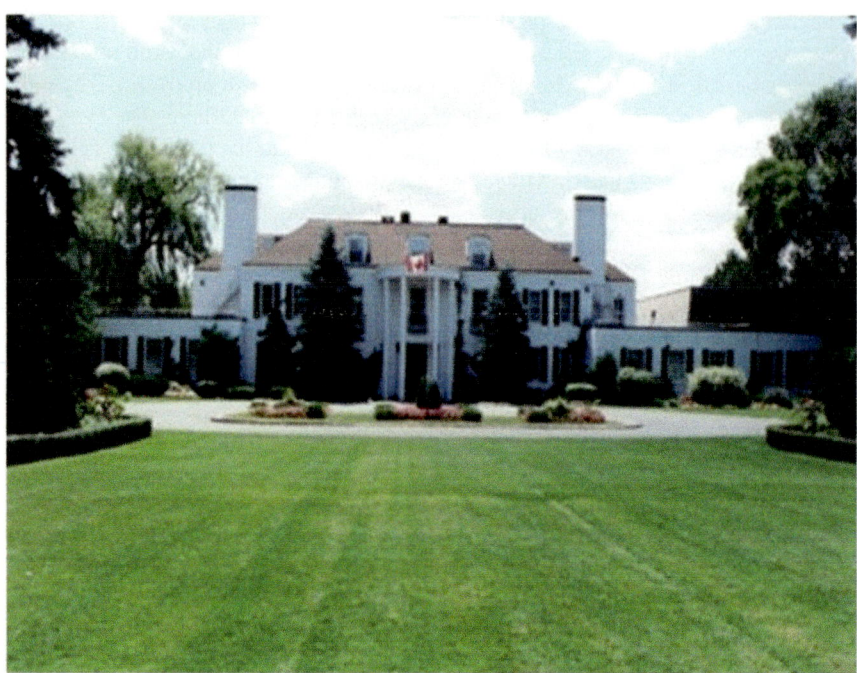

Fig. 2.8 Shouldice Hospital. This striking picture of the hospital reveals its patient-centric culture. The surgical hospital and clinic are hidden inside a beautiful luxurious well-maintained country estate with lush landscaping. For some patients we interviewed, it evokes feelings of comfort, safety, and confident expectations. The picture is the antithesis of a distant bureaucratic institution

Fig. 2.9 Dining and Sitting Areas. This is a view into the dining hall from a sitting area

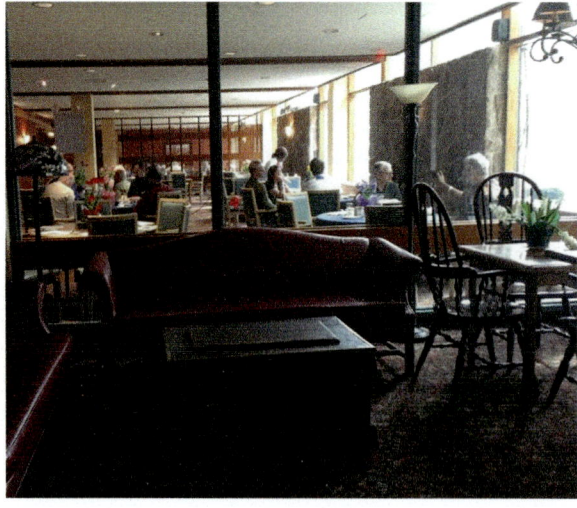

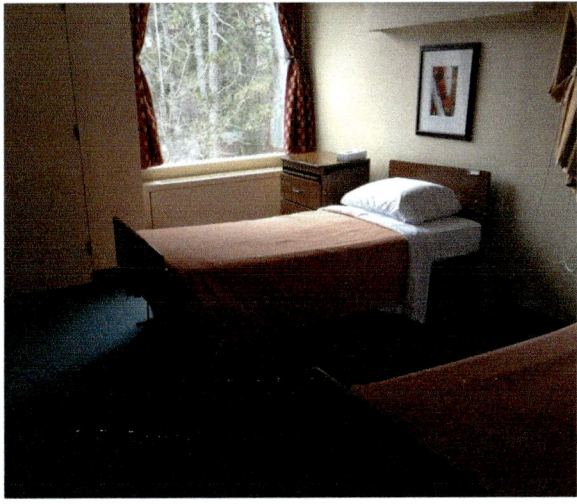

Fig. 2.10 Shouldice Semi-Private Room. The rooms are intentionally stoic to get patients to walk to the dining hall, recreation rooms, lounge and the grounds. Some patients said it was liberating to not be cloistered in a cluttered room

support patient recovery with light exercise. The facility has a solarium for reading and reflection, exercise rooms, and a game room with billiards and card tables. There is even a music room with a guitar and piano lounge. On the grounds are lovely walking paths, shuffleboard, and putting greens. Patients can decide to play billiards or use the exercise equipment. Alternatively, weather permitting, they can go outside for a walk, play shuffleboard, or golf.[50]

Caregiver and Staff Echoes and Voices: Value Creation for Employees

Observations and interviews at Shouldice revealed that everyone understood the importance of a patient-centered service attitude and the systems and care processes that support that mindset:

> Once I started working here, I realized that Shouldice Clinic had been designed to meet all the needs of every patient. Every employee and every part of the system is patient centered. Nurses and dieticians and other staff counsel patients and do not change bedpans. (Shouldice caregiver)

Interviews with other caregivers revealed the true appeal of a patient-centered health clinic:

> When I came here, I liked the Shouldice concept. The attention they give to patients is awesome–the dining rooms, the patient rooms. The clinic caters to the patients… (Shouldice employee)

---

[50] In 2016, the land was sold and the hospital has a 20-year lease on 2.7 acres. The rest of the property surrounding the hospital is scheduled for further real estate condo development. In the past, the hospital had built an independent living facility on the grounds. That facility was sold in 2000.

One surgeon spoke of how value is created for patients:

> The whole system is designed to manage patient expectations. They are guided each step in the process by everything and everyone in the hospital. From the video they watch in the waiting room to every encounter with hospital employees. Just by coming here, patients know they are cared for by the best hernia surgeons in the world.

Another surgeon spoke of the value created by the reputation and culture.

> I love the rich tradition. The Shouldice technique was developed by surgeons, and the procedure and care process evolved over time to become a much better set of medical practices. The outcomes are durable and recurrence rates are rare events. Finally, the patients treat me with great respect. They believe that they are being seen by the best hernia surgeon in the world. Shouldice is totally new and different from anything else I have done in my life as a physician. (Shouldice surgeon)

The genuine enthusiasm at Shouldice is not explained by compensation but by witnessing every day that the hernia patients they operated on are eating in the dining hall, socializing in the lounge, and having fun on the putting green. There is primarily an internal labor market for promotion, and employees who deliver good service have the security of a lifetime job.

Shouldice has been successful at establishing and maintaining an outstanding surgical record. Patients are very satisfied with the care and treatment and with the staff's strong service attitude. Based on these interviews, the surgeons believe in the care program and enthusiastically communicate their beliefs to non-clinical staff.

Next, we will evaluate performance including financial aspects, quality, social impact, current challenges, and future demand.

End Results and Performance at Shouldice

Shouldice has always argued that the cost per procedure is substantially lower than at other institutions and though they are a private hospital, their prices are significantly lower.[51] One prospective randomized study at a Spanish hospital in 2005 compared hospital costs when surgeons used the Lichtenstein versus Shouldice methods. They found Lichtenstein to be significantly more expensive than Shouldice (235 Euro versus 180 Euro) with comparable outcomes [54]. The next section will look closely at price and payment systems.[52] A description of all the price components and a summary of costs are shown in Table 2.1.

---

[51] In Ontario in 2017 the average general hospital cost per comparable hernia surgery case was $1639, compared to that funded to Shouldice of $1072. The difference is made up by the semi-private room and out-of-province fees.

[52] Payments made by third parties (which include government or insurers) for health services are called a reimbursement. If there are no out-of-pocket charges to the patient, the amount reimbursed is the effective "price" paid for a service in health care.

Financial Aspects

Reimbursement to Shouldice for a hernia repair is complicated. There are hospital fees and professional practice fees that comprise Shouldice's price structure.

Hospital Fees There are two charges for the hospital: a facility fee and a per diem charge. The facility fee is set by the provincial government and based on a volume (in 2021) of 6480 cases.[53] That flat fee was $1072 per patient and includes the operating room, food services, housekeeping, nursing, etc. The other fee is a per diem charge of $305 for each night they stay at the hospital.[54]

Professional Fees Next, there are professional practice fees that include: the original surgical consult, surgeons and anesthetist's fees, post-operative follow-up fees, and a day of discharge fee. The surgeon's fee is $357, the surgical assistant is (approximately) $120, the anesthetist is $180, the surgical consult fee is $92 and the general practitioner's fee is $77.[55] There is a post-operative consult fee of $34.10 for days 1 and 2. On the day of discharge, there is a fee of $60. The average reimbursement (or price to the provincial government) is $2950.00 per hernia repair. In 2021, the operating costs for 6480 cases were between $17,500,000 and 18,800,000.

At $2950 (Canadian dollars) Shouldice continues to have lower costs per procedure than hospitals in the United States and in Canada.[56] The average price of a single hernia repair surgery in the United States is $7750 (US dollars). Prices can range from $3900 to $12,500 depending on location, which procedure is done—open or laparoscopic, and what type of facility (outpatient or inpatient).[57] As discussed previously, in Ontario, Canada the average general hospital's OR cost per comparable hernia surgery case was $1639, compared to $1072 for Shouldice. Adding in physician fees, the average price for a hernia is closer to $4000 (Canadian dollars) compared to Shouldice's $2950. The cost of a laparoscopic case in Ontario

---

[53] According to the Managing Director, the government gave them a budget of $6,946,560 for the facility fee. That was based on a day-center rate for extra post-operative days (89%) and an inpatient rate (11%). If they had more than 6780 hernia repairs, they would not get more reimbursement. If they did fewer than 6280, they would get less than $6,946,560.

[54] Most rooms are semi-private, and there is a ward rate option that is covered by the provincial health care plan. Most patients want a semi-private room and stay an average of 3.2 nights. As mentioned, their insurance covers the per diem charges. Patients with bilateral hernia surgery require a 5–6 day stay and most Canadians carry insurance that pays the $305 per diem.

[55] About 60% of patients that come to Shouldice are scheduled for surgery. About 4000 patients are given a complete physical examination by the general practitioner, and checked for a hernia by the surgeon (surgical consult), but are not scheduled for surgery. The clinic can bill for the GP examination and surgical consult. About 10% of the Shouldice patients request a 30-min massage, for which the clinic will bill $75.

[56] The data for Canada came from a 2014 research study [55] and the data from the US are from New Choice Health, [56].

[57] In the United States, the average price for an inpatient hernia repair is $11,500 USD, while the average price for an outpatient procedure is $6400 USD. Those estimates came from New Choice Health [56].

would be even higher.[58] As mentioned earlier, a Toronto ambulatory care center sent a quote in writing that a laparoscopic hernia procedure would cost between $6500 and $9000 in 2022.

The variable OR costs are $130 and total fixed costs (both direct and indirect) per patient are between $2574 to $2774. The total cost per patient for the hospital and clinic is between $2704 and $2904. The excess of hospital and clinic revenue ($2950) against the total per patient expense is between $46 to $246.

Next, we will discuss the quality of care in five dimensions [2]. First, we will review the outcomes literature comparing Shouldice with the alternatives on recurrences, complications, and post-operative pain.

Incidence of Recurrent Hernias: Shouldice Versus Mesh

One of the most important complications of hernia surgery is a hernia recurrence. One study of three databases in the United States challenged the finding that hernia recurrence rates following tension-free mesh repair were between 1 to 5% [57]. Calling those statistics "overly optimistic they found the recurrence rates to be 10.5% (2015), 11.2% (2014), and 11.5% (2014).

Shouldice wants to achieve a permanent repair with zero defects. One independent 14-year research study of all the hospitals in Ontario, Canada performing primary inguinal hernia repairs (excluding Shouldice) found that the age-standardized recurrence rate ranged from 4.79% to 5.63%; whereas the age-standardized recurrence rate at Shouldice hospital was 1.15% [58]. That is not zero defect, but it is close.

Over many years, Shouldice published superior end results in non-comparative retrospective studies. A 10-year study of Shouldice hernia patients found a .13% recurrence rate. A 17-year follow-up of all 6773 repairs performed at Shouldice in 1985 found a .6% recurrence rate [4].

A measure of the learning performance of a hernia surgeon is the reduction in recurrences after repeating the same surgery over time. Figure 2.11 shows the number of hernia recurrences after 409,229 hernia surgeries for Shouldice from 1945 to 2020. There is a nearly exponential decrease in recurrences from 1945 (20% recurrence rates) to 1952 (1% recurrence rate). An asymptote of 1% was sustained with small fluctuations until 2020. It took Shouldice surgeons about 10 years to learn how to achieve mastery at that near-perfect level of recurrence.[59] They continue to aim for zero defects.

---

[58] The $4000 estimates are conservative. The Chief of Surgery at Shouldice conducted a hernia cost study in a Toronto general hospital comparing open versus laparoscopic hernia surgery from 2011–2009 [55]. He found that operating room and total hospital costs for open inguinal hernia repair were lower than for laparoscopic, (median cost, $3207 vs $3724). Over the last 8–10 years, it is likely that these costs have risen much higher than $4000.

[59] Shouldice found several innovative ways to conduct longitudinal follow-up studies with patients. For 50 years, Shouldice had an annual reunion of patients with a celebration and dinner and at those events, thousands of Shouldice patients were checked for hernias. They also reach out to patients for whom they had performed surgeries and conduct monthly traveling clinics in Ontario, and now across western Canada.

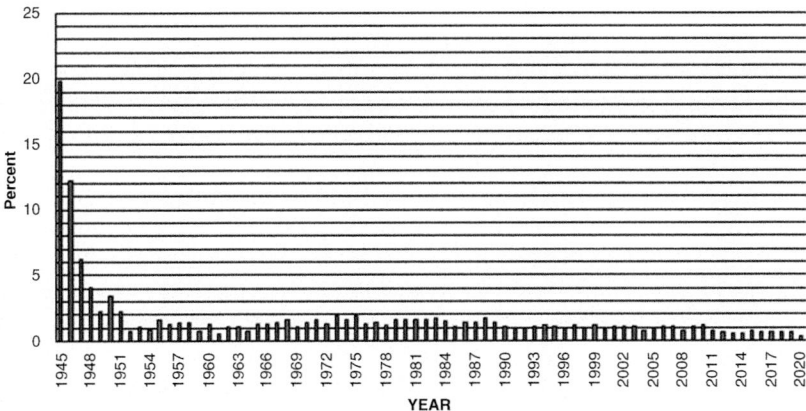

Fig. 2.11 Shouldice Recurrence Rate 1.2% from 1945 to 2020. This graph displays the recurrence rates from the beginning. There were 4934 recurrences after 409,229 surgeries. Eyeballing the data one can make two observations. First, there was a learning curve during the first 8–10 years. Second, although the recurrence rate dropped below 1.2% it reached an asymptote

Chronic Post-Operative Pain and Complications

Throughout the world, studies report anywhere from 8% to 54% of patients with hernia repairs experience a level of postoperative chronic pain that not only interferes with daily life but also can be disabling [59, 60]. Post-hernia pain is associated with lowering one's quality of life, interfering with social activity and interpersonal connections, and leading to suicidal ideation [60]. More prevalent than hernia recurrences, chronic pain is the most common adverse event.

One retrospective study of 76,173 mesh hernia repair patients demonstrated the prevalence of pain to be 20%, and the year pain was diagnosed resulted in a 1.75-fold increase in inpatient/outpatient costs, and a 2.26-fold increase in pain prescription versus the next 9 years [60]. This is value destruction.

Another retrospective cohort study of emergency department (ED) visits and hospital admissions from 2014–2018 in Ontario in the three days after ambulatory surgery found that of 14,950 patients who visited the ED 4440 (29.7%) had had a hernia repair [14]. Complications such as hemorrhage, hematoma, and acute pain were among the top reasons for the ED visit and admission to the hospital. All of these hernia surgery patients had an outpatient procedure that was not performed at Shouldice and reveals the hidden costs of mesh surgery and the high price society pays.

Shouldice's standardized open groin repair and early ambulation are associated with comparatively lower complication rates. There is a .15% hematoma rate (seven in 5000 cases, and a .05% urinary retention rate [4]. Only mild and superficial infections occur in .6% of the cases, and the testicular atrophy rate is .02% in primary repairs [4]. Patients operated on by Shouldice surgeons rarely experience chronic pain; rather a few may report some mild discomfort from time to time.

On the other hand, there has been a strong association between the utilization of mesh in herniorrhaphy and the escalation of serious chronic pain syndromes. The literature has reported that after mesh repair there is a high incidence of inguinodynia, dysejaculation, pain during sexual activity, and other types of nerve damage and complications. One meta-study of mesh complication rates found: 3.1% for dysejaculation; 10.9% for sexual pain; 10% hernia recurrence rate; and 13% chronic post-inguinal herniorrhaphy pain [61]. A recent randomized clinical trial in four Dutch hospitals comparing two mesh procedures found the recurrence rates were greater than 5% and the incidence of pain after 1 year was greater than 7% [62].[60]

Studies of post-operative complications when mesh is used suggest there is value destruction, not value creation. There are three implications. First, there is no trade-off between cost and quality. Post-operative complications are associated with poor quality and escalating health care costs. Procedures done at Shouldice are associated with higher quality and lower costs and lower prices [59–61].

A second implication is the proliferation of poor-quality mesh studies. Most of the studies are retrospective cohort studies and cover short time periods; longitudinal studies would be better. Moreover, very few studies are randomized clinical trials. The third implication is that when comparing different surgical mesh techniques researchers should consider outcomes such as chronic pain, hernia recurrences, and the annual and cumulative inpatient and outpatient costs over longer time periods. This should be a required area of focus for meaningful hernia research publications.

Social Impact of High-Performance Care at Shouldice: Value Creation

At the outset of this chapter, we defined value as offering the highest quality to patients for a relatively lower price, and at a reasonable cost to the organization. Quality, as defined here, has five dimensions [2, 64]. The first dimension is the outcome, whether the surgery shows an improvement in health status and quality of life (absent any complications or a recurrence). The second is decision-making efficiency, Was the right mix of clinical activities and resources used to obtain a good outcome? The third dimension is the overall patient experience and satisfaction with the care processes. The fourth is the amenities and convenience of the care program. The fifth dimension is the quality of the relationships between the caregivers and the patients, in terms of information, emotional support, and respectful interactions. To create value, Shouldice had to deliver on all five dimensions of quality with fair or relatively lower prices.

---

[60] A recent study of the utilization of mesh in hernia repair from 2014–2018 found most studies (81%) had one or more authors who had received payments from any one of 8 major mesh suppliers but did not declare a conflict of interest accurately [63]. The open payments database was used [63].

Excellent Outcomes/Strong Clinical Reputation	Decision-Making Efficiency
• No mesh used in surgery • Low recurrence rates: less than 1% over the last 10 years • Complication rates: less than .5% • On average patients back to work in 7 days	• Quick diagnosis to treatment: combining primary care, lab testing, surgery, and rehabilitation in one care process • Rapid turnaround of lab tests, medications, OR rooms etc • Optimal involvement of the patient in the care process • Sutures removed the second day after the surgery • Immediate and early ambulation reduces complications
Overall Patient Experience: Extremely High Patient Satisfaction	Amenities and Convenience
• 98% extremely satisfied (5/5); 2% satisfied (4/5) • Less time in pain • 99% willing to recommend the service again • Repair has a lifetime guarantee	• Walk-in clinic no appointment needed • Admission takes 2 visits with short waits • Excellent dining services • Semi-Private rooms have no: showers, telephones, televisions, or electric beds. • Staying at Shouldice is fun not boring (lounges, putting green, exercise machines, etc)
Excellent Relationship, Psychological Support, and Information	Lowest Price Hernia Repair with 3 to 4-day Length-of-Stay
• High touch clinical work (surgeon walks with patients into clinic, in and out of the operating room) • High degree of trust • Nurses, Dietician and Surgeons answering questions & teaching patients • Membership in the Shouldice network	• In the United States the average cost per case is $7,750 USD, compared with $2,700 (in Canadian$) • Historically, Shouldice is @42% of the price per case in any hospital in Ontario, Canada.

Fig. 2.12 Price and Five Quality Dimensions as Strategic Factors for Shouldice. This figure illustrates why Shouldice has been successful. Patient value is created in nearly every dimension of quality and price

Figure 2.12 displays that Shouldice not only challenged the pricing model of the industry by being low-cost, but they have also been able to deliver on the five dimensions of quality at competitive prices. The technical outcomes are excellent with lower recurrence rates, complications, and less time in pain. We see patient experience and satisfaction are also very high, with a lifetime guarantee, and 99% willing to recommend the service. There are trusting relationships between patients and staff with information conveyed to offer psychological support with carefully planned social interactions. The walk-in clinic and admissions process is simplified and convenient. The patient is admitted with a hernia and is discharged feeling that the hernia was permanently repaired, knowing that the surgeon discovered the weak areas and prevented future occurrences.

Past success does not guarantee future success. As Kim and Mauborgne state, there are no permanently successful organizations [36, 37]. We asked the leadership about problems and opportunities they are facing.

Challenges for the Coming Years

Discussions with Dr. Shouldice and the Managing Director revealed 4 problems. The first problem they face is the need to break away from old assumptions about who has been coming to Shouldice to understand the future potential demand. One assumption is about referrals from family and friends. As one Shouldice surgeon said:

> It is common to meet patients that come to Shouldice because family members have been there before. In some instances, I met a third-generation patient, where their grandfather and father were there before them.

One 14-year study found that Shouldice performed 27.7% of all abdominal wall hernias in Ontario, Canada, some 167,274 patients went to competing hospitals [58]. There are several possible reasons why they went elsewhere such as (1) lack of capacity at Shouldice, (2) an emergent or overweight case, (3) being unsuitable owing to their co-morbidities, (4) the referring physician or patient not understanding the benefits of natural tissue repair, or (5) for other health or attitudinal reasons.

The Managing Director and others hypothesized there are at least four hernia patient segments that come to Shouldice:

- Those who do not want mesh or general anesthesia.
- Those who want a "home-like, family" setting.
- Those who trust the Shouldice brand and care program.
- Those referred by former patients (friends, relatives, coworkers), or by a physician.

They know that after a patient spends three or four days at Shouldice, virtually everyone discharged becomes a fierce advocate. The Shouldice experience creates an enduring emotional and trusting relationship with nearly all their patients. That "strong brand" hypothesis has been tested year after year for decades, eliminating the need for advertising and marketing on social media.

They hasten to add that the brand is very powerful in what they called "Old Toronto," and that reputation translated into new patients who heard about Shouldice from a very loyal patient network of family and friends. However, people have been emigrating to Toronto from all over the world. That is creating important new communities in Toronto. The leaders at Shouldice said it could take years to build networks in these new communities. They also realize the need to take advantage of social media, and the powerful "word of mouse" when people look for caregivers not on official websites, but from on-line patient communities.

The second problem is the changing mix of medical tourists—local versus international patients. Many years ago, the hospital claimed that only 56% of its patients are Canadian, while 42% are from nearby, English-speaking United States (42%), while the remaining 2% come from Europe [5]. Medical tourism has been dramatically reduced by US Medicare changing rules on foreign coverage as well as the Ontario Hospitals being required to focus on Ontario patients. The local health authority reminded hospitals in Ontario that they are funded by a mandate to care for residents of Ontario and medical tourism must stop.[61] Since 2016, the hospital

---

[61] According to the Managing Director, it was further fueled by a newspaper headline from the nurses' union "Ontario health dollars going to the US." That resulted in less medical tourism. In the US, when Senator Rand Paul came to Shouldice and paid for his hernia procedure, the newspaper headline said "Kentucky Sen. Rand Paul, one of the fiercest political critics of *socialized medicine*, will travel to Canada later this month to get hernia surgery." Today Shouldice would charge a patient who is not a Canadian citizen approximately a total of $5500 for the surgery and 4-day hospital stay.

has focused on serving the residents of Ontario and now performs surgery on non-Ontario patients less than 10% of the time.

A third challenge is how to continue to position the Shouldice Care Program as an in-patient, holistic medical experience with a pure-tissue and suture repair that comes with a lifetime guarantee, in a hernia repair world that has gone 90% to mesh in an ambulatory setting.

A fourth and final challenge is that the hospital facility is more than 54 years old and it must be maintained. Given that the funding model does not include capital expenditure items, operating fees must cover all facility maintenance. Recently, they installed a new elevator costing $265,000, a new boiler system that cost $180,000, and are investing in a proprietary electronic medical record. The historical appeal of Shouldice was being a comfortable, home-like family setting. Will that advantage become a disadvantage?

In Ontario, Canada the Shouldice brand has always been strong. In 2021, they performed 20% of the 32,000 hernia repairs [58]. Management is concerned that this market share will not continue unless inroads are made in the new communities of Greater Toronto and surrounding areas. The next section will explore ways to analyze future demand.

Future Demand for Hernia Repairs

Patient demand for hernia repairs is very high—hernia repairs are among the top major ambulatory and inpatient surgeries for general surgeons as well as health systems throughout the world. Globally, each year more than 20 million patients have a groin hernia repair [8]. In the United States, alone, more than 965,000 patients underwent abdominal hernia repairs in 2019 [65] at an annual direct cost of more than $2.5 billion [6]. In Canada, there are about 50,000 hernia repairs annually, and more than 32,000 in Ontario. The universe of hernia patients seems large. Next, we explore how Shouldice can bring some of that future demand to Shouldice.

The Four Tiers of Shouldice Patients

We described a large pool of hernia patients above. To determine the size of a target market for Shouldice requires precise ways to catalog current and potential patients. Kim and Mauborgne argue that the way to target new patient segments is by categorizing patients by their demographic and psychographic characteristics[62] and their proximity to the current patients [36, 37].

Based on interviews with senior leadership at Shouldice, we defined and identified four categories of patients. Tier zero is the current tier of loyal patients. Tier 1

---

[62] Psychographic segmentation clusters patients by their attitudes, interests, opinions, personalities, sentiments, and values.

includes some of the current patients who may leave if a better opportunity is offered. Tier 2 are the patients who have refused the Shouldice care program. The third tier is patients and payors who are unaware of Shouldice but could be potential patients. Each tier will be described.

Tier Zero Patients

Shouldice patients have a referral through their general practitioner, the internet, a friend, colleague at work, or a family member These are the most loyal hernia patient. They are somewhat stoic and are not looking for a 5-star hotel. They select Shouldice by choice and after they go, they are extremely satisfied believing they have chosen the right care program. They urge other patients to go there.

Another group in tier zero believes that results and the patient experience are excellent. The fact that Shouldice guarantees the repair for life seals the deal. These extremely satisfied patients will tell everyone about this experience and as we have seen in this chapter, the network of patients has grown.

There are several patient segments and sub-populations in Canada and the United States who have chosen Shouldice. For example, there is a community of Mennonite patients from Pennsylvania in the US who have historically patronized Shouldice. They travel to Shouldice because they do not want mesh and they believe they will get the best care. They also like the fact that it is a lifetime guarantee, unlike when a hernia patient has a recurrence in the US.

Some patients are practicing physicians who know this surgery is superior [17],[63] and some are patients who have had a hernia repair that failed. Another group of patients goes to Shouldice not only because they believe this surgical technique is better, but even more importantly they do not want a foreign device, mesh, in their body. These patients may have heard about complications with mesh or plug and patch. Since 90% of surgeons around the world use mesh, Shouldice may be their only choice. Finally, there are patients who had a mesh repair with post-operative complications and want it removed and to have the guarantee of a Shouldice repair.

Tier One Patients

In the future, some patients in tier zero may disappear and go elsewhere. As mentioned, Toronto is changing, and new subpopulations are emerging. In the past, patients were given a referral from a trusted friend, co-worker, and/or relative, but newcomers will not know about Shouldice. In the future, they will rely on multiple sources of information. Shouldice needs to get ahead of this problem.

Another part of this group got a referral from a friend or family and thought about going to Shouldice, but they have different personalities, values, and attitudes. They are not sure about an open surgical procedure and a natural or pure tissue repair. Being with a group of strangers and staying as an inpatient (with little to do) is a concern. If they find a better alternative, they will go there.

---

[63] One study of 165 young German surgeons, median age 33, found that 36% would choose a pure tissue repair for their own hernia repair [17].

Tier Two Patients

The patients in this group thought about going to Shouldice but immediately changed their minds. They may ask only one or two questions. They might ask how much pain will there be? They are told there is only mild pain that is treated with Acetaminophen (such as Tylenol). Or they might ask when can I get back to work? They are told on average 7 days. However, when they learn that they will be conscious during the procedure and the procedure requires 4 days in the hospital with little to do, they immediately reject going there.

The fact that these Tier Two patients investigated Shouldice and made a rational choice, suggests that some persuasive arguments and a better understanding of their pain points may have reversed their refusal [37]. If Shouldice can understand the pain points of that patient, it could result in a new type of Shouldice patient.

Tier Three Patients

These patients are unlike any from the past. They do not understand the difference between natural (or pure) tissue versus mesh, or laparoscopic versus open surgeries. Their needs are taken care of by alternatives or other health care organizations. They may also include people who have health anxiety or a fear of hospitals and surgery. Other segments in tier three have been trying alternatives to surgery. They wear a corset or truss to ease the pain and discomfort. They may try to reduce the hernia manually, and/or use ice packs. These uninvestigated patients are health avoiders and need better information, counseling from trusted sources, and more emotional support.

In addition to these patients, there are non-governmental payors or corporations like Walmart, looking for low prices and excellent outcomes. For example, there are payors, like Blue Cross of Massachusetts, who have begun Alternative Quality Contract (AQC) programs. The program was introduced in 2009 to pay for better patient experiences and better technical outcomes, instead of fee-for-service payments for doctor visits, tests and hospital admissions. The Shouldice model would have great appeal to these large-scale payors. A final example is situations when patients have deductibles, co-pays, and co-insurance; these patients may not realize that their insurance plan does not cover the entire cost and their out-of-pocket payments might be lower if they go to Shouldice.

In the next section, we discuss what accounts for their success. We begin with positioning and the strategic landscape.

Discussion and Conclusions

This chapter has attempted to explain a mystery—the success of Shouldice as a modern health care organization, especially compared with the apparent satisfactory underperformance or malperformance of many general hospitals in recent years. To understand its success, we summarize some of the advantages of the focused clinic.

Being a focused clinic means that they set expectations for what they will do and will not do.[64] As a focused clinic, the mission, and results at Shouldice are brought into sharp relief—to deliver the world's best surgical outcomes and patient experience in hernia treatment. However, management is not only focused on the external market for hernia patients, but also on the internal organization, values, and relationships that enable the caregivers and staff to achieve their objectives. Adopting a focused clinic strategy puts both the patient and the caregivers at the center. They clearly defined their clinical practice and the activities necessary to implement the focused clinic strategy.

They have learned how to respectfully refuse patients they are unable to treat, while they learned how to meticulously serve every aspect of care their patients' experience. They do this by adopting some important managerial practices: (1) strategic positioning; (2) leveraging value to patients and employees in relation to the cost of care; (3) an integrating culture; and (4) value innovation [23, 36, 37, 66].

Positioning and the Strategy Landscape

Positioning identifies how to turn the targeted patient and employee segments into external and internal "customers." It answers the questions "what would create value for patients and employees" and "how is their value proposition unique"? In 1945, Dr. E.E. Shouldice clearly understood that there were many pain points in hernia repair at a hospital: poor outcomes, weeks of recovery in the hospital, and a boring, forgettable patient experience.

Patients in a traditional hospital or ambulatory center experience many pain points before, during, and after day surgery. For example, there is no choice, they must accept a mesh repair. The cost is high, and the experience is not fun. Preadmission is complex, requiring many separate visits that are somewhat inconvenient and inefficient. Post-operative care does not really exist other than removing sutures a few weeks later. There are complications with mesh and sometimes higher recurrence rates depending on the surgeon and technique used.

Shouldice, in contrast, offers a durable non-mesh natural tissue repair with very low recurrence rates, significantly lower postoperative complications, less chronic pain, and an overall cost saving to society. Their hernia repair comes with a lifetime guarantee—correcting any recurrence is free of charge.[65]

Our research surfaced three findings of the internal value added for both caregivers and for non-clinical staff. First, Shouldice offers its employees challenging goals with high standards, continuous learning, and opportunities to achieve by doing "productive work."[66] Second, Shouldice offers patients and employees a blend of centralized

---

[64] They have chosen hundreds of diagnoses and procedures that they will never do.

[65] They do fewer than 50 recurrences a year on patients who previously had their hernia repair performed at Shouldice.

[66] The term "productive work" implies that managers continuously eliminate anything that diverts caregivers and staff from patient care and performance. Removing unnecessary paperwork and unproductive meetings will improve caregiver and staff productivity and their job satisfaction.

clinical goals, and standardized procedures along with the requisite autonomy to make important choices. Third, the leadership and the caregivers take time to explain the rationale behind important clinical, non-clinical, and staff decisions, which creates a perception of fairness in the workplace. When employees perceive fairness in the workplace they feel a sense of pride, they become more connected and attached to the patients and other employees, and more loyal to Shouldice [67].

With respect to the first value-added, Shouldice hires and trains employees for the three-pronged approach of (1) educating, (2) counseling and (3) caring for patients. They look for people who can take responsibility for outcomes and who can contribute to the mission and goals. More specifically, we found that they look for:

> *knowledge workers and service workers* with service attitudes and growth mindsets, energized and willing to take responsibility as part of a team delivering the world's best surgical outcomes and patient experience in hernia treatment.

Knowledge workers, a term coined by Peter Drucker, are highly trained professionals who not only concentrate on their job, but they also know how to use their skills and experience to be very productive, never straying from performance [68]. The caregivers, administrative staff and senior managers are all well-educated knowledge workers who can manage themself. Non-clinical service workers do food preparation, housekeeping, maintenance, clerical, and support work. They can also manage themselves when the tasks, goals and standards are clear.

What brings both clinical and non-clinical employee groups together at Shouldice is a desire to help patients and to contribute to a "world-class" patient experience. The clinical and non-clinical service staff are not "know-it-alls" or in competition, but instead are people who see each surgery and every patient encounter as an opportunity to learn and improve their coordination and performance—that requires growth mindsets [69].

Shouldice recognized that compensation must be perceived as "fair." Fair compensation means employees doing the same tasks should be paid in line with their colleagues and equivalent to what others are paid in similar organizations. However, compensation does not motivate employees [70]. Caregivers and other staff are motivated by a belief in the organization's mission and values, which creates very high employee satisfaction. There is annual turnover at Shouldice, however, it is low compared to similar hospitals.

Leveraging Value to Patients and Employees over the Cost of Care

Shouldice positioned its service concept to simultaneously focus on offering a low price, high quality, and an "unwavering focus" on patient experience and caregiver/staff experience. However, that is not enough to achieve financial sustainability. As Heskett argues:

A properly positioned service concept has to be provided at a margin that allows for adequate employee salaries, investment, and return on investment. [23, p. 36]

This requires offering the services efficiently leveraging value to patients over the cost. We observed 4 management practices that Shouldice used (1) standardization in the backstage and customization on the frontstage; (2) managing patient demand; (3) optimizing patient co-production; and (4) creating a loyal patient base.

Standardization in the Backstage and Customization on the Frontstage

Another advantage of a focused clinic is learning better ways to perform clinical and non-clinical work. Over time, the clinical leaders and managers found standardized ways to accomplish work to obtain the best outcomes while using the fewest resources. In this chapter, we observed that leadership standardized the following areas (1) communicating with patients in detail about what to expect; (2) explaining the benefits of the semi-private room; (3) preparing surgical instruments and sutures; (4) preparing the operating room for the surgery; (5) preparing and administering medication; (6) performing the hernia surgery; (7) cleaning and disinfecting rooms.[67]

Standardized work does not mean that it is done exactly the same way by every nurse and physician. There is often small variation, such as making adaptive responses when encountering uncertainty during the surgery. However, standardization is key to success, and when a standardized procedure is not followed, the patient can be at risk.

Outside of the operating room, there is a customization of the care program to meet patient needs. For example, patients can begin the process of booking their surgery by going to the walk-in clinic. Admitted patients are matched up with someone in a semi-private room. Post-surgery recreation is always customized. Patients choose to walk to the game room, or lounge and pick up a guitar or play the piano. Depending on their recovery, patients can request an earlier discharge.

While the people who work at Shouldice matter and help to customize the patient experience, they can only be successful if the outcomes are excellent. And while the outcomes matter, so does the patient's experience, their relationships with caregivers and staff, simplicity and convenience, and efficient care processes [2].

Managing Patient Demand and Coordinating Patient Flow

Focused clinics can reduce unexpected demand and uncertainty for some diagnoses and procedures. Repairing abdominal wall hernias is a case in point. It is an elective procedure, so there is little uncertainty. Shouldice does have excess demand, but the

---

[67] Although not discussed in this chapter, there are protocols for cleaning and disinfecting rooms.

wait list is only several weeks. They can manage their demand with superb scheduling and a care process managed by a cross-functional team of people.

Once a patient is admitted there are standardized steps that must be followed. The result is a care pathway or value stream, defined as the entire care process (from admission to discharge) crossing over and coordinating with multiple caregivers and staff. They manage patient demand in the following way.

Every day (from Sunday to Thursday) 25–30 patients are admitted. As noted in the chapter, the average length of stay is 3.2 days. Since there are only 89 acute beds, they will reach capacity by Tuesday or Wednesday. Part of their success is not taking more patients than their staff can manage. This also reduces the stress and strain on the caregivers and other staff. However, to reduce the surgical backlog due to Covid-19, Shouldice started admitting patients on Friday and performing Saturday surgeries.

Figures 2.13, 2.14, 2.15, and 2.16 show a high-level service process flow chart that breaks the care process down into activities and identifies the interdependencies with other caregivers and staff and departments. The boxes represent different departments, caregivers, or steps in the process. The black boxes are patients' wait times (which are very short). Figure 2.13 is the diagnosing & scheduling process. Figure 2.14 is the admission process. Figure 2.15 shows day two which includes the surgery. Figure 2.16 shows post-operative days three and four, as well as day five, which is the typical day of discharge. All these care processes have standardized solutions, so there is little variation.

Overall, we observed very smooth flow times. There were very few repetitions for any one of the steps in the process since they were done "right first time." We also observed people working in parallel, one team ending a care process while another team is starting the cycle again. For example, a great deal of pre-processing work is accomplished before a patient arrives—checking for co-morbidities, verifying insurance or an address, or listing allergies (see Fig. 2.13).

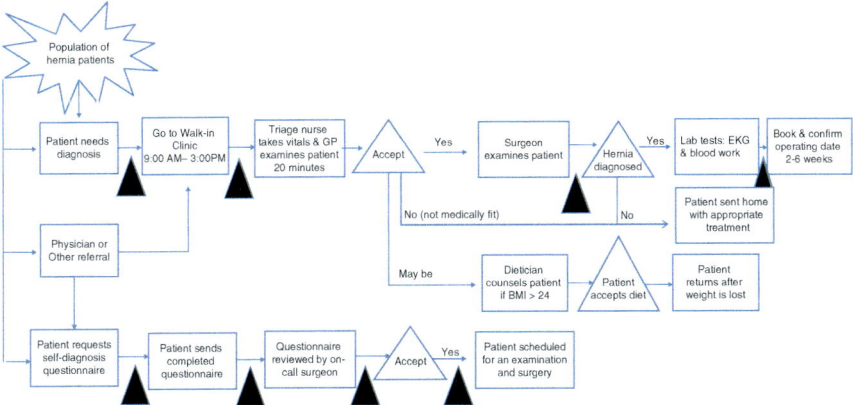

Fig. 2.13 Diagnosing and Scheduling the Surgery. Several elements of the care process are illustrated in the flow maps (Figs. 2.13, 2.14, 2.15, and 2.16)

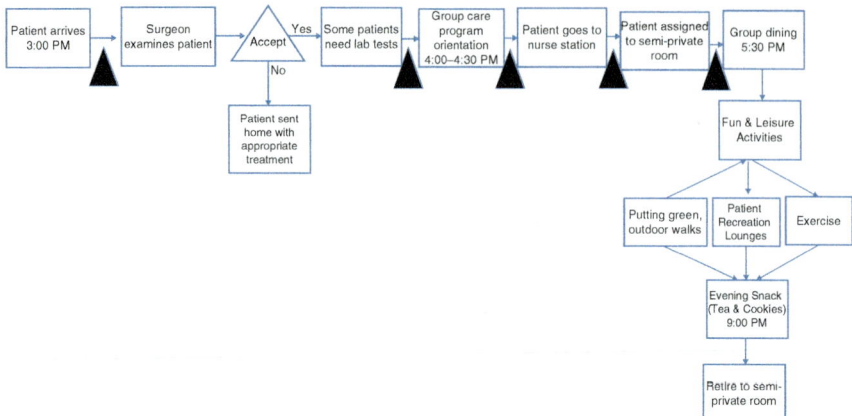

Fig. 2.14 Admission Process Day One

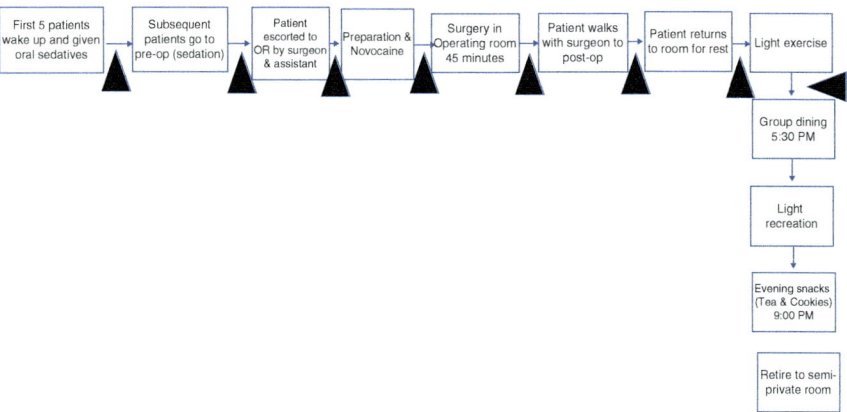

Fig. 2.15 Surgery Day Two

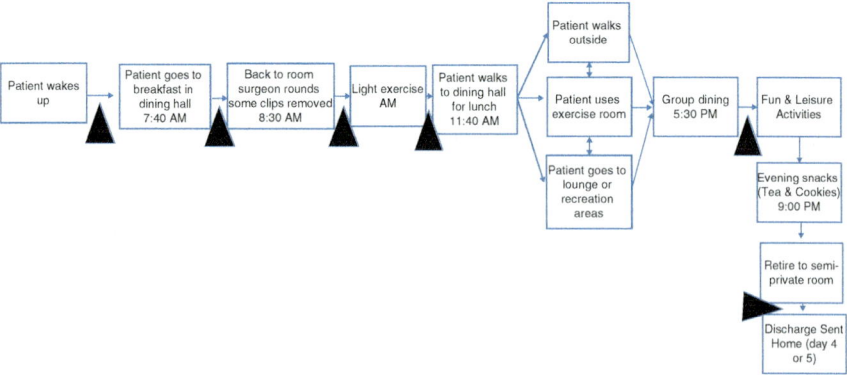

Fig. 2.16 Post Operative Day 3, 4 and 5

We observed that the flow in and out of the operating room is smooth. Every surgeon follows the standardized protocols, so the actual surgery is approximately 45 min, with very little variation. Although the members of the team rotate, they are dedicated to one activity—concentrating on the repair of hernias. That increases the speed and quality of the surgery, in contrast to clinical teams working on many different surgeries with rotating team members. Finally, when we observed the surgery, we noted that the patient, surgeon and assistant arrive and enter the operating room on time (with very little variation in the inter-arrival rate) because (by design) they walk in together (see Fig. 2.15).

After performing their 1000th surgery, the typical Shouldice surgeon becomes very efficient. As we noted in the case, the team works in parallel. The surgeon and assistant have "four hands carefully taking care of each patient." When the surgeons are closing the wound, the nurses get everything ready for the next patient. Immediately, after the patient walks out of the room with the physicians, the "scrub" nurse goes to the central sterilization area and soaks the surgical tools. Another nurse takes the linens to the central laundry 15 feet away.

In parallel a "relief" team is opening all the tools and supplies for the next procedure, as the next patient is brought into the room, less than 5 min after the previous patient walked out. While the next patient is being prepped the surgeon and assistant dictate surgical notes. They re-enter the room with the next patient and the process starts again. The result is productive efficiency and value creation for Shouldice.

Optimizing Patient-Caregiver Co-production

Patients are not passive recipients of care; they play an active role in the care program as co-producers in the care processes. They are encouraged (and they agree) to take part in their own care and recovery in the following ways.

Patients fill out a medical questionnaire and self-diagnose their hernia. Based on careful screening, patients are scheduled for surgery based on their ability to work with the caregivers and staff and take responsibility for self-care. They are motivated and committed to the care program, but they may feel insecure in this new situation. Consequently, patients need some coaching and counseling, which physicians and staff are trained to provide. Incoming patients receive a detailed orientation that includes videos.

Throughout the stay, patients are given information and have re-assuring conversations with other patients about what to expect. The patient and caregivers walk into the operating room together. Moreover, patients are awake and can talk with the surgeons during the surgery.

After the surgery immediate ambulation helps with the recovery process.[68] A few hours after the surgery, patients are told to do light exercise. They take themselves

---

[68] Before Covid19, patients were invited to get off the operating table and walk (with the help of the surgeon) to the post-operative room.

to the dining room and toilets. They have the freedom to go almost anywhere and to do almost anything that they want. In this way, they become willing and able partners and leave feeling extremely loyal to the clinic.

A Loyal Patient Base: The Lifetime Value of Shouldice Patient

Another advantage of focus is the ability to carefully select patients who will most likely get an excellent outcome. By improving the likelihood of an excellent result, they can focus more attention on customized care (meeting individual patient needs) and designing standardized service processes to meet general patient needs. The result is that patients become Shouldice advocates.

The retention of loyal patients is a critical success factor at Shouldice. For decades, Shouldice has maintained a continuing and active relationship with its patients. They track discharged patients and invited a small cohort to attend the annual "commemorative" alumni reunions.[69] At the reunions, they checked more than 1500 people for hernias. Patients received an invitation:

> You are cordially invited to attend our annual reunion to be held in the Royal York Hotel in downtown Toronto. The gala event will include dinner, entertainment, camaraderie, and an examination of your hernia repair.

Shouldice leaders learned several lessons from these reunions. For nearly 50 years, their patients have been motivated to attend reunions of 1500+ patients. That fact alone redefines extreme patient satisfaction. Second, after checking tens of thousands of patients the caregivers learned that their four-layer hernia repair was not only long-lasting but also eliminated the burden of a future hernia and any risk of recurrence—in short, it was both a repair and prevention. Third, they discovered that patient gratitude translated into a family, friend, and co-worker referral network that eliminated the need to build referral networks with primary care physicians. When former patients share their knowledge and experience by making positive referrals, there is a large future payoff. This has been described as the "lifetime value" of a patient [66].

The lifetime value of a Shouldice patient is the number of positive referrals they help to generate because they believe in the outcome and the patient experience. According to Dr. Shouldice, once a patient is admitted, has the hernia repair, and the post-operative care, there is a transformation—

> We send everyone out as a life-long advocate for the clinic. They tell everyone who needs a hernia repair to go to Shouldice.

Research suggests that when customers have an outstanding experience a small percentage tell their caregivers [66]. Less than one-third of truly dissatisfied patients tell

---

[69] While they no longer have reunions, they still contact patients annually and offer free examinations.

the original caregivers; however, they do tell dozens of other people about a poor outcome or experience [66]. In this age of social media and posts going viral, it is no longer dozens of people, but an order of magnitude above that. Therefore, when patients are asked "how likely are you to recommend this hospital to a family member or friend" only the "top box" (or extremely likely) scores matter in health care [66].

An Integrating Culture

Shouldice Hospital was created for a purpose—to deliver the best surgical outcomes and patient experiences in hernia treatment. The fundamental (though invisible) aspects of an organization are the shared assumptions that emerge around how to achieve the mission, accomplish the goals, and get work done. Once people find a way to achieve the purpose a culture emerges and evolves [71]. It is a shared product of shared learning as the group began solving external patient problems and internal operating problems [71].

The Shouldice culture evolved through the leadership of Dr. E.E. Shouldice and the other surgeons, using their influence to frame clinical and care management problems, experiment, propose solutions, and facilitate learning. The first problem they had to solve was identifying large groups of hernia patients with common characteristics that could be helped by their open surgical repair technique.

In the previous section Fig. 2.11 showed how the accumulation of knowledge, skills, and experience in the operating room over the first 8–10 years led to a rapid decline in failures (recurrences). They learned that their pure tissue surgical technique, with local anesthesia and immediate ambulation, was delivering the best outcomes for large groups of patients. However, they had to select the right hernia patients with consideration to patient safety given documented co-morbidities and obesity. They would never take a case to "fill the beds."

Next, they experimented with different ways of offering the highest quality patient experiences. They accomplished this by asking employees to focus on identifying and satisfying unmet patient needs. Every caregiver and many staff became a subject matter expert on the functional and emotional needs of hernia patients during every phase of care from precondition and admission, surgery, and post-operative care to achieve rapid and durable recovery.

By listening and interacting with patients, they learned how to deliver excellent patient services. As Schein argues, once a solution obtains a reasonably good result, it is approved by the senior leaders and taught to new members as the correct way to perform a task and behave [71]. This learning process is how culture evolves.

Patient-Centered Focus

One way to understand organizational culture is to visualize the basic assumptions using a cultural paradigm. A cultural paradigm is a way to display the underlying

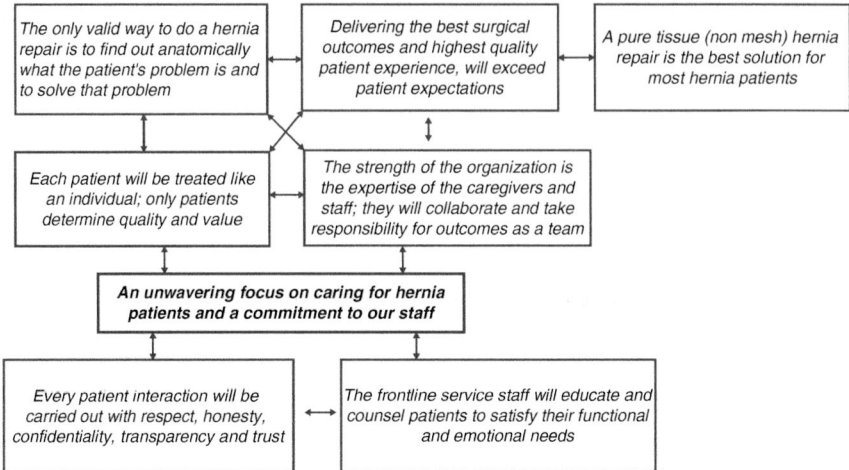

Fig. 2.17 Shouldice's Cultural Paradigm (basic assumptions). To understand how Shouldice's stated beliefs and values influence caregiver and staff behavior, Schein argues that the researchers must decipher the cultural paradigm by revealing the underlying premises and assumptions [71]. This figure is our interpretation of what we believe unconsciously enacts Shouldice's values and reduces variation in employee behavior and supports self-management and teamwork

clinical assumptions, ways of thinking, and premises, deeply embedded at Shouldice (see Fig. 2.17). Their cultural paradigm is a mix of clinical and managerial assumptions, reflecting the group's values, beliefs, methods and techniques. The culture at Shouldice is patient-centered, employee-centered, and team-based. As the caregivers and staff interact and counsel patients daily, they enact the organizational values of excellent quality, integrity, and compassion.

The fundamental assumption puts both the patient and employee at the center. The seven assumptions surrounding the fundamental assumption help us see how the Shouldice culture integrated the delivery system with the operating strategy.

They recognized that each patient is an individual with a unique hernia that can only be repaired by a 4-layer incision and a pure tissue repair. If every patient interaction is carried out respectfully, with transparency and honesty, the patient will not only have an excellent technical outcome but also a very good experience. However, they assume that only a patient can determine quality and value. That means they must measure and track performance to fulfill their mission.

Managing Patient Expectations

Patient-focus means conscientiously knowing and serving the needs of patients. When patients do not know what to expect, they experience uncertainty, which is dissatisfying. A patient's experience is what happens in relation to what they expect [66]. One of the underlying reasons that patients have a poor service experience is uncertainty–the lack of knowledge about what happened, what is happening, or what will happen next [72].

At Shouldice patients are not only told what to expect, they are given step-by-step instructions and counseling. They see a daily itinerary posted on bulletin boards throughout the areas they travel. During the orientation, a nurse prepares them for every phase pre- and post-surgery. They are told when they must fast, and the importance of being able to get on and off the operating room table. They are taught how to sit up, reassured that their bowels will move, and when the sutures will be removed.

Team-Based and Patient-Centered Culture

Interviews with employees revealed that caregivers and staff felt they were, as individuals and working in teams, contributing to Shouldice's success. There was a strong perception of fairness in the employment relationship. This perception is one way that Shouldice integrates the operating strategy and the delivery system.

The second way is by creating a patient-centered culture. Having discovered a purpose that everyone agrees is more important than self-interest, the culture supports the focused strategy.

Value Innovation at Shouldice

Kim and Mauborgne offer a four-action framework to analyze innovative value. The four actions lead a health organization to simultaneously pursue higher quality and low prices by asking probing questions [36, 37][70]:

1. What strategic activities do not add value and can be eliminated without harming quality?
2. What strategic activities do not add value and can be reduced below current standards without harming quality?
3. What strategic activities can be raised well above the current standards to improve quality?
4. What new strategic activities can be created that have never been offered and will improve quality?

Eliminating and reducing medical practices that do not add any value but will reduce the cost of care enable strategic options that will create and raise value for patients, caregivers and staff, and for the organization. In other words, it allows a reallocation of existing resources to create better quality at a lower cost. This framework will be used to make some analytic comments about Shouldice.

Figure 2.18 is the eliminate-reduce-raise-create grid for Shouldice Hospital. It reveals how value is created for patients and forces us to reconsider factors or practices that the health care industry competes on. Shouldice eliminated several factors

---

[70] This tool is called the eliminate-reduce-raise-create, or ERRC grid [36, 37].

Eliminate	Raise
• Mesh • Any procedure or diagnosis that is not an abdominal wall hernia • No direct marketing or advertising • High risk patients & emergency and urgent care • Private rooms, TV, showers in rooms	• Patient contact with physicians • Patient counselling & reassurance • Patient engagement, participation & independence • Park-like aesthetics & grounds • Longer stay
Reduce	Create
• Difficult check-in and wait times • Patient dependency on dietary, housekeeping, and nursing staff • Prices for self-pay patient • Look and smell of a hospital and bureaucratic rules • Variations in surgical outcomes: surgical site infections	• Hyperspecialized surgeons who achieve the world's best results • A lifetime guarantee for the surgery • Customized roommates • Recreational areas for exercise and fun

Fig. 2.18 Value Innovation at Shouldice. This shows how Shouldice is able to create patient value with no trade-off between low prices and quality. This tool is called the eliminate-reduce-raise-create, or ERRC grid. To raise and create value for patients, they found ways to reduce or eliminate some of the costs that do not create value. This links innovation with the value it offers patients. This way of thinking does not fall into the trap of adopting the next new ingenious expensive technology or that conveys the symbolic look of a hi-tech hospital. Note—this figure only displays value for patients. In addition, there is an ERRC grid to create value for caregivers and staff, and value for the enterprise

offered by hospitals and outpatient clinics such as the use of mesh, high-risk patients, emergency cases, private rooms, and direct marketing. They reduced: difficult check-in procedures; dependency on dietary workers serving food, housekeepers changing linen and nursing staff at the bedside; and variation in surgical outcomes. By eliminating and reducing those factors they could offer a much lower price and raise and create factors that add value for patients.

Patient value is raised by increasing the frequency and amount of contact with physicians; involving patients with their own care; offering patients the freedom to walk about and exercise indoors or outdoors on the park-like grounds. While most hernia procedures are "in and out" in less than one day, Shouldice raises the post-operative length-of-stay to a more comfortable four days, at a much lower price than the "treat em' and street em'" outpatient facilities.

They create clinical value by employing hyper-specialized surgeons who achieve the world's best results and offer a lifetime guarantee for their surgery. By using a unique algorithm to connect patients to a compatible roommate and offering recreational areas for light exercise and fun even more value is created.

Conclusions: Lessons from Shouldice

The Shouldice hernia repair and care process has consistently produced excellent outcomes for more than 75 years. They perform about 6480 abdominal wall hernia repairs each year. The surgery is durable with very low recurrence rates, significantly lower postoperative complications, less chronic pain, and an overall cost saving to society. All hernia repair comes with a lifetime guarantee—any recurrence is done for free.[71] They offer exceptional patient experience.

Shouldice is an example of a well-managed organization [38]. By breaking away from the competition, Shouldice has found what Kim and Mauborgne [36] call a "blue ocean." Competing for hernia patients does not seem to enter either into their strategic thinking or their lexicon. They are focused on creating value for their patients, implementing their mission and patient care goals, with a relentless pursuit of high-performance standards.

Shouldice has a set of clear and measurable goals. Patient care processes are standardized procedures monitored by clinical and managerial leadership. Their care processes are steadily and continuously improved.

Clinical outcomes, productivity, costs, patient experience and staff turnover are relentlessly tracked over decades. Performance is not only tracked but also reviewed so problems can be addressed quickly. Talented, high-performing surgeons are retained, and poor or under-performing caregivers are dealt with quickly.

This chapter is an account of our investigation, research, and findings of a highly effective health care organization. It is based on depth interviews, careful observations, facts, anecdotes, interpretations, concepts and analysis. We conclude this chapter with five lessons for health care organizations.

Lessons for Health Care Organizations

Lesson One
- *Working as a focused clinic, Shouldice not only cares deeply about their patients, but they also partner with their patients, and they set clinical targets and establish performance standards that are well-defined, measured, and clearly understood*

Shouldice is a focused clinic specialized in abdominal wall hernias. This allows them to understand each patient as an individual and to fine tune the process of care delivery in ways that add patient value. By understanding patients as individuals, they learned that the only way to improve value in health care is by creating a true partnership between the patients and the caregivers. Productivity at Shouldice requires continuous learning and self-improvement. The best way for caregivers, patients, and staff at Shouldice to be productive is for them to play the dual role of

---

[71] As previously stated, Shouldice has fewer than 50 recurrences a year on patients who previously had their hernia repair performed at Shouldice.

learner and teacher for other caregivers and patients.[72] Senior surgeons teach incoming surgeons. Patients who had the surgery the day before teach the incoming patients what to expect. Nurses and other staff counsel and educate patients.

Lesson Two
- *The care program and surgical workflow have been scientifically studied with standards and protocols to achieve excellent end results.*

A focused health care program that wants to offer the best surgical outcomes and best patient experience at the lowest prices must be supported by efficient care processes that reduce unproductive work. The care program had 4 components (1) diagnosing and scheduling (2) admission and day one; (3) surgery and day two; and (4) post-operative care and discharge days three to five. All four processes had standardized protocols to facilitate patient flow with little variation and congestion. These care processes were designed so each team member would get the right information to perform their function or task and be able to identify emergent patient problems and customize solutions.[73] When the workflow is structured efficiently, caregivers and staff spend most of their time on patient care activities; reducing unproductive work creates a strong people proposition for employees.

Lesson Three
- *A health care organization's culture is the de facto competitive strategy.*

The focus on the market for hernias and the care program are integrated by a patient-centered, self-directed, and team-based culture. There are so many stakeholders in health care (government, insurance, primary care physicians, etc.) that often we ask, "who is the customer?" At a focused clinic, everyone knows the hernia patient is the external customer, and the clinical caregivers and staff are the internal customer.

The 142 employees plus 18+ FTE physicians work together for a long time. They have learned how to solve problems and take advantage of opportunities. Their values are strongly held and have become an unconscious cognitive map of where to focus attention, how to feel about a patient situation, and what actions to take when patients have unmet needs.

The cultural paradigm not only enacts their values but also activates their collective purpose and identity as a working team, partnering with patients. They know that their performance is greater than the sum of the individuals and everything is centered on the patient outcomes and experience. Shouldice designs processes that

---

[72] The classic model for training physicians was described as "see one, do one. Teach one." Though some have called this practice old-fashioned, the benefits of teaching others include improving communication skills and feelings of self-efficacy while building leadership skills.

[73] Patients get information from the staff, nurses and physicians, as well as other patients. In the operating room, the surgical team gets information from the patient and the situation. The chief of surgery and the administrator gets information from the nurses, and assistant surgeons, about underperformance or concerns, and so on.

allow the caregivers and staff to learn from each other and avoid processes that pit employees against each other.

Lesson Four
- *Health care organizations need a strong people proposition.*

People are at the center of every health care organization. In most hospitals, studies reveal that some clinical caregivers have low productivity because they do not spend most of their time on patient care. A good deal of time is spent on workarounds, administrative paperwork, logging into medical records, waiting for patients, queueing in the operating or exam rooms, looking for other caregivers, looking for supplies, etc.

Shouldice offers their employees challenging goals, continuous learning, and an opportunity to achieve while doing productive work. They take a profound sense of responsibility for their people. The workflow is structured so efficiently that they spend most of their time on patient care activities that create value. Every employee (surgeons, nurses, staff, and patients) is both a learner and a teacher, focused on listening to patients and offering outstanding quality, learning, and new ways to reduce costs. They may not always achieve the goal that employees feel fulfilled, but they aim to send people home believing that their abilities and talents are being used to help patients at the end of every workday.

Lesson Five
- *There is a system of accountability, with no extra layers of management.*

Shouldice has found a way to reduce the cost of administrative overhead[74] and middle management, by balancing an individual's autonomy with their team interdependence. They do this by hiring people who can (1) identify with the mission; (2) learn and believe in the Shouldice methodology and protocols; (3) become committed to the goals; and (4) learn to be team players. They thrive at Shouldice by taking responsibility for their own productivity and achievement while holding each other accountable for the goals and standards.

Finally, before setting expectations, the leadership and the caregivers take time to explain the rationale behind important clinical, non-clinical, and staff decisions, which creates a perception of fair process and justice at Shouldice. When employees identify with the mission and perceive fairness in the workplace, they become more committed to the goals and expectations and more allegiant to Shouldice. Consequently, caregivers and staff do not need to be managed; they manage themself. In the words of two former senior leaders:

---

[74] Larger hospitals often lose money on patient care because of their total cost structure—direct plus indirect costs. First, they may have higher direct costs. Second, their indirect costs (e.g., administrative overhead) are substantially higher. Even if their direct costs are competitive, most large hospital systems have crushing indirect overhead costs.

Every patient and every staff member, doctor, nurse, administrator, and housekeeper knows exactly why he or she is there. Each of them knows exactly what to expect at every moment…all feel the effects of being cared for in a facility designed, built, and staffed exclusively for the purpose of caring for people with their condition. The result is confidence… [5, p. 631].

This final quote summarizes the indispensable quality of Shouldice as a well-managed organization—having an inspirational organizational purpose. A higher purpose becomes a greater good and a source of pride for employees. It is more important than individual self-interest. To conclude this chapter, we submit that our facts, assertions, and theory cannot fully describe or explain a complex health care organization, like Shouldice.[75]

On that note, we invite others to continue to study this fascinating organization. It is far from a perfect medical care organization, but the people at Shouldice believe that it is perfectible. This organization like every organization can be improved.

References

1. Female patient posting on Facebook, see. https://www.facebook.com/ShouldiceHospital/photos/here-is-dr-michael-alexander-performing-his-30000-hernia-surgery-at-shouldice-ho/1157567120966286
2. Chilingerian JA. Who has star quality? In: Herzlinger RE, editor. Consumer-driven health care: implications for providers, payers, and policymakers. San Francisco: Jossey-Bass; 2004. p. 443–53.
3. Chan CK, Chan G. The Shouldice technique for treatment of hernia. J Minim Access Surg. 2006 Sep;2(3):124–8. https://doi.org/10.4103/0972-9941.27723.
4. Shouldice EB. The Shouldice repair for groin hernia. Surg Clin N Am. 2003:1163–87.
5. Urquhart DJB, O'Dell A. A model of focused health care delivery. In: Herzlinger RE, editor. Consumer-driven health care: implications for providers, payers, and policymakers. San Francisco: Jossey-Bass; 2004. p. 627–34.
6. Hori T, Yasukawa D. Fascinating history of groin hernias: comprehensive recognition of anatomy, classic considerations for herniorrhaphy, and current controversies in hernioplasty. World J Methodol. 2021 July;11(4):160–86.
7. Bendavid R. Biography: Edward Earle Shouldice (1890-1965). Hernia. 2003;7(4):172–7.
8. The HerniaSurge Group. International guidelines for groin hernia management. Hernia. 2018;22(1):1–165. https://doi.org/10.1007/s10029-017-1668-x.
9. Millikan KW, Cummings B, Doolas A. The Millikan modified mesh-plug hernioplasty. Arch Surg. 2003;138(5):525–9.; discussion 529-30. https://doi.org/10.1001/archsurg.138.5.525.
10. Destek S, Gul VO. Comparison of Lichtenstein repair and mesh plug repair methods in the treatment of indirect inguinal hernia. Cureus. 2018;10(7):e2935. Published 2018 Jul 6. https://doi.org/10.7759/cureus.2935.

---

[75] We are not the first to write a case study on Shouldice. In 1983, James L. Heskett wrote a business School case study [73]. That case brought this fascinating hospital into the management curriculum of virtually every business school worldwide. We owe a debt of gratitude to him for that well-written, nicely framed original case study. Although we have added more clinical details, new facts, and updates, the narrative told in the original case has not changed much. Dr. Atul Gwande also visited Shouldice, observed surgeries, and talked about the distinct repair method and clinical efficiency [74].

11. Frey DM, Wildisen A, Hamel CT, Zuber M, Oertli D, Metzger J. Randomized clinical trial of Lichtenstein's operation versus mesh plug for inguinal hernia repair. Br J Surg. 2007 Jan;94(1):36–41. https://doi.org/10.1002/bjs.5580.
12. Bendavid R. The Shouldice technique: a canon in hernia repair. Can J Surg. 1997;40(3):199–205. 207
13. Nordin P, Bartelmess P, Jansson C, Svensson C, Edlund G. Randomized trial of Lichtenstein versus Shouldice hernia repair in general surgical practice. Br J Surg. 2002;89(1):45–9.
14. Sawhney M, Goldstein DH, Wei X, Pare GC, Wang L, VanDenKerkhof EG. Pain and haemorrhage are the most common reasons for emergency department use and hospital admission in adults following ambulatory surgery: results of a population-based cohort study. Perioper Med (Lond). 2020 Aug;19(9):25. https://doi.org/10.1186/s13741-020-00155-3.
15. Gohel J, Naik N, Parmar H, Solanki B. A comparative study of inguinal hernia repair by Shouldice method vs other methods. IAIM. 2016;3(1):13–7.
16. Köckerling F, Brunner W, Mayer F, Adolf D, Lorenz R, Zarras K, Weyhe D. Assessment of potential influencing factors on the outcome in small (<2 cm) umbilical hernia repair: a registry-based multivariable analysis of 31,965 patients. Hernia. 2021;25:587–603. https://doi.org/10.1007/s10029-020-02305-4.
17. Lorenz R, Arlt G, Conze J, Fortelny R, Gorjanc J, Koch A, Morrison J, Oprea V, Campanelli G. Shouldice standard 2020: review of the current literature and results of an international consensus meeting. Hernia. 2021 Oct;25(5):1199–207. https://doi.org/10.1007/s10029-020-02365-6.
18. Latenstein CSS, Thunnissen FM, Harker M, Groenewoud S, Noordenbos MW, Atsma F, de Reuver PR. Variation in practice and outcomes after inguinal hernia repair: a nationwide observational study. BMC Surg. 2021 Jan 20;21(1):45. https://doi.org/10.1186/s12893-020-01030-0.
19. Chilingerian JA, Glavin MP. Temporary firms in community hospitals: elements of a managerial theory of clinical efficiency. Med Care Rev. 1994. Fall;51(3):289–335. https://doi.org/10.1177/107755879405100303.
20. Simons MP, Aufenacker T, Bay-Nielsen M, Bouillot JL, Campanelli G, Conze J, de Lange D, Fortelny R, Heikkinen T, Kingsnorth A, Kukleta J, Morales-Conde S, Nordin P, Schumpelick V, Smedberg S, Smietanski M, Weber G, Miserez M. European hernia society guidelines on the treatment of inguinal hernia in adult patients. Hernia. 2009;13(4):343–403. https://doi.org/10.1007/s10029-009-0529-7. Epub 2009 Jul 28
21. Amato B, Moja L, Panico S, Persico G, Rispoli C, Rocco N, Moschetti I. Shouldice technique versus other open techniques for inguinal hernia repair. Cochrane Database Syst Rev. 2012 Apr 18;2012(4):CD001543. https://doi.org/10.1002/14651858.CD001543.pub4.
22. Graban M, Toussaint J. Lean hospitals: improving quality, patient safety, and employee engagement. 3rd ed. Productivity Press; 2016. https://doi.org/10.4324/9781315380827.
23. Heskett JL. Managing in the service economy. Boston, MA: Harvard Business School Press; 1986.
24. Herzlinger RE. Consumer-driven health care: implications for providers, payers, and policymakers. San Francisco: Jossey-Bass; 2004.
25. Chilingerian JA, Savage GT. The emerging field of international health care management: an introduction. In: Savage GT, Chilingerian JA, Powell M, Xiao Q, editors. International health care management (advances in health care management, Vol. 5). Bingley: Emerald Group Publishing Limited; 2005. p. 3–28. https://doi.org/10.1016/S1474-8231(05)05001-9.
26. Skinner W. The focused factory. Harv Bus Rev. 1974;May/June:112–21.
27. Skinner W. Manufacturing–the formidable competitive weapon. New York: Wiley; 1985.
28. Skinner W. Manufacturing strategy on the "S" curve. Prod Oper Manag. 1996;5:3–14. https://doi.org/10.1111/j.1937-5956.1996.tb00381.x.
29. Carey K, Mitchell JM. Specialization as an organizing principle: the case of ambulatory surgery centers. Med Care Res Rev. 2019;76(4):386–402.
30. Bredenhoff E, van Lent WA, van Harten WH. Exploring types of focused factories in hospital care: a multiple case study. BMC Health Serv Res. 2010;10:154. Published 2010 Jun 7. https://doi.org/10.1186/1472-6963-10-154.

31. Diwas Singh KC, Terwiesch C. The effects of focus on performance: evidence from California hospitals. Management science. INFORMS. 2011;57(11):1897–912.
32. Casalino LP, Devers K, Brewster LR. Focused factories? Physician-owned specialty facilities. Health Aff. November/December 2003;22(6).
33. Cook D, et al. From 'solution shop' model to 'focused factory' in hospital surgery: increasing care value and predictability. Health Aff (Millwood). 2014;33(5):746–55.
34. Wasenhove LV, How "Focused Factories" deal with disruption. INSEAD Knowledge. 2015. https://knowledge.insead.edu/operations/how-focused-factories-deal-with-disruption-4357. Accessed 12 December 2020.
35. Intelligence Unit, Specialization and standardization: value-Based health care at Canada's Shouldice hospital. The Economist. 2016. https://knowledge.insead.edu/operations/how-focused-factories-deal-with-disruption-4357. Accessed 12 December 2020.
36. Kim WC, Mauborbne R. Blue Ocean strategy. 2nd ed. Boston: HBS Press; 2015.
37. Kim WC, Mauborbne R. Blue Ocean shift. Boston: Hachette; 2017.
38. Sadun R, Bloom N, Van Reenen J. Why do we undervalue competent management? Harv Bus Rev. 2017;September–October:120–7.
39. Porter M. How competitive forces shape strategy. Harv Bus Rev. 1979, March-April;57(2):137–45.
40. Liu JH, Etziono DA, O'connel JB, Maggard MA, Ko CY. The increasing workload of general surgery. Arch Surg. 2004;139(4):423–8. https://doi.org/10.1001/archsurg.139.4.423.
41. AAMC. Physician specialty data report. 2020. https://www.aamc.org/data-reports/workforce/interactive-data/active-physicians-us-doctor-medicine-us-md-degree-specialty-2019. Accessed 16 October 2021.
42. Dow T, McGuire C, Crawley E, Davies D. Application rates to surgical residency programs in Canada. Can Med Educ J. 2020;11(3):e92–e100. Published 2020 Jul 15. https://doi.org/10.36834/cmej.58444.
43. Grand View Research. Hernia Repair Devices Market Size, Share & Trends Analysis Report By Product Type (Hernia Mesh, Hernia Fixation Devices), By Surgery Type (Inguinal, Incisional), By Procedure Type, By Region, And Segment Forecasts, 2021–2028. Published September 2021. https://www.grandviewresearch.com/industry-analysis/hernia-repair-devices-market. Accessed January 17, 2022.
44. DePietro MA. Does Medicare cover hernia surgery? Medical News Today. 2020, October 28. https://www.medicalnewstoday.com/articles/does-medicare-cover-hernia-surgery. Accessed January 17, 2022.
45. Ishikawa S, Kawano T, Karashima R, Arita T, Yagi Y, Hirota M. A case of mesh plug migration into the bladder 5 years after hernia repair. Surg Case Rep. 2015;1(4) https://doi.org/10.1186/s40792-014-0004-2.
46. Bendavid R. The Shouldice repair. Oper Tech Gen Surg. 1999;1(2):142–55.
47. Bendavid R. L'operation de Shouldice. In: Encyclopédie médico-chirurgicale. Techniques chirurgicales appareil diges-tif. Paris: Encyclopédie médico-chirur-gicale. 40112 4.11.12:5 pages.
48. Campbell EB. Anesthesia in the repair of hernia. Can Med Assoc J. 1950;62:364–6.
49. Teboul J. Service is front stage. New York: Palgrave Macmillan; 2006.
50. Sanjay P, Jones P, Woodward A. Inguinal hernia repair: are ASA grades 3 and 4 patients suitable for day case hernia repair? Hernia. 2006;10(4):299–302. https://doi.org/10.1007/s10029-005-0048-0. Epub 2006 Apr 1
51. Katzenbach JR, Smith DK. The wisdom of teams: creating the high-performance organization. Boston, Mass: Harvard Business School Press; 1993.
52. Bassini E. Nuovo metodo operativo perla cura radicale dell'ernia inguinale. Padova (Italy): R. Stabilimento Prosperini; 1889.
53. Hirshberg KL, Mattox KL. Top knife: the art and craft of trauma surgery. Castle Hill Barns: TFM Publishing; 2005.
54. Porrero JL, Bonachía O, López-Buenadicha A, Sanjuanbenito A, Sánchez-Cabezudo C. Reparación de la hernia inguinal primaria: Lichtenstein frente a Shouldice. Estudio prospectivo y aleatorizado sobre el dolor y los costes hospitalarios [repair of primary inguinal hernia:

Lichtenstein versus Shouldice techniques. Prospective randomized study of pain and hospital costs]. Cir Esp. 2005;77(2):75–8. Spanish. https://doi.org/10.1016/s0009-739x(05)70811-3.
55. Spencer Netto F, Quereshy F, Camilotti BG, Pitzul K, Kwong J, Jackson T, Penner T, Okrainec A. Hospital costs associated with laparoscopic and open inguinal herniorrhaphy. JSLS. 2014 Oct-Dec;18(4):e2014.00217. https://doi.org/10.4293/JSLS.2014.00217.
56. New Choice Health. https://www.newchoicehealth.com/hernia-repair-surgery/cost. Accessed March 15, 2022.
57. Murphy BL, Ubl DS, Zhang J, Habermann EB, Farley DR, Paley K. Trends of inguinal hernia repairs performed for recurrence in the United States. Surgery. 2018;163(2):343–50. https://doi.org/10.1016/j.surg.2017.08.001. Epub 2017 Sep 15
58. Malik A, Bell C, Stukel T, Urbach D. Recurrence of inguinal hernias repaired in a large hernia surgical specialty hospital and general hospitals in Ontario, Canada. Can J Surg. 2016 Feb;59(1):19–25. https://doi.org/10.1503/cjs.003915.
59. Andresen K, Rosenberg J. Management of chronic pain after hernia repair. J Pain Res. 2018 Apr 5;11:675–81. https://doi.org/10.2147/JPR.S127820.
60. Elsamadicy AA, Ashraf B, Ren X, Sergesketter AR, Charalambous L, Kemeny H, Ejikeme T, Yang S, Pagadala P, Parente B, Xie J, Pappas TN, Lad SP. Prevalence and cost analysis of chronic pain after hernia repair: a potential alternative approach with Neurostimulation. Neuromodulation. 2019;22(8):960–9. https://doi.org/10.1111/ner.12871. Epub 2018 Oct 15
61. Bendavid R, Mainprize M, Iakovlev V. Pure tissue repairs: a timely and critical revival. Hernia. 2019;23(3):493–502. https://doi.org/10.1007/s10029-019-01972-2. Epub 2019 May 20. Erratum in: Hernia. 2019 Aug 6
62. Bökkerink WJV, Koning GG, Vriens PWHE, et al. Open Preperitoneal inguinal hernia repair, TREPP versus TIPP in a randomized clinical trial. Ann Surg. 2021;274(5):698–704. https://doi.org/10.1097/SLA.0000000000005130.
63. Sekigami Y, Tian T, Char S, Radparvar J, Aalberg J, Chen L, Chatterjee A. Conflicts of interest in studies related to mesh use in ventral hernia repair and Abdominal Wall reconstruction. Ann Surg. 2021 Jan 11; https://doi.org/10.1097/SLA.0000000000004565. Epub ahead of print
64. Chilingerian J. Evaluating quality outcomes against best practice: a new frontier. In: Kimberly J, Minivelee E, editors. The quality imperative. London: Imperial College Press; 2000p. p. 141–67.
65. McDermott, KW, Liang L. Overview of major ambulatory surgeries performed in hospital-owned facilities, 2019. AHRQ. Healthcare Cost and Utilization Project, Statistical Brief #287. https://www.hcup-us.ahrq.gov/reports/statbriefs/sb287-Ambulatory-Surgery-Overview-2019.pdf. Accessed on February 19, 2021.
66. Heskett JL, Sasser W, Schlesinger LA. The value profit chain. New York: The Free Press; 2014.
67. Miles JA. Management and organization theory. San Francisco: Jossey Bass; 2012.
68. Drucker PF. Post-capitalist society. New York: Harper; 1993.
69. Dweck C. Growth mindset: the new psychology of success. New York: Penguin Random House; 2016.
70. Pink D. Drive. New York: Penguin; 2009.
71. Schein EH. Organizational culture and leadership. Hoboken, New Jersey: Wiley; 2017.
72. Chilingerian J. The discipline of strategic thinking in health care. In: Jones R, Jenkins F, editors. Management, leadership and development in the allied health professions. Oxford: Radcliffe Publishing, Ltd; 2006.
73. Heskett JL. Shouldice hospital ltd. HBS case number 9–683-068. Boston: HBS Publishing; 1983.
74. Gawande A. Complications: a Surgeon's notes on an imperfect science. New York: Picador; 2002.

Improving Leadership and Business Structures in a Rural Emergency Department

3

Guy Nuki

Key Learning Points
- Physician engagement requires a strong culture, support for physicians and the information that they need to understand what changes are necessary
- Relational coordination can help to improve cultures even without formal authority across disciplines
- Validated data that everyone agrees with helps physicians and leaders understand and drive needed improvements
- Keeping the focus on quality patient care allows individuals and teams to work together to improve
- Stabilizing senior leadership across disciplines is essential for long lasting cultural change

Background

Critical Access Hospitals (CAH) face many of the same issues common to rural hospitals, such as serving an older population with high rates of substance abuse, mental illness, and chronic disease, and having an impoverished payer mix. The Emergency Department (ED) at the hospital at the focus of this study had a total of six beds and the majority of payments were received through either Medicare or Medicaid payments as illustrated in Table 3.1 supplied by the CFO of the hospital. The rural location of the hospital presents significant difficulties in recruitment of physicians and those with hospital management expertise.

In July of 2009, the hospital entered into receivership after concerns over the care delivered by the ED resulted in investigations by CMS (Personal communication

G. Nuki (✉)
BlueWater Health, Brunswick, ME, USA
e-mail: gnuki@bluewaterhealth.com

Table 3.1 Payer Mix

Source	Year			3-year Average
	2012	2013	2014	Avg
Medicare	29%	31%	29%	30%
Medicaid	35%	34%	31%	33%
Anthem blue cross blue shield	9%	7%	8%	8%
Other commercial insurance	18%	18%	20%	18%
Uninsured & Other	9%	11%	12%	11%

Source: [Provided by Hospital CFO]

with hospital CFO). Since then, the hospital has been able to come out of receivership but has continued to struggle with management and staffing of ED physicians. In February of 2016, the hospital sought technical assistance from BlueWater Emergency Partners (BWEP), a private Emergency Medicine LLC, to provide physician staffing and management of the ED. The main objective of the project with BWEP was to bring values, concepts, and tools to the hospital to improve the hospital's financial situation and quality of care delivered. In particular, the project was built on the assumption that bringing a new business structure and leadership to the ED at the hospital would improve the quality of care, enhance efficiency, and increase the ED's net profit. This was expected to be achieved by decreasing the left without being seen rate (LWBS); improving the time spent for a patient to be seen in the ED and either discharged, admitted, or transferred (throughput time); and improved reimbursement through more accurate coding (measured through relative value units).

BWEP was contracted for this task based on their expertise in improving clinical quality and enhancing finances in non-urban ED settings. Headquartered in Brunswick, Maine, the organization was made up of 11 physician partners, 9 employed physicians, 18 employed advance practice clinicians, and 20 contracted per-diem providers. In addition to this project at the hospital, the organization staffed and managed three EDs and one walk-in clinic in Maine and provided temporary staffing for three other EDs in the state (Personal communication).

Prior to the engagement by BWEP, the hospital had faced multiple issues in the ED pertaining to patient safety, quality of care, and hospital efficiency and finances. First, the facility was very outdated. It was originally built in 1964 with an ED renovation completed 27 years prior to this study. Second, the position of ED Nursing Director was vacant and during the same week that the project with BWEP began, the Chief Nursing Officer (CNO) was asked to step down, requiring both positions to be filled by locums. Additionally, the ED faced significant human resource constraints (Table 3.2). Much of the ED nursing staff was made up of travelers. The ED was staffed by only one full time physician, who had little emergency medicine experience. The remaining physician shifts were staffed by per diem physicians, each covering up to four shifts per month, and who could often withhold taking on shifts until the hospital was forced to increase the rate for the shift at the last minute. With per diem rates increasing up to two-fold to cover these shifts, this was a considerable expense to the hospital (Personal communication with hospital CFO).

3 Improving Leadership and Business Structures in a Rural Emergency Department

Table 3.2 The hospital staffing prior to project start

Role	# of Physicians	Desired by The Hospital Administration to Keep
Director	1	0
Full time	1	0
Locums	1	0
Per diem	18	13

Table 3.3 Patient statistics at the hospital prior to project start

Year	ED Volume	Number of Patients Admitted	Admit Rate	Number of Patients Transferred	Transfer Rate	LWBS
2012	9209	770	8.4%	442	4.8%	0.6%
2013	8844	700	7.9%	461	5.2%	0.5%
2014	9035	642	7.1%	479	5.3%	1.0%
2015	9223	765	8.3%	342	3.7%	1.5%

Source: The Hospital Database

Table 3.2 shows the staff make-up of the ED prior to the project start, including the number of staff desired by the hospital leadership to keep for the project, as articulated by the hospital administration at the beginning of the project.

In terms of ED performance, there was a higher-than-expected rate of patients who left without being seen (LWBS rate, Table 3.3); coding was performed by in-house general medical coders rather than emergency medicine specialized coders; and there were no standard-work protocols in place, such as stroke, ST-elevation myocardial infarction (STEMI), or sepsis protocols. Prior physician staff and the hospital's Director of Quality reported that the quality improvement plan was largely reactionary, having been developed as the result of prior state inspections, and had poor staff acceptance.

The project with BWEP began on February 1, 2016 when BWEP provided the role of ED Medical Director. On April 1, 2016, BWEP began the process of staffing the ED, outsourcing coding to a company specializing in emergency medicine, and onboarding a new ED Medical Director. Because of the broad nature of issues facing the ED, it was seen as important to address the challenges facing the ED from multiple stakeholder perspectives. As such, priority was given to establishing nursing and physician leadership and improving provider performance. Physician staffing was also stabilized into a core permanent group of physicians, after which standard-work processes and clinical protocols could be developed.

Overview of BWEP Engagement & Methodology

This paper discusses the process of BWEP's engagement with the hospital and the successes and challenges that were faced through the project period. Using the author's observations during the project period, as well as qualitative and quantitative data measuring BWEP's impact, this paper aims to draw out the leadership and business management principles that proved successful in achieving positive results for both the hospital ED and BWEP. By cataloguing these activities, this paper aims to highlight processes on improving clinical quality and hospital finances that could be implemented in other similar contexts.

BWEP took a multifaceted approach to improving the performance in the hospital ED. Based on the initial assessment of challenges facing the ED and discussions with hospital staff, there needed to be changes in both structure and function of the facility in order to improve the finances and the quality of care. Furthermore, in order to implement and sustain these changes, robust cultural changes would also be required. Each area that was addressed through the project is described below.

Emergency Department Structure and Equipment

The ED had six beds with an annual volume of 9223 patients, an average length of stay of 166 min, and a LWBS of over 2.4% in the month prior to the initiation of this project. As relayed to BWEP by the hospital administration, the limited space in the ED had created bottlenecks and plans were already in place for a renovation to expand the capacity to ten beds. This renovation also provided the opportunity to standardize the lay-out of the patient rooms and allowed for a review of equipment to facilitate the delivery of quality patient care. Prior to this, frequently used equipment and supplies were inconsistently stocked in patient rooms thus increasing inefficacies of provider and staff workflows. BWEP also worked with the hospital to add an additional workstation for clinicians and provided them with access to dictation software, embedded into the electronic medical record to increase physician efficiency.

Staffing & Finance

Prior to the engagement by BWEP, the hospital had a very large number of physicians staffing the ED (See Table 3.2). All of the physicians were contracted and had additional positions elsewhere, which resulted in the hospital having to use increasing financial incentives to ensure that shifts were covered. To address these staffing inefficiencies and to reduce the hospital's expenses for clinical compensation, BWEP hired five full-time physicians with a standardized pay scale, which was based upon an hourly rate with a small component to incentivize productivity. Recruitment was supported by the hiring of Physician Assistants to support the physicians. Having PAs staff along with physicians at night allowed the physicians to have 24-h shifts. In the evening and at night the PA would be the point person in the ED. This allowed for an expanded recruitment pool of physicians that did not need to live locally. There were no financial incentives for meeting quality metrics. It was made clear that all providers would work towards these goals as a cultural expectation. This was created through processes that began through recruiting and hiring and extended through leadership techniques that go beyond the scope of this chapter.

Critical Access Hospitals are reimbursed on a cost basis by CMS. To participate in the program the hospital is required to have an emergency medicine provider available at all times. However, in low volume hospitals, that provider is often unable to generate billing when there are not patients to see. Therefore, CAHs are able to be reimbursed for the cost of a physician during this down time. Many CAHs underestimate the amount of this time thus missing appropriate CMS reimbursement. *Centers for Medicare and Medicaid Services* (CMS) allows for multiple ways to measure this. BWEP worked directly with CMS to develop a method that allowed for a more realistic measure that was financially advantageous to the hospital.

Relative value units (RVUs) are a method of defining the value of specific services or procedures relative to other services and procedures and are used by CMS and private providers to determine physician payment [1]. RVU generation is dependent upon accurate and complete documentation of services performed, as well as accurate coding of that documentation to arrive at an appropriate fee for the service. It is important that patients are neither charged more than the value of the care that they received nor are they undercharged. In order to address this and enhance the revenue collected at the ED, BWEP moved the coding to a specialty specific vendor and provided training to the providers to fully document the care that they provided, including giving providers feedback on their performance.

Quality Work

BWEP worked with the hospital leadership to establish a comprehensive Quality Improvement Plan. This was divided into three components including: (1) an 18-month ED Performance Plan, (2) a shared Departmental Dashboard, and (3) individual clinician performance tracking. This plan also resulted in the development of multiple clinical and process improvement projects. Lean process improvement methods were used to create flow maps, identify areas for improvement, and make changes through rapid small Plan-Do-Study-Act (PDSA) cycles.

Through tracking multiple performance measures and reporting them on a shared dashboard, system process issues and challenges at both the departmental level as well as at the individual clinician level were found and addressed. For example, there was a particular physician who struggled with throughput times and was an outlier in terms of having a high LWBS. Through coaching and mentoring, this physician was able to make substantial improvements to match his colleagues.

Relational/Cultural/Political

Developing a quality patient-oriented culture that also supported ED staff was likely the single most important area to improve. Physicians previously worked there as moonlighting opportunities for high pay. There was no sense of team or orientation towards improving care. An example was the complete lack of physician participation in department meetings. According to hospital leadership, there was only one physician that would attend. This issue was addressed both at the leadership level and the level of frontline workers. This required the development of accountable leadership on all levels including administration, providers, and nursing leadership. Recruiting and onboarding, and the management of front-line staff, with the aim of creating a culture that could address the needed improvements was a priority.

At the start of the project, there was a lack of nursing leadership and the hospital team was limited to the author and the hospital's Director of Quality. Realizing that many issues with the nursing team could not be addressed without leadership in place, BWEP began with the development of a performance improvement plan with the Quality Director. Relational coordination concepts were used to develop a leadership team that included the CNO, Nursing Director, Quality Director, and Medical Director. Emphasis was made on putting processes in place to allow for issues to be addressed in a proactive and congenial manner, while still holding members of the group accountable. Specific tools were developed to help in communication and transparency. Stoplight reports were posted in the ED, where all staff could see what had been accomplished as well as what projects were in process. Leadership also had access to HIPAA-compliant file sharing, where all ED data was made available with shared responsibility for data acquisition and reporting. Last, morning huddles which involved the entire ED team were instituted and monthly department meetings were opened to everyone, in order to help establish a sense of team mentality.

The hospital hired an interim CNO, an interim Nursing Director and BWEP hired a new Medical Director. All three of these individuals were experienced and skilled. BW presented relational coordination concepts, and these were enthusiastically accepted which facilitated a functional leadership team. The next several months resulted in rapid progress, however, all good things must come to an end. The permanent CNO arrived but there was a 2-month gap again with no full-time Nursing Director. Once the new Nursing Director was chosen, BWEP met and at our first meeting she outlined her plans as the new director to ignore prior leadership plans and to focus entirely on pride in nursing. The author realized the leadership team development was going to need to start over. Shortly after this the Quality Director announced she was leaving. The disruption brought about by changing leadership was a major challenge in this project.

BlueWater Emergency Partners Internal Changes

In order to effectively support the hospital ED, BWEP also had to make enhancements to its company structure and reassess its resources. This included hiring additional staff and redistribution of workload. Initially, the Regional Medical Director for BWEP assumed both the roles of Department Director and for overseeing the implementation of the contract with the hospital, in addition to their existing role. Given the considerable workload that this placed on the Regional Medical Director, these roles were handed over to the permeant Medical Director after 3 months into the contract. BWEP also hired a Director of Quality and an Executive Director in order to increase attention to tracking and addressing quality issues, as well as hiring and human resource concerns, respectively. Distributing the workload in this

3 Improving Leadership and Business Structures in a Rural Emergency Department

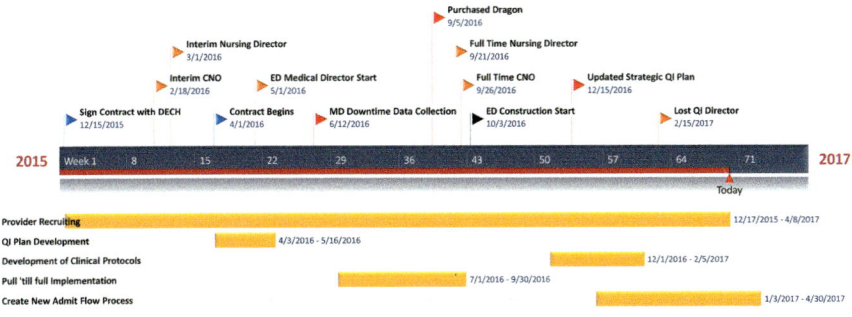

Fig. 3.1 Timeline for project

Table 3.4 Metrics used to evaluate project and baseline figures

Metrics Evaluated	Measures Used	Baseline Figures
Patient satisfaction scores	NRC picker data	Top box overall rating: 60
Complaint rate	Complaints per 1000 visits	1.5 complaints per 1000 ED visits
LWBS rate	Reduction in rate of patients that LWBS	2.4%
RVUs produced	Total work relative value units per month (wRVU/mo)	8995 visits 1.9 wRVUs per visit
Physician stand-by time	% stand-by time on cost report	16%
Throughput times	• Door to doctor time for all patients • LOS for admitted patients	• Door to doc: 32 min • LOS for admitted: 420 min
Sepsis bundle	CMS 3 and 6 h sepsis bundles	No sepsis protocol or data collection

way was intended to free-up the local Medical Director and Regional Medical Director to prioritize work on cultural and leadership issues at the hospital. BWEP also hired an outside vendor to take on information technology issues, which had also been previously handled by the Regional Medical Director.

A timeline of the project is displayed in Fig. 3.1.

In order to evaluate the project's impact, BWEP relied upon direct observations during the project period, interviews with hospital staff and leadership, and several qualitative and quantitative metrics collected at the ED. Specific metrics evaluated, measures used, and baseline figures at the start of the project are listed in Table 3.4.

In improving the quality and financial situation of the ED, it was critical to develop a culture that focused on patient safety, acceptance of standard-work, and a patient-centered approach. Having a stabilized physician group was critical to developing and maintaining this culture, as the physicians could reinforce this consistently in the ED, on a daily basis. Leadership from BWEP also worked with the hospital's senior leadership team to improve capture of physician downtime cost reimbursement. Despite multiple changes to the core leadership of the ED during this period, the hospital nursing and administration departments worked well with BWEP in order to focus on the broad goal of improving the ED.

Results

Overall, the project showed strong results. Patients reported better experiences in the ED, there was improved income generation, standard-work protocols were developed, clinical quality measures universally improved and, although not reported here due to the sensitivity of the data, a staff survey was conducted and all staff reported a much-improved workplace environment.

In particular, the project resulted in the following improved outcomes:

1. Patient satisfaction scores improved from 64.1% to 75%
2. The LWBS rate decreased from 2.4% to 0.8%
3. Net revenue generated increased by $612,139 per year
4. Average door-to-doctor time decreased from 32 to 28 min
5. Improvements were made in clinical quality metrics for pain medication in long bone fracture*, and antibiotic use in bronchitis*
    *not reported in study see addendum

Finances

Revenue generation was significantly increased through multiple channels. Work RVUs per patient increased from 1.9 to 2.52. The enhanced clinical abilities of the team resulted in an ability to keep more patients that needed hospitalization and prevent unnecessary transfers. The admit rate rose from 8.0% to 9.0%. Physician standby time went from 16% to 59% allowing for a more appropriate cost report savings. The LWBS rate also dropped from 2.4% to 0.8%. These changes resulted in increased net revenue of $612,139 per year. (Figs. 3.2 and 3.3).

Quality Work

Quality was measured through the results of patient experience scores, patient-oriented process measures and clinical quality metrics.

Patient satisfaction was measured through NRC Health surveys and individual patient complaints and comments. Data for this project was collected prior to the end of construction. Top box overall scores improved from 60 to 75 from first quarter of 2016 to the first quarter of 2017. The new scores beat the NRC database, the critical access hospital database, and the database from Maine hospital's averages. Complaints dropped by 25% until construction of the new ED started. This resulted

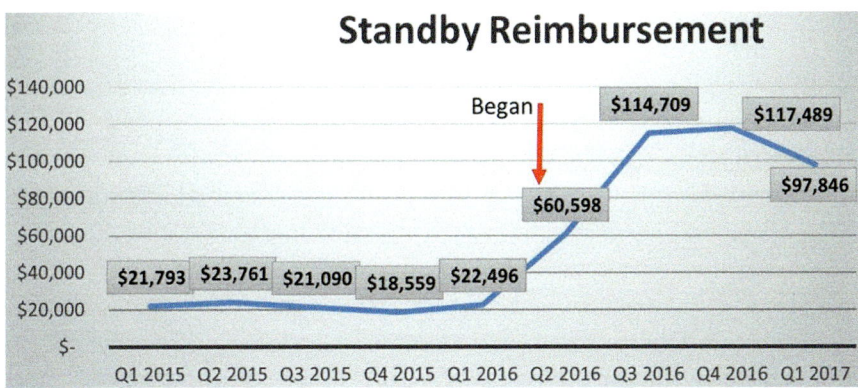

Fig. 3.2 Improvement of reimbursement on cost report using more accurate documentation of standby time for physicians in the ED

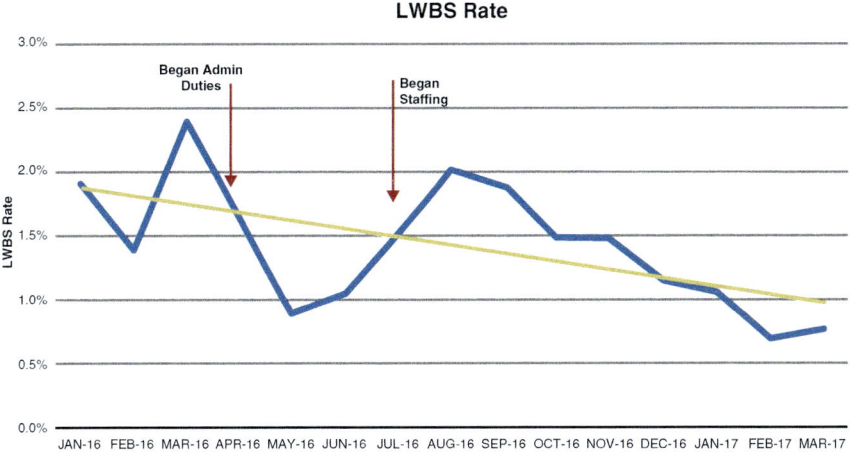

Fig. 3.3 Improved rate of patients leaving prior to being seen by a provider

in an increase in complaints around privacy as physical space suffered during construction. (Figs. 3.4 and 3.5).

Door-to-doctor time measures the amount of time patients are waiting to be seen by a physician in the ED. This not only impacts the patient's experience but also directly effects the clinical quality of their care. Over the 1 year of data collection, the door-to-doctor time decreased by 13% (from 34 min to 30 min). Throughput time for patients discharged home dropped by 31% from 174 mins to 120 mins. The improved throughput times contributed to a drop in LWBS from 2.4% to 0.8%. There was also a slight increase in the length of stay for admitted patients from 420 min to 480 min. (Figs. 3.6, 3.7 and 3.8).

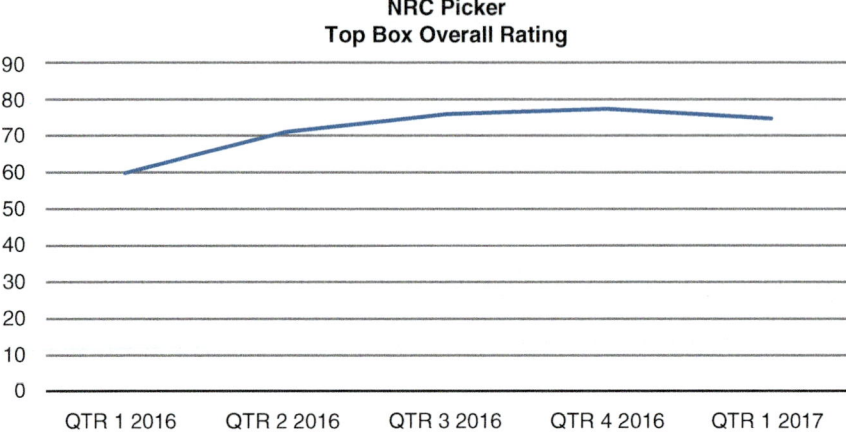

Fig. 3.4 Improvement of the Overall Rating by patients as answered on the NRC patient experience survey

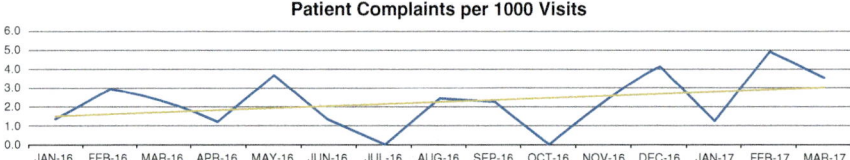

Fig. 3.5 The number of complaints made by patients seen in the ED

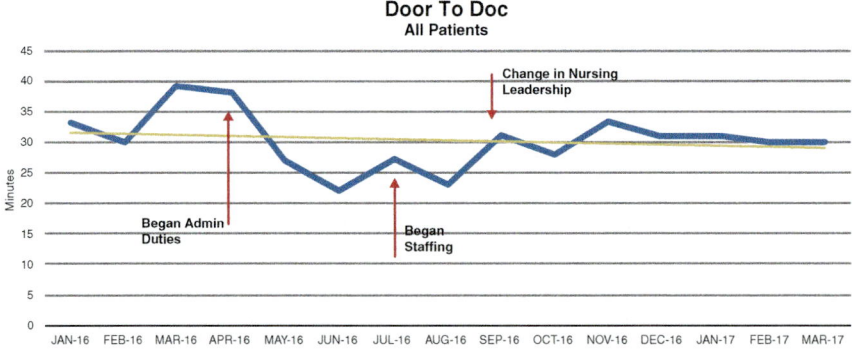

Fig. 3.6 The time for patients to be seen by a provider in the ED from the time that they arrive

To monitor quality of care delivered, clinical quality metrics were developed. These included measures on the prescribing of antibiotics for bronchitis, which is appropriate in limited situations and is marker of good antibiotic stewardship. The baseline figure for the percentage of patients who were prescribed antibiotics for

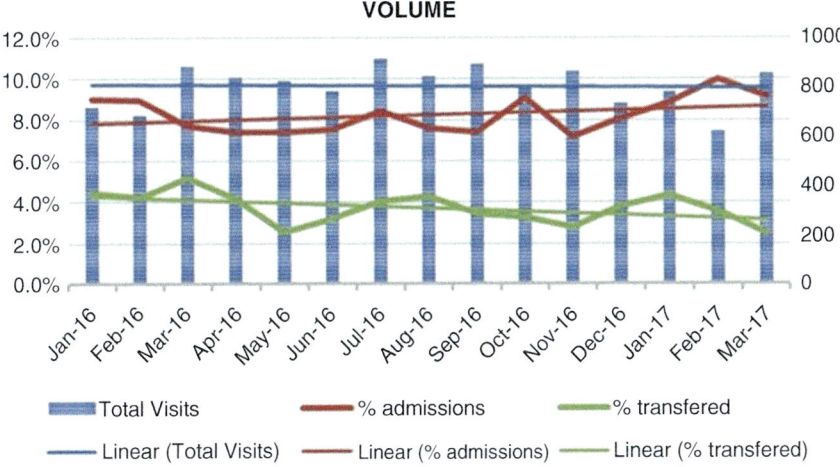

Fig. 3.7 The total number of visits by month seen in the ED and the percentage either admitted to the hospital, or transferred to another hospital for a higher level of care

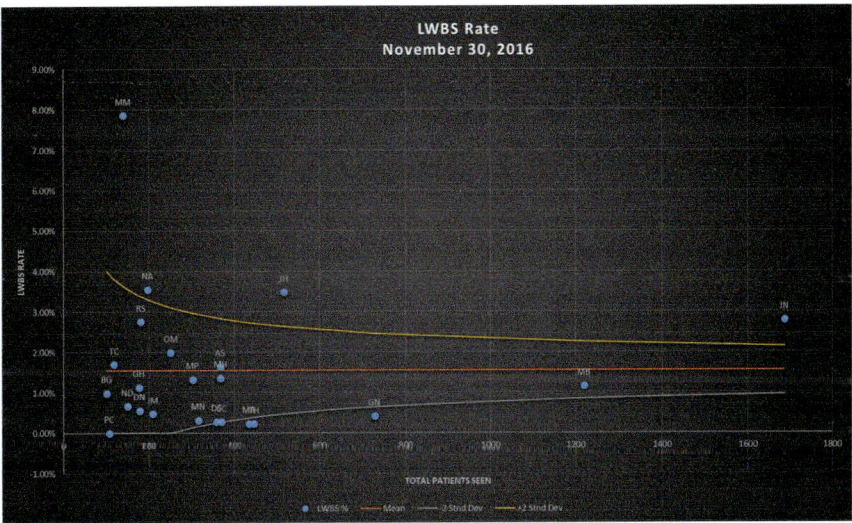

Fig. 3.8 A funnel plot comparing each provider's rate of having patients leave prior to being seen while on duty

bronchitis was 28%. This improved to just under 5% by the project end. Similarly, sepsis was also identified as an area of focus. After a clinical protocol was developed, education was provided, and buy-in from staff was achieved, outcomes were measured using the CMS 3-h bundle. Compliance to sepsis protocols rose from 20% to 60% for the 3-h bundle. (Fig. 3.9).

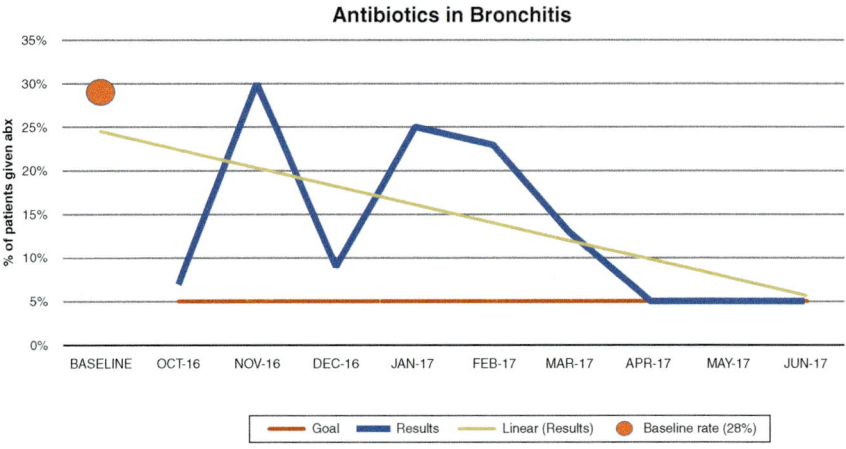

Fig. 3.9 The percentage of patients with bronchitis that were given antibiotics. This was the baseline rate of 28%

Discussion

It is important to understand that while BWEP was brought in from the outside to facilitate change within the organization, the organization was tasked with creating change without any formal authority except for the ED clinicians. Therefore all projects and changes needed to be accomplished through collaboration and influence.

Although the hospital had recognized that they had quality issues, it was critical that bottom-line finances were not strained by awarding BWEP the contract. Therefore, financial performance with immediate returns needed to be part of the implementation. This was accomplished through improved physician downtime cost reporting, increasing admissions, and decreasing left without being seen rate. The hospital desired to utilize marketing in local media to promote the enhanced service as well as to develop understanding of the patient's needs. To this end, hospital staff and leadership were interviewed by local newspapers and television and attendance at local sporting events and health fairs was also promoted by the BWEP.

The hospital had been run by the nursing department and hospital administration with little physician input. The general tone of management had also not been collaborative, especially in the ED. This was further exacerbated by the fact that the nursing leadership was in flux throughout this project period. Upon initiation of this project, the CNO and nursing directors were classified as only interim positions. Unfortunately, this was followed by the appointment of an inexperienced, permanent Nursing Director who was given a large workload and was often drawn away from her leadership duties to fill clinical shifts due to a shortage of staff. This resulted in the Nursing Director feeling overwhelmed and being largely unable to follow through on the rest of the nursing team's plans. She was also not accustomed to physician input. Relational coordination mapping helped to open discussions to slowly improve leadership teamwork.

Creating a culture that was patient-oriented and team-focused among the ED clinicians was a critical step that was needed before making any other improvements.

By hiring staff for core values and working with the clinicians to show that they were valued members of a team, the group coalesced and transitioned into a supportive and forward-thinking team.

There was one development with a particular physician with which exemplified this. This physician had less experience in emergency medicine and was having trouble keeping up with the pace of work in the ED, as shown by his high LWBS rate. This posed a significant problem for the management of the ED as well, as the department was unable to meet its goals for this metric and several nurses reported being frustrated when working with this provider. As a result, the ED management was under pressure from the leadership at BWEP, the CEO of the hospital, and from nursing to ask him to leave. However, despite these challenges, he was very good to patients, was knowledgeable in medicine, and was kind to other staff. Additionally, he was one of the few physicians that had been chosen to stay on from the initial group of physicians that had been working at the hospital at the start of the project. Over the course of this project, leadership worked with this physician to improve his performance and help him to identify ways to become more efficient through individual physician coaching. This proved very effective and his LWBS rate dropped.

However, an additional obstacle he faced was the reputation that he had developed with the nurses. If he was working, nursing reported being more likely to tell patients that there was going to be a long wait and any delay in decision-making was seen as typical for him. To combat this negative reputation, he was urged to join the nursing sign-out meeting each morning that he worked. During these sign-outs, he informed the nurses that he would be setting a goal for himself during the day and asked them for their help in fulfilling this goal and for their suggestions. These relational processes helped him to repair damaged relationships with the nursing team and ultimately increase his efficiency so that his throughput times and LWBS rate matched that of his colleagues. He also became a favorite physician of the staff.

Conclusion

Emergency departments of critical access hospitals provide a crucial service to rural communities. However, many CAHs are struggling financially. This can often coincide with a lack of physician engagement, a less than optimal culture across disciplines and subsequent quality of care issues. Expertise in rural ED management can not only improve the quality of service but also contribute to significant financial improvements. In this incidence it was done by stabilizing leadership and staffing, creating physician engagement, providing rigorously validated data to teams and leaders, and working to create a culture that was patient focused. This project demonstrates how this can be done by small physician owned democratic group that does not have formal authority within the hospital but the support of hospital senior leaders.

Addendum

Figure 3.10 shows the time it took after arrival for patients with a long bone fracture to be given pain medication.

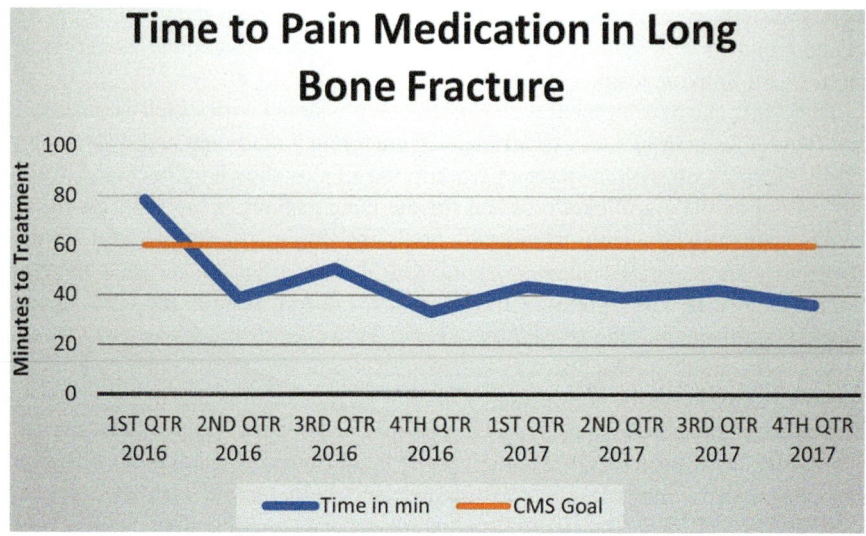

Fig. 3.10 The time it took after arrival for patients with a long bone fracture to be given pain medication

References

1. AAPC: advancing the Business of Healthcare. What are relative value units. https://www.aapc.com/practice-management/rvus.aspx
2. Chipp C, Dewane S, Brems C, Johnson ME, Warner TD, Roberts LW. "If only someone had told me ...": lessons from rural providers. J Rural Health. 2011;27(1):122–30. https://ruralhospitals.chqpr.org/

Part II

Physicians Leading and Implementing Change: Improving Operating Strategy and Changing Culture While Overcoming Organizational Inertia

Improving the Operating Room Efficiency through Communication and Lean Principles

4

Roni Tomashev, Jonia Alshiek, and S. Abbās Shobeiri

Key Learning Points
- Lean thinking is focused on the creation of value through the elimination of seven wastes, including overproduction, inventories, defects, motion, transportation, waiting, and processing.
- Six Sigma is a methodology whose target is to increase customer satisfaction and reduce costs.
- Relational coordination, defined as "communicating and relating for task integration," has been found to contribute to quality treatment and patient safety.
- A hospital is not merely a factory, but it comprises multiple subsystems that function as self-organizing complex adaptive systems.
- Integration of relational coordination into lean–six sigma evaluation considers the human factor involved in operating room process improvement.

R. Tomashev
INOVA Women's Hospital, Falls Church, VA, USA

Assaf Harofe Medical Center, Zrifin, Israel

J. Alshiek
INOVA Women's Hospital, Falls Church, VA, USA

Department of Obstetrics and Gynecology, Holy Family Hospital, Nazareth, Israel

S. A. Shobeiri (✉)
Professor of Medical Education, The University of Virginia, Charlottesville, VA, USA

Faculty of Bioengineering, George Mason University, Fairfax, VA, USA

Women Service Line, NOVA Health System, Falls Church, VA, USA
e-mail: abbas.shobeiri@inova.org

Executive Summary

The new operating rooms at the hospital were experiencing increased surgical volume. The first case start-time had dropped to 56% in January 2016, and the turnaround time had increased. We gathered a team of Ob/Gyns and breast surgeons, anesthesiologists, nurses, and the other support staff to manage increased volume better and decrease resource utilization using relational coordination and six sigma principles.

Introduction

In 2015, hospitals accounted for 32% of U.S. health care expenditures, and this rate is increasing [1]. The hospitals' most expensive and complex part is perioperative services, which account for about 27% of discharges and 52% of inpatient spending and represent a significant opportunity for productivity improvement [2]. Many methods used to improve hospital and perioperative services productivity and quality of care have assumed that the hospital is essentially a factory, and therefore, that industrial engineering and manufacturing derived redesign approaches such as Six Sigma and Lean can be applied to hospitals and perioperative services just as they have been applied in factories [3]. Six Sigma identifies and aligns improvement initiatives with strategic objectives and business goals and looks at critical processes across the System. Six Sigma examines the quality, as defined by the customer, to focus on the requirements and expectations that are genuinely critical and measurable. Disciplined methodologies and aggressive variation reduction have been shown to speed improvement efforts and sustain gains in factory settings [3]. Lean Six Sigma or Lean Sigma is a particular pattern to follow, referred to as define-measure-analyze-improve-control (DMAIC) that leads in a rigorous way towards generalized improvements. Many tools can be used during the five DMAIC stages [4].

1. Define (D) the problem within a process.
2. Measure (M) the defects.
3. Analyze (A) the causes of defects.
4. Improve (I) the process performance to remove causes of defects.
5. Control (C) the process to make certain defects do not recur.

Lean Six Sigma is a fusion of two essential and robust management systems.

First, Lean thinking is focused on the creation of value through the elimination of seven codified and well-known wastes, including [5]:

1. Overproduction
2. Inventories
3. Defects
4. Motion

5. Transportation
6. Waiting
7. Processing

Six Sigma is a methodology whose target is to increase customer satisfaction and reduce costs. Each Six Sigma project is based on the DMAIC pattern, and usually, a team formed by a Black Belt and several Green Belts manages the five stages. The Black Belt is a typical team leader who knows all the Lean Six Sigma tools well and gets an external certification for the scope. Green Belts are participants that have less deep knowledge about Lean Six Sigma. Green Belts are also usually certified. Using the six sigma process aims to improve the first case starts has shown promise in improving the metrics [2, 6]. A hospital is not merely a factory, but it comprises multiple subsystems that function as a self-organizing complex adaptive system. There is no hierarchy of command and control in a complex adaptive system. The System is continually self-organizing through the process of emergence and feedback [2].

Perioperative care is a subsystem with features of a complex adaptive system and factory-like processes [2]. In surgical teams, health professionals are highly interdependent and work under time pressure. It is of particular importance that teamwork is well-functioning to achieve quality treatment and patient safety. Relational coordination, defined as "communicating and relating for task integration," has been found to contribute to quality treatment and patient safety [7]. Relational coordination has also been found to contribute to psychological safety and the ability to learn from mistakes. Four different types of collaboration in interdisciplinary surgical teams in contexts of variable complexity have been identified, representing other communication and relationship patterns:

1. Proactive and intuitive communication,
2. Silent and ordinary communication,
3. Inattentive and ambiguous communication,
4. Contradictory and highly dynamic communication [2].

In this chapter, we highlight how we incorporated relational coordination evaluation into the traditional six sigma process to improve team functioning that led to improved first case start time.

The Environment

In 2016, Inova Health System ("IHS") was a not-for-profit health care system serving Northern Virginia, Washington, D.C., and parts of Maryland and offered a comprehensive array of services at multiple access points. IHS included five hospitals with over 1700 acute care beds to provide inpatient services and provided other outpatient health services, including emergency and urgent care, senior services, home care, mental health, and blood donor services. Services ranged from health promotion and disease prevention to the most advanced treatment services, with notable distinctions in several areas, including cardiology, neuroscience, orthopedics, women's and children's services, and cancer care. IHS also owned and operated *INTotal Health*, a Medicaid health plan licensed in Virginia with approximately 58,000 members. The System's mission was to provide quality care and improve the health of the diverse communities it served. The main competitors in the area were Medstar, Kaiser Permanente, and Centra Health. Only Kaiser Permanente had facilities within Inova service areas, and they did not have their own hospital.

The new Inova Women's Hospital, which opened in January 2016, was a hospital devoted solely to women's care. Many aspects of the patient process, such as admission to pre-op to surgery to postoperative and discharge planning, were readdressed with the move to the new hospital. With the change in healthcare regulations, decreasing reimbursements, and a competitive healthcare delivery environment, it is essential to remove the System's waste and maximize patient processing while adhering to lean principles.

The strategic plan called for coordination of human, financial, and material capital amongst the hospitals. The five hospitals include Inova Fairfax Hospital, Inova Fair Oaks Hospital, Inova Loudoun Hospital, Inova Alexandria Hospital, and the Inova Mount Vernon Hospital. The IFH is the hospital system flagship where the high acuity cases are performed. The Inova Women's Hospital at the IFH complex is the only dedicated women's hospital in the region. The following section describes the methods of the study we implemented at the Inova Women's Hospital.

Methodology

Problem Definition

Inefficient operating rooms affect all aspects of care, including but not limited to patient satisfaction, provider satisfaction, quality metrics, safety metrics, and financial metrics. The operating room efficiency is directly related to scheduling, staffing, nursing, environmental services, cleaning services, and supply chain management.

Preliminary Hypothesis

Operating room first case start can be made more efficient by identifying problem areas, bottlenecks, and lean principles. Our primary aim was to improve the first case On Time Start Percentage, Overall On-Time-Start Percentage and Average Case Turnover Time.

Project Plan

Process Improvement Tools

In a one-year project, we proposed a team consisting of a lean expert, admissions, pre-operative, operating room, postoperative care, and anesthesia. Additionally, we proposed to systematically dissect the processes, perform root cause analysis (RCA), identify performance metrics through a Kaizen event, create a value stream map (VSM) of the processes (first four months), relational coordination assessment (RC), and conduct a healthcare failure mode and effect analysis (HFMEA) to set long-term achievable goals (the following eight months).

The root cause analysis is adapted from the high-risk industries such as power plants and adapted for use in the healthcare industry. RCA is not a single technique, broadly understood as a method of structured risk identification and management in the aftermath of adverse events. Instead, it describes a range of approaches and tools drawn from fields including human factors and safety science used to establish how and why an incident occurred to identify how it, and similar problems, might be prevented from happening again [8]. The root cause analysis consisted of a couple of components. First direct observations and time studies by a Lean consultant of the following processes; Pre-Surgical Services patient and chart ready process, day of surgery Pre-Op Process, OR room set up and turnover process. All processes were developed into process maps with waste/non-value-added steps identified and categorized. Additionally, updates were made to the data collection process to obtain more accurate "case delay reasons" agreed upon by all stakeholders.

There are numerous performance metrics applied to the performance of the operating room. The metrics can include the number of canceled cases, average turnover time, the average time to the operating room ready and patient in the room, number of delayed first case starts, average induction time, average extubation time, the average time to recovery room arrival to discharge, performance feedback from other providers, and compliance to various protocols [9].

Kaizen is a Japanese word that translates to "change for the good." The kaizen event is the "implementation arm of a lean manufacturing program" and notes that events typically are carried out in one week. In other words, it's all about action. The most critical stage of any kaizen event is preparation. Yet correctly defining the problem, goal and scope can be very challenging. Try this simple but effective approach. First, team leaders should ask:

What is the purpose of the event? What process or value stream will be targeted? What are the desired outcomes? Who should be on the team? Answering these questions helps ensure planning and scoping are done properly, goals and objectives are realistically determined, and the right people participate. Next, the team creates a problem statement. Answer these questions to define the problem: What is or isn't occurring, and to what degree? Where in the process or product does it occur? Who does the problem affect? When did it occur, and has it happened before [10]? In the manufacturing sector, a Kaizen event can last five days. In the healthcare sector, it isn't easy to conduct a 5-day workshop, and they are generally conducted over ½ day to 3 days.

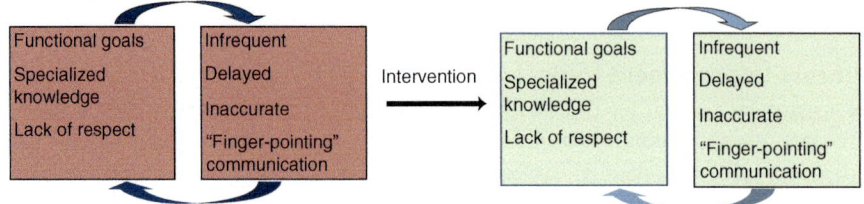

Fig. 4.1 Communication and relationship building for task integration using relational coordination

Value stream mapping (VSM) is a beneficial technique to visualize and quantify the complex workflows often seen in clinical environments. VSM brings together multidisciplinary teams to identify parts of processes, collect data, and develop interventional ideas. Value stream map (VSM) is a visual, simple, but powerful tool and an essential component of a Lean production system. In VSM, a few efficiency indexes of process operation are used to compare the efficiency or estimate the waste between different processes. Process cycle efficiency (PCE) is often used and described as follows:

$$PCE = VA\ time\ /\ total\ lead\ time$$

where VA time, value-added time, is the necessary activity time for products or services based on the customer's viewpoint. Total lead time is the time spent from the beginning to the end of the whole process [11].

Relational coordination (RC) theory helps healthcare providers enhance the quality of communication and relationships among providers to better coordinate care [12] (Fig. 4.1). According to RC theory, high-quality communication (frequent, timely, accurate, and problem-solving) reinforced by high-quality relationships (shared goals, shared knowledge, and mutual respect) enables providers to effectively coordinate work, with positive implications for quality, efficiency, and workforce satisfaction [7, 13].

To conduct a healthcare failure mode and effect analysis (HFMEA) procedure, five main steps are adopted and described as follows:

1. Define the HFMEA topic.
2. Assemble the team.
3. Describe the process graphically.
4. Conduct a hazard analysis
5. Define actions and outcome measures [9, 11].

For each sub-process, all potential failure modes are listed and illustrated. The severity and probability of the listed possible failure modes are determined based on pre-set criteria. The severity score is used to measure the levels of potential failures that can negatively affect patients or patient care in terms of four degrees:

1. Catastrophic (4 points),
2. Major (3 points),

3. Moderate (2 points),
4. Minor (1 point).

The probability score is used to evaluate the frequency of possible failure. Based on the definitions in a previous report from the National Centre for Patient Safety in 2001, this score is rated as follows:

1. Frequent (several times in 1 year, 4 points),
2. Occasional (several times in 2 years, 3 points),
3. Uncommon (sometimes in 2 years to 5 years, 2 points),
4. Remote (sometimes in 5 years to 30 years, 1 point).

The scores of severity and probability are multiplied together to obtain the hazard score. By considering the hazard score and criticality, controllability, and detectability, an HFMEA decision tree is generated to determine the actions of improvement to be taken in the succeeding steps. HFMEA, as classically described, did not pertain to this project, and only some elements were adapted.

The Project Initiation

Our group created an A3 form to identify problems (Fig. 4.2). A3 is a structured approach to problem-solving that utilizes the talent of all staff. The A3 can be used

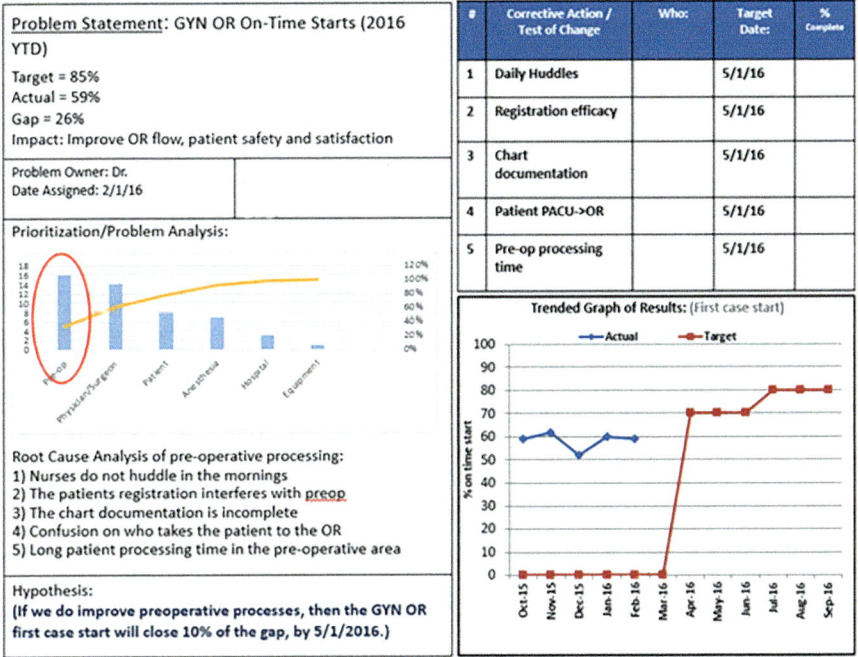

Fig. 4.2 A3 of the on-time start process. The names of responsible parties are whited out for privacy

to update leaders and stakeholders. It is also meant to be updated as the team progresses and learns more through the problem analysis and tests of change.

- A **Problem Statement** was created by asking: Have you defined the target/actual gap? What dates apply to the target and actual? Impact- Why do we care? Patient Safety? Cost? Employee Engagement? Is your problem statement free of blaming, assumptions, symptoms, causes, and solutions?
- A **Problem Owner** was identified by asking: Is the owner someone other than the manager? Have you considered front-line staff owning or co-owning the problem?
- A **Problem-Solving Team** was determined by asking: Do you have the right team members? What other stakeholders should be involved?
- The **Problem Analysis/ Root Cause Investigation** was carried out by asking: Have you gone to see the problem? Was the team involved in determining the root cause? What techniques did you use? (Process Map, Value Stream Map, Pareto, Fishbone, 5Y, Barrier Analysis, Is/Not-Is, etc.).
- A **Hypothesis** was created by asking: What are you trying to achieve? How much of the gap do you plan to close by addressing the root causes selected? What is the impact of the corrective action plan? Did you involve the team in building the hypothesis? The **Corrective Actions** were taken as follows: Did you involve the team in developing the corrective actions? Do corrective actions address the root cause? How do you know? How will you communicate your plan to encourage trust and engagement? What is the impact of each corrective action? How much will the gap close? Immediate Containment Actions (if applicable). If rapid containment is necessary, how is it implemented and communicated? What is the plan for removal?
- **Trended Graph of Results** was created emphasizing: Should tie directly to Problem Statement- trended results- is the gap closing? How will the team check results? Are results posted in a visible location? Can you see cause and effect on the verification chart? How will the team sustain the gains? How will the team check any new standard work? How will the team adjust if the process and/or outcome did not meet expected results?

During weekly meetings, the A3 was revisited to fill gaps and assess progress. During this time, the group leader also considered the relational coordination of the group. The health care providers face pressure to transform healthcare systems, achieve better outcomes for patients *and* do it more efficiently with fewer resources. The relationships amongst the healthcare workers shape the communication through which coordination occurs. Groups can have varying degrees of interpersonal or relational coordination, which is communication and relationship building for task integration (Fig. 4.3).

The stakeholders in the process were identified as:

- Pre-Op nurses
- Pre-Op nurse manager
- Operating room nurses

4 Improving the Operating Room Efficiency through Communication and Lean... 119

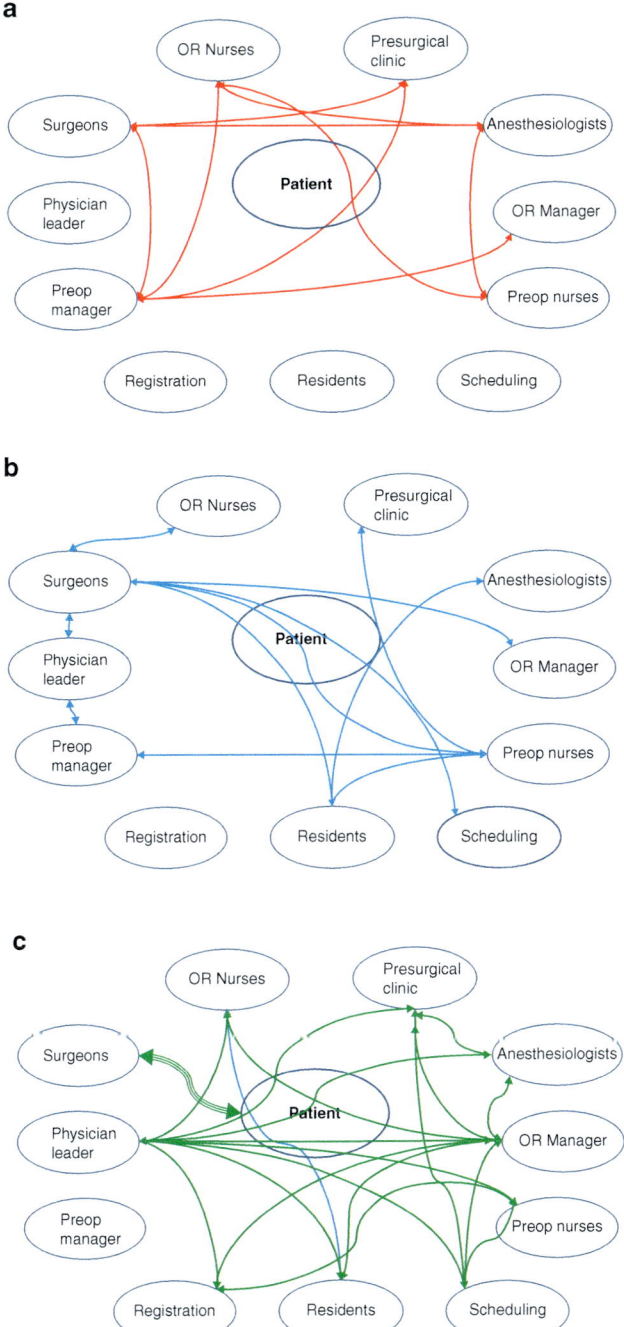

Fig. 4.3 (**a, b, c**) Details the patient in relation to all the team members that are in charge of her well-being. The relationship between various team members is noted with lines. A red line denotes strained **a**, a green line a positive **c**, and the blue line neutral interactions **b**

- Operating room nurse manager
- Anesthesia (MD and anesthetists)
- Surgeons
- Residents
- Scheduling
- Registration

Data Gathering

By February 2016, we had identified and engaged the team members. Identified bottlenecks in the processes and performed root cause analysis in the pre-operative area. We had collected some preliminary metrics as part of the root cause analysis. The targeted metrics were the first case On-Time Start Percentage, Overall On-Time-Start Percentage, and Average Case Turnover Time. The hospital had committed a lean manager and a data manager for the project. Because this was a quality improvement project, it did not require IRB approval. We engaged all the stakeholders, including the physicians.

The communication and interaction amongst team members should enhance the care of the patient. The relationship between the pre-op nurses/leadership and operating room nurses/leadership was stained (Fig. 4.1a). The relationship between the surgeons and almost everyone else was also strained, as noted by the graph's red lines. The green lines denote an excellent working relationship (Fig. 4.1b), while the dark blue lines denote a neutral interaction (Fig. 4.1c). It was hypothesized that improving the relationships will improve performance and push the first case on-time start time to 85%.

Then a matrix (Table 4.1) was created to investigate various relational coordination domains between parties. The questions were guidelines for success in problem-solving and incorporating teamwork, empowerment, engagement, and trust. The physician leader for the operating rooms, scheduling, pre-surgical services, registration, pre-operative nurses, the operating room nurses, and the anesthesia were given a clean version of this matrix and asked to rank each group for each domain between (1, very weak, 2, weak, 3, neutral, 4, strong, 5, very strong). The numbers seen in Table 4.1 are the average from all rankings by the participants. A score of 1 and 2 were low and colored in red, 3 was average and colored in blue, and 4–5 were deemed acceptable target relational coordination between the team members and colored in yellow.

Additionally, the participants were asked to assess the overall environment in the following categories by choosing a yes or no answer: selection for teamwork, teamwork training, shared for accountability of outcomes, shared conflict resolution process, fitness for job design, leadership relationships, boundary spanner roles, shared meetings, shared protocols, and shared information systems. A reply of YES had a score of one, and a NO answer had a score of zero. There was a significant variation in each group (Table 4.2). The most significant areas of improvement, below 40%ile were: Shared meetings "Shared protocols & job design" Boundary spanner roles / shared conflict resolution process / shared accountability for outcomes.

Table 4.1 A survey of the group at before intervention revealed significant opportunities for improvement in relational coordination for all the team members

	Please score the following person or group as 1–5 with: 5 as superior 4 is above average performance 3 is expected level of performance 2 is below expected performance 1 being low performance	Physician Leadership	Scheduling	PSS	Registration	Pre-Op	OR	Anesthesia	Breast & Plastics
Frequent communication	How **frequently** does this person or group communicate with you or your group about (focal work process)?	2	2	3	3	1	3	1	NA
Timely communication	How **timely** is this person or group communication with you or your group about (focal work process)?	2	3	3	4	2	3	2	NA
Accurate communication	How **accurate** is this person or group communication with you or your group about (focal work process)?	2	2	2	3	1	3	2	NA
Problem solving communication	When there is a problem with (focal work process), does this person or group blame others or work you and your group to **solve the problem**?	3	2	2	2	1	2	2	NA
Shared goals	Do people in this person or group share your and your group's **goals** for (focal work process)?	2	3	2	3	2	3	1	NA
Shared knowledge	Does this person or group **know** about the work you or your group does with (focal work process)?	2	2	2	3	1	3	1	NA
Mutual respect	Does this person or group **respect** the work you and your group do with (focal work process)?	2	3	3	4	1	3	2	NA
	Total score 5–35	15	17	17	22	9	20	11	0

Table 4.2 Fitness of environment for teamwork: The table details the percentile of the groups that had an "acceptable" score of 1

Organization Structures Analysis Template	Physician Leadership	Scheduling	PSS	Registration	Pre-op	OR	Anesthesia	Total	Relative Number	%
Selection for teamwork	1	0	0	1	0	1	0	3	3/7	43%
Training for team	1	1	1	0	0	1	1	5	5/7	71%
Shared accountability for outcomes	1	0	0	0	0	1	0	2	2/7	29%
Shared rewards for outcome	1	0	0	0	1	1	0	3	3/7	43%
Shared conflict resolution process	1	1	0	0	0	0	0	2	2/7	29%
Relational job design	1	0	0	0	0	0	0	1	1/7	14%
Relational leadership	1	1	1	1	0	1	0	5	5/7	71%
Boundary spanner roles	1	0	0	0	0	0	0	1	1/7	14%
Shared meetings/huddles	0	0	0	0	0	0	0	0	0/7	0%
Shared protocols	0	0	0	0	0	0	1	1	1/7	14%
Shared information systems	1	1	1	1	1	1	1	7	7/7	100%
Total									31/77	**40%**

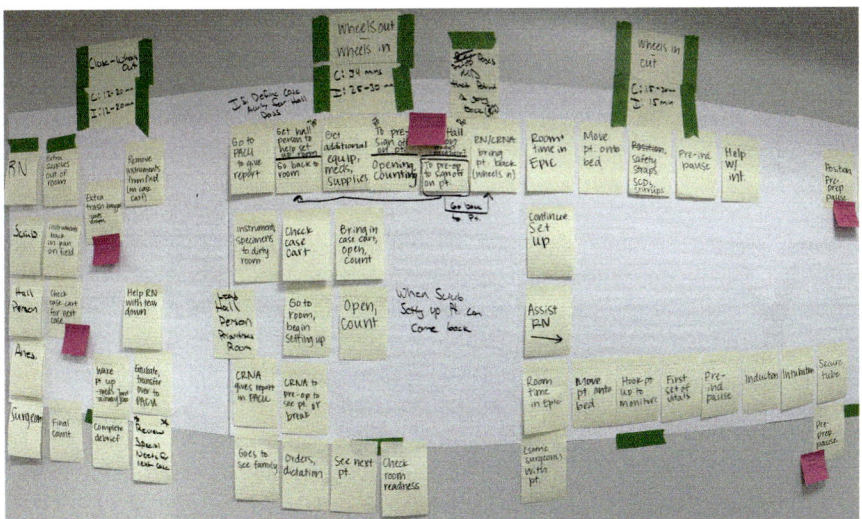

Fig. 4.4 Six sigma Kaizen event sticker board with a continuous improvement engineer taking notes

A cross-functional group with representatives of all stakeholders (Presurgical Nurses, Pre-Op Nurses, OR Nurses, Anesthesia, Surgeons) were brought together in a Kaizen event in a conference room for one day to develop a value stream map of the surgical process from the start (patient identified as needing surgery) through completion of surgery and next patient in the room. Barriers or wastes in the process were identified by the group and denoted with red sticky notes atop the process step. Individual process step times and wait times were included from the time studies conducted for the day of surgery flow to show bottlenecks in the process (Fig. 4.4).

Enhanced frequent, timely, accurate, problem-solving communication between all parties was seen as essential to enhance shared goals, knowledge, and mutual respect. The enhanced relational coordination was seen as critical in order to measurably change the first case on time start time in the operating rooms. The team was meeting on a biweekly basis to achieve shared goals.

At the onset of the intervention and again at 3 months after the intervention, the team members were surveyed. Based on Table 4.1, if the domain reached an acceptable relational coordination range of 4–5 (yellow), a numerical value of 1 was given, and if the relational coordination score was 1, 2 (red), or 3 (blue), a numerical value of 0 was given. In general, the group felt the group and people were engaged but remained some System-related deficiencies that prevented the group from achieving its relational coordination goals. The group identified the areas in the pre-operative processing that were associated with delays. Besides the emphasis on culture, there was a heavy emphasis on the process (Table 4.2). During the group meetings, our lean specialist broke down the process to its essential elements per participants' suggestions. Each point of the process was placed on a board with yellow sticky notes and the sub-processes in blue and orange notes (Fig. 4.4). The areas of opportunity were highlighted with red notes. The information thus derived was placed in a graph format to assess pre-operative delays areas of improvement (Fig. 4.5).

We documented "5 why" root cause analysis conducted for the day of surgery Pre-Op delays. After completing the value stream mapping and five why sessions, the team evaluated all barriers and waste and developed an Ideal State process for On-Time Starts. This included defined roles and responsibilities, implementing parallel processing steps, and agreed-upon time goals for each phase. Based on the information gathered, the desired state for on-time surgical start time was created (Fig. 4.6). Likewise, a value stream map was created for all the areas or groups involved in the on-time start process: Pre-Op, PACU, Anesthesia, Pre-surgical services (PSS), and Environmental Services (EVS) (Fig. 4.7). Additionally, for each process, time studies were performed to determine the time required for patient processing. Standard work was developed to improve handoff times between OR and Pre-Op nurses. The purpose was to enhance handoffs' quality to reduce quality errors and drive quicker turnaround times (Table 4.3).

4 Improving the Operating Room Efficiency through Communication and Lean... 125

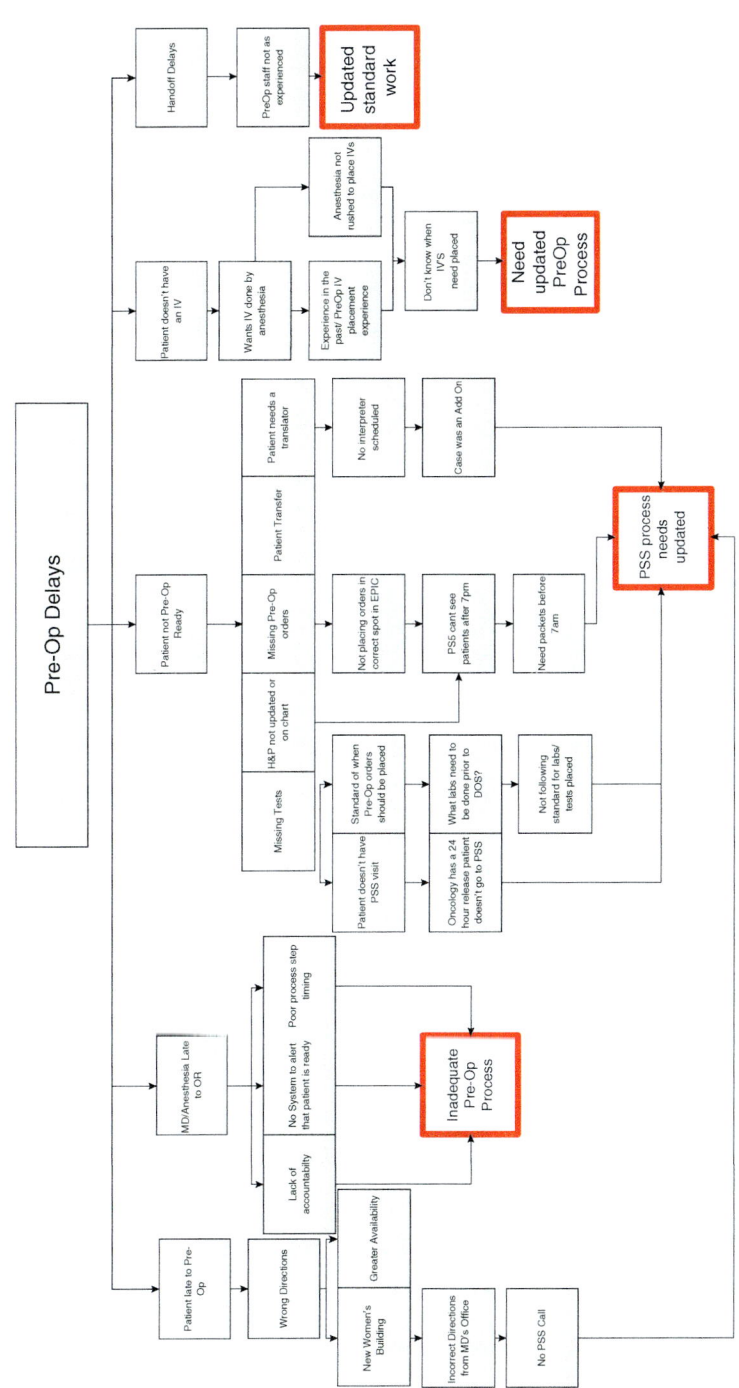

Fig. 4.5 The process map detailing the area of improvement

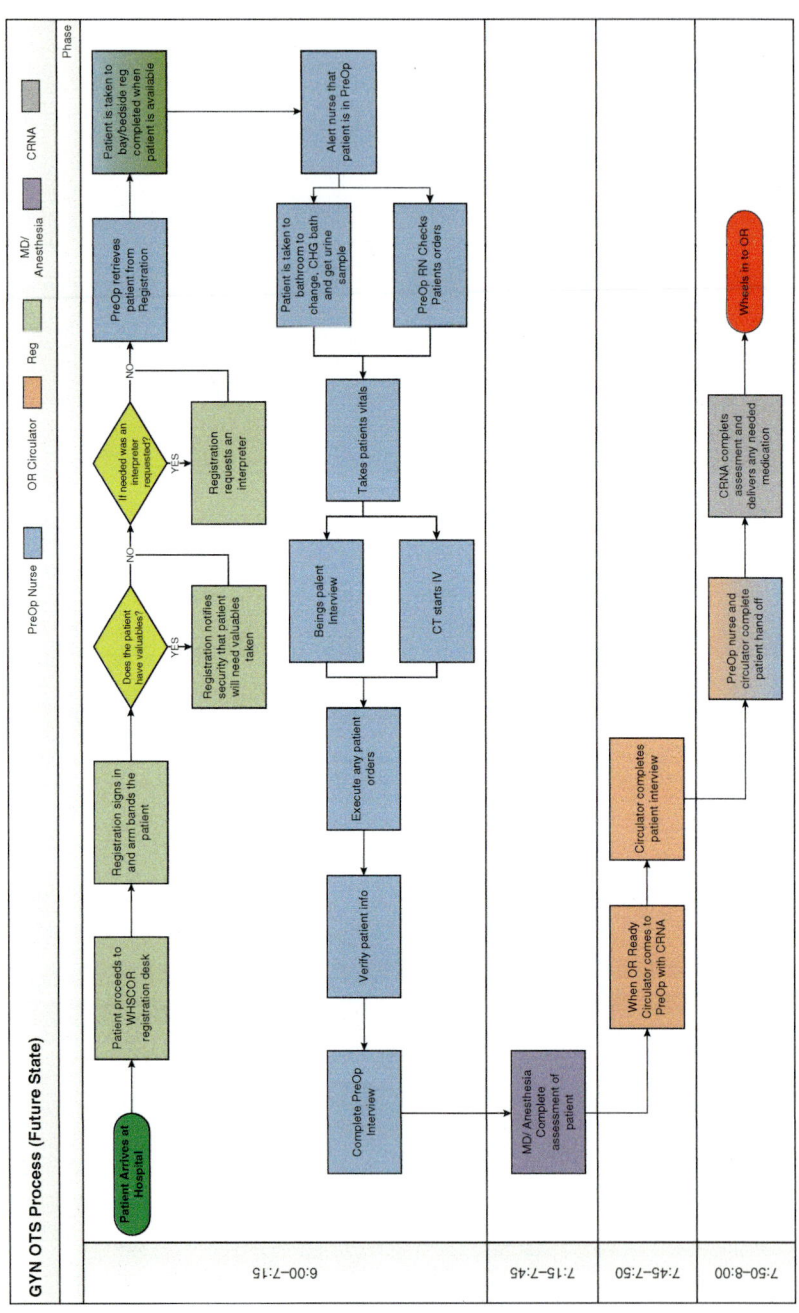

Fig. 4.6 The desired state for on-time surgical start time

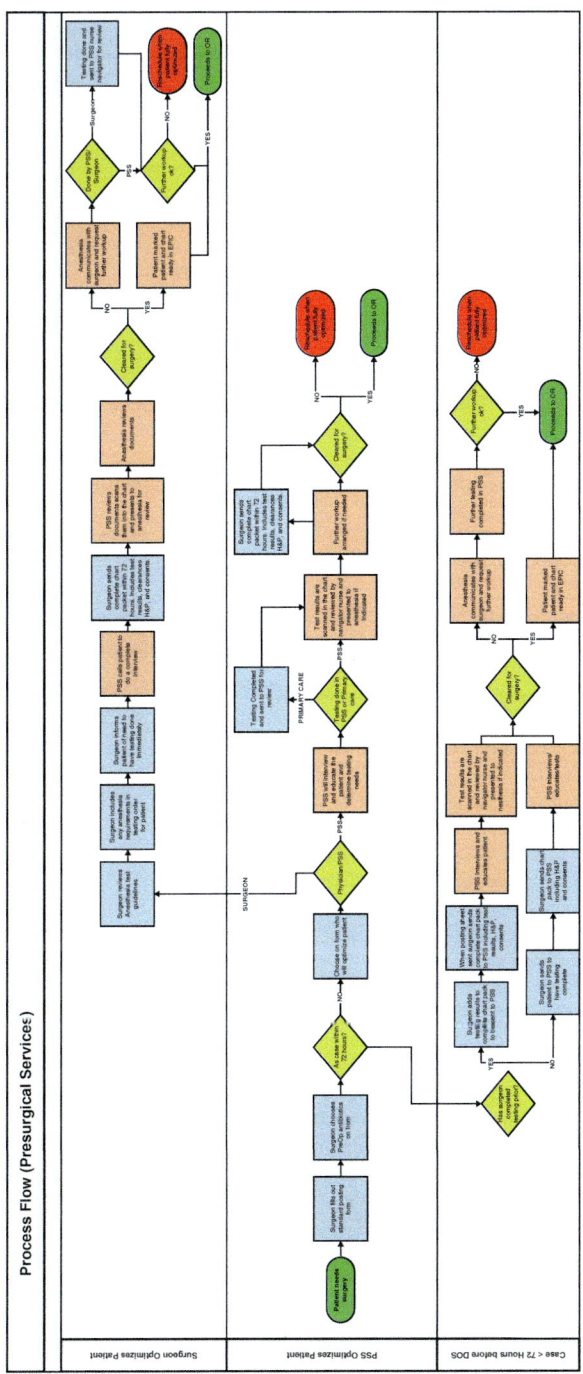

Fig. 4.7 Value Stream Map for presurgical services

Table 4.3 Standard work was developed to improve handoff times between OR and Pre-Op nurses

Operating Unit	Process Name	Process Location	Target Time	Created	Reviewed/Revised	Author
Pre–Op	Pre-Op handoff	Pre-Op		10 minutes	04/01/16	

PURPOSE: Provide necessary patient info from pre-Op to the OR
EXPECTED OUTCOME: Effectively communicate needed patient information from pre-op to OR and ensure patient safety

Step	Process step	Responsible	Time goal	Critical notes on steps
1	Patient band is read to pre-Op RN	OR CIRC	30 sec.	Name, DOB, CSN MR#
	Pre-Op RN confirms patient identification	Pre-Op RN	30 sec.	
2	Pre-Op RN reads allergies from EPIC	Pre-Op RN	30 sec.	Verify on band
	OR confirms allergies	OR circulator	30 sec.	
3	Confirm NPO states with patient	Pre-Op RN/ OR circulator	30 sec.	PT vocalizes last time the patient ate
4	Communicate special needs (take verbiage off sheet)/issues with patient	Pre-Op RN	30 sec.	Glasses Dentures Body jewelry
	Communicate special needs /issues with patient	OR circulator	30 sec.	
5	Communicate patient comorbidities	Pre-Op RN	30 sec.	BP Diabetic status
	Take notes on any comorbidities	OR circulator	30 sec.	
6	Communicating any pending labs/tests	Pre-Op RN	30 sec.	CBC Txx Pregnancy
	Take notes of any pending labs/tests	OR circulator	30 sec.	
7	Show medication doses and times in EPIC to OR circulator	Pre-Op RN	30 sec.	Beta blockers Antibiotics And band
	Takes notes on medication doses and times	OR circulator	30 sec.	
8	Verify skin integrity with patient, Verify ROM with patient	Pre-Op RN/ OR circulator	30 sec.	
9	Communicate to OR circulator where patient belongings are located	Pre-Op RN/ OR circulator	30 sec.	
10	Visually verify all components of the boarding pass	Pre-Op RN/ OR circulator	90 seconds	Verifying surgical, anesthesia and blood special consents Site marking, H&P

Results

According to the graph in Fig. 4.8, the first-case start improved significantly and increased from 59% to 93%. Historically the on-time starts had been around 75% with an occasional increase to 82%. Three months after the initiation of the process, the group had significantly improved relational coordination (Fig. 4.9). The preoperative area, pre-surgical services, and anesthesia had opportunities in timely communication, but overall, many responses had turned favorable (Table 4.4).

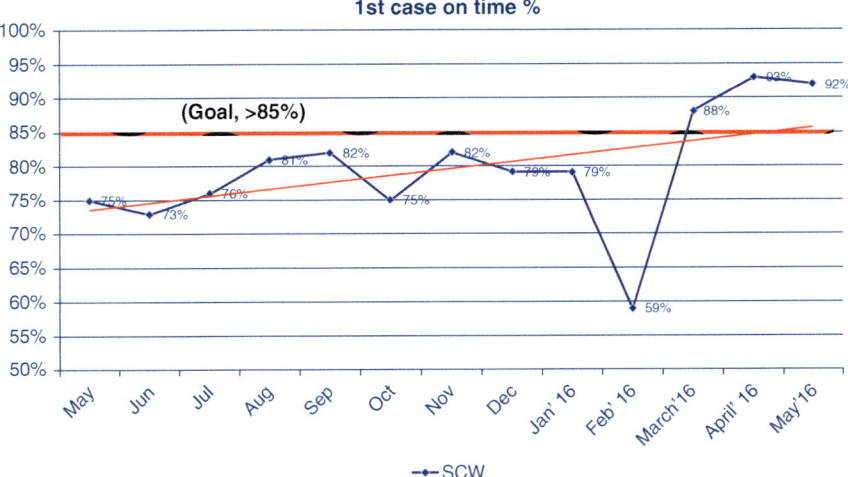

Fig. 4.8 The graph illustrating the improvement in the on-time start after the initiation of the Lean process intervention

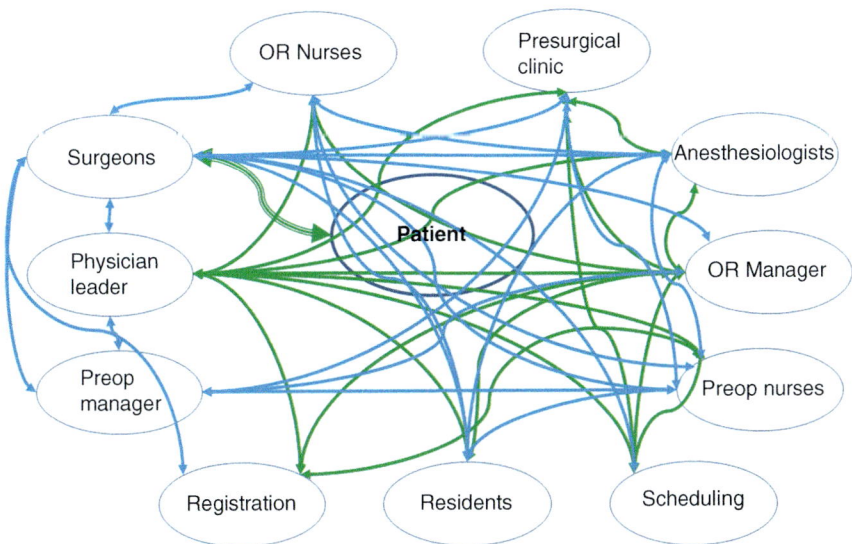

Fig. 4.9 The relationship between all the groups had improved significantly to serve the patient

Table 4.4 A three-month survey of the group at six months post-intervention revealed significant improvement in relational coordination for all the team members

Please score the following person or group as 1–5 with: 5 as superior 4 is above average performance 3 is expected level of performance 2 is below expected performance 1 being low performance	Physician Leadership	Scheduling	PSS	Registration	Pre-Op	OR	Anesthesia	Breast & Plastics
Frequent communication How frequently does this person or group communicate with you or your group about (focal work process)?	4	4	3	4	3	4	4	NA
Timely communication How timely is this person or group communication with you or your group about (focal work process)?	4	5	3	4	2	3	2	NA
Accurate communication How accurate is this person or group communication with you or your group about (focal work process)?	3	3	2	3	3	3	3	NA
Problem solving communication When there is a problem with (focal work process), does this person or group blame others or work with you and your group to **solve the problem**?	4	4	4	3	3	4	4	NA
Shared goals Do people in this person or group share **your and your group's goals** for (focal work process)?	5	4	4	4	4	4	3	NA
Shared knowledge Does this person or group **know** about the work you or your group does with (focal work process)?	4	4	3	3	3	4	3	NA
Mutual respect Does this person or group **respect** the work you and your group do with (focal work process)?	4	4	4	4	4	3	3	NA
Total score 5–35	28	28	23	25	22	20	22	0

In June 2016, INOVA Women's hospital added two additional operating rooms and assimilated the breast and plastic cases. The resulting inflow disrupted the standard operations, and the first case start went back down to 82% during the integration process. To measure the effect of our interventions, the group gathered on a weekly basis and reported on their area's true north board to review metrics.

Discussion/Lessons Learned

What was unique about our approach was combining the lean principles with elements of relational coordination to affect operating room key metrics. By early December 2016, we had improved perioperative processes for the entire INOVA women's operating rooms. In November of 2016, a weekly working group meeting with the new breast and plastics surgeons was instituted as a pathway to address multiple issues in addition to on-time start. We addressed other problems, which included:

1. Equipment processing.
2. Appropriate anesthesia for outpatients.
3. Appropriate anesthesia for inpatients (ERAS protocol).

By mid-November 2016, we had an action plan as follows and assigned appropriate individuals to the tasks. In addition, we created an ERAS group that met separately weekly. One of the biggest challenges for coordinating processes and creating new processes for breast / plastic surgery was the ERAS (Enhanced Recovery After Anesthesia) protocol. This required the creation of a joint task force between the OR physician leader, anesthesia, the nursing, and the breast surgeons. Once this process was created we started working on two fronts: (1) We started working and finalized ERAS pathways for Gynecology, Gynecologic Oncology, and Urogynecology. (2) We worked with EPIC EMR leadership to incorporate these pathways into the electronic medical records to use the patient outcome metrics. Some of our initial gains were lost during the introduction of the breast and plastic surgeries, which necessitated further reappraisal, assessment, and revision of our processes.

We looked for further improvement opportunities to procure and install a system-wide inventory management system within the perioperative setting and improved staffing, financials, material flow, and tracking. The inventory system is expected to manage and automate inventory replenishment activities across the inventory continuum, from owned and consigned to tissue and other regulated products. The inventory management system may provide the necessary framework and infrastructure to standardize inventory management practices across the health system. The long-term goal is to expand the infrastructure to include inpatient, outpatient, and procedural settings.

The staffing can be a challenge in a high-demand area such as Northern Virginia. The areas of improvement are increased staff scheduling accuracy, increasing nursing staff skill level and defining the metrics required for assessing performance, clarifying roles and accountability, and growing job allocation responsibilities.

Operating room financials heavily rely on material flow and track by ordering the suitable material to be placed in the right cart and be charged accurately. The right product relies on inventory tracking, inventory visibility, automated orders, and appropriate staff with the required expertise, expiration management, and meeting compliance requirements. The right product relies on pick case carts, specialty items, valid and complete preference cards, picking correct items, case cart auditing, and a standardized return process. The accurate billing relies on documentation of all supplies, implants in EMR.

Hospitals and health systems routinely perform gap analysis for opportunities to improve order management, case carts, and billing. These processes that run in the background can have a profound impact on first case start time.

Conclusion

The first case on-time start metric is used as one of several indicators of the health of the operating room. We made a measurable improvement in our first case start times objectively by measured dramatic improvement. Of significance, the operating room health and the key metrics fluctuate. The operating room leaders need to institute a durable method of governance responsive to the ever-changing operating room environment.

References

1. Martin AB, Hartman M, Washington B, Catlin A, Team NHEA. National health spending: faster growth in 2015 as coverage expands and utilization increases. Health Aff. 2017;36(1):166–76.
2. Mahajan A, Islam SD, Schwartz MJ, Cannesson M. A hospital is not just a factory, but a complex adaptive system—implications for perioperative care. Anesth Analg. 2017;125(1):333–41.
3. Sehwail L, DeYong C. Six sigma in health care. Leadersh Health Serv. 2003;
4. Bowerman J, Antony J, Downey-Ennis K, Antony F, Seow C. Can six sigma be the "cure" for our "ailing" NHS? Leadersh Health Serv. 2007;
5. Chiarini A. Risk management and cost reduction of cancer drugs using lean six sigma tools. Leadersh Health Serv. 2012;
6. Phieffer L, Hefner JL, Rahmanian A, Swartz J, Ellison CE, Harter R, et al. Improving operating room efficiency: first case on-time start project. J Healthc Qual. 2017;39(5):e70–e8.
7. Gittell JH, Fairfield KM, Bierbaum B, Head W, Jackson R, Kelly M, et al. Impact of relational coordination on quality of care, postoperative pain and functioning, and length of stay: a nine-hospital study of surgical patients. Med Care. 2000:807–19.

8. Peerally MF, Carr S, Waring J, Dixon-Woods M. The problem with root cause analysis. BMJ Qual Saf. 2017;26(5):417–22.
9. Gabriel RA, Gimlich R, Ehrenfeld JM, Urman RD. Operating room metrics score card—creating a prototype for individualized feedback. J Med Syst. 2014;38(11):144.
10. Nino V, Claudio D, Valladares L, Harris S. An enhanced kaizen event in a sterile processing department of a rural hospital: a case study. Int J Environ Res Public Health. 2020;17(23)
11. Hung S-H, Wang P-C, Lin H-C, Chen H-Y, Su C-T. Integration of value stream map and healthcare failure mode and effect analysis into six sigma methodology to improve process of surgical specimen handling. J Healthc Eng. 2015;6:517429.
12. Kyriakidou O, Èzbilgin M. Relational perspectives in organizational studies: a research companion. Edward Elgar Publishing; 2006.
13. Gittell JH, Weinberg D, Pfefferle S, Bishop C. Impact of relational coordination on job satisfaction and quality outcomes: a study of nursing homes. Hum Resour Manag J. 2008;18(2):154–70.

Implementing Change in Surgical Culture

Mike K. Chen

Key Learning Points
- Organizational culture requires management.
- Decision making requires transparency.
- Boundary spanner roles facilitate honest communication as a third party to stakeholder groups.
- Early buy-in from leadership helps to facilitate change management.
- All stakeholder groups must be present when designing policy.

Executive Summary

Hospital culture predicts work engagement, job satisfaction, and staff burnout. This paper uses Relational Coordination (RC), a theory of organizational behavior, in conjunction with stakeholder interviews to diagnose a dysfunctional culture in a pediatric surgical ward. We found that RC between surgeons and hospital administration was generally poor. As a result, nurses were often put in the position of informing surgeons of changes to hospital policy, which proved ineffective and harmful to group dynamics. These findings informed the creation of a physician of the day (POD), a boundary spanner role designed to enforce policy and resolve conflict between workgroups. This intervention was associated with a 3.8% increase in on-time start to surgeries, and an 8.3 min reduction in turnover time between surgeries. The fact that the POD role had buy in from leadership made the project particularly successful and durable over time.

M. K. Chen (✉)
Department of Surgery, Children's of Alabama Hospital, Heersink UAB School of Medicine, Birmingham, AL, USA
e-mail: mike.chen@childrensal.org

Introduction

The operating theatre may be the most intimidating environment in the hospital. This is a place where egos and pride can run amok and overwhelm the ecosystem. It is a stressful environment with an unpredictable ebb and flow. It is also a sanctum where lives are saved and miracles happen. Cultivating a culture and fostering a system that enhances the vitality of this environment can lead to better patient care, boost job satisfaction, as well as improve the bottom line [1, 2]. Building quality relationships between roles involves mutual respect, shared goals, and shared decision making.

In our children's hospital, the surgical theater is one of the busiest and most profitable areas. From early morning to late evening, elective procedures are churned through as safely and efficiently as possible. Much of this work is unpredictable and time sensitive, driven by an emergency or other urgent procedures. Scheduled procedures may have to be delayed as emergent conditions take priority. The downstream effect of this can significantly stress the system, affecting patients, operating room (OR) personnel, perioperative services, and other members of the hospital.

In a finely tuned and cohesive ecosystem, the unpredictability is expected and managed as a part of the routine in surgery. Patients are kept informed and workers are empowered to make adjustments as needed to minimize the disruption. To achieve a highly functional system requires the culture to be one that provides the participants with the tools to perform their tasks. Communication and relationships are inherently part of the job design for workgroups that function in the OR.

We chose to apply Relational Coordination (RC) theory to diagnose the challenges facing our organizational culture because it incorporates measures of both communication and relationships between roles. RC is a theory of organizational behavior developed by Gittell [1] that is supported by these two mutually reinforcing constructs of relationships and communication. The theory posits that the quality of relationships is measured across the three domains of shared goals, shared knowledge, and mutual respect. The quality of communication is assessed across the four domains of frequency, timeliness, accuracy, and ability to problem solve.

RC as a validated construct has been studied in several health care settings, from private clinics to large academic hospitals. In the context of surgical care, increased RC between clinical staff was shown to predict psychological safety [3], work engagement, job satisfaction, and decreased burnout [4]. Regarding efficiency, increased RC between providers predicted lower total cost of hospital care [2], and shorter length of stay [1, 2]. RC between providers was further shown to predict several safety outcomes, including reduced medical errors, fall related injuries, and hospital-acquired infections [4], as well as wrong site surgeries [5]. RC between providers was also shown to predict several patient reported outcomes such as patient satisfaction [6, 7]. The theory posits that RC is positively affected by organizational structures that facilitate communication between workgroups [8], which leads to the hypothesis that adding a boundary spanner role will increase RC, which will increase work engagement and decrease medical errors.

This project first used relational coordination mapping as a diagnostic tool to understand the quality of relating and communication between workgroups in our surgical ward. We then used the theory of relational coordination to guide the development of an intervention.

Methods

Our mixed methods project involved two consecutive steps. We started by diagnosing the pain points in our hospital's culture using qualitative interviews. This research was used to guide the formation and rollout of the key intervention, establishing a new managerial position designed to cross workgroups.

This project started with interviews. I asked staff open ended questions on the broad theme of "how can I help you do your job better". I also asked people to explain their assumptions regarding (1) how management makes decisions, (2) how policy decisions are communicated, and (3) how disputes are handled. This information was recorded and coded for themes.

We then constructed a Relational Coordination stakeholder map. We took time to understand who the stakeholders were, how they interacted among themselves, and how they engaged with other stakeholders.

After constructing the relational map, our team performed an organizational structures analysis. We broke down the data produced from this tool and identified a current state and desired state for our organization.

We then developed a change management team involving representatives from each stakeholder group. This started with an initial meeting where we articulated the rationale for this project and each group expressed key goals for culture change that would help their workgroup. We worked hard to reach a consensus surrounding the value of the organization, the goals that would achieve this value, and the implementation. As part of our relational intervention we broadcasted the notion of a 'safe space' where blaming individuals was not tolerated. Surgeons were not treated differently in this regard. We worked together with stakeholders to create an intervention that would help to support a safe and fair environment.

The intervention that we agreed upon was creating a physician of the day (POD). The hope for this role was to manage within and between group competitions by allowing stakeholders to seek outside counsel from a third party to handle disputes. Each stakeholder was then asked to explain the intervention to their respective workgroups. We met frequently with members of each workgroup to check in and iterate goals.

We determined the effects of the POD intervention using two efficiency measures of on-time start to surgical procedures and OR turnover time as indicated by administrative log records. The effects of this intervention were measured a year after baseline using a pre/post quasi-experimental design without a control group.

Results

There are numerous participants in the OR with a wide range of skill sets. Contribution from the variety of team members is vital to achieve the singular goal of doing the best we can to provide safe and efficient care for the surgical patients. Interviews indicated that the culture of the surgery unit involved six main stakeholder groups including nurses/staff, private surgeons, academic surgeons, anesthesiologists, OR administration, and hospital administration. We conducted stakeholder interviews which informed the following themes.

Nurses as Boundary Spanners

A central theme that surfaced from interviews was the role of nurses as boundary spanners between administrators and surgeons. We found that administrators were effective at communicating with the nursing staff but ineffective at communicating with surgeons. Hospital administration consist of only one practicing physicians. In practice this meant that nurses were responsible for informing surgeons about decisions made by hospital administration. We noted several instances where nurses were made to feel as if they were personally responsible to administrators for policy compliance in the OR. We found examples where a surgeon learned about a new policy from a nurse, and then used the inherent power differential between themselves and nurses to overlook the policy change. This put nurses in the difficult position of managing up to adhere with policy changes, which resulted in a large variation in compliance and deterioration of between-group relations.

We found that variation in compliance was in part caused by multiple workarounds that the hospital used to accommodate dysfunctional processes and hotheaded personalities. We found that this resulted in perceptions that some surgeons could get away with poor behavior. Hospital personnel were left to try to manage disruptive incidents with one-off interventions instead of using policies that were intentional. Effectively we were reactive rather than proactive, constantly playing catch up. A second observation was that several physicians indicated that they had the option of taking their patients to a competing hospital, which gave them leverage that resulted in immunity to retribution from administration. These practices resulted in a general lack of accountability which added a layer of inconsistency to the clogged communication channels that were already kneecapping effective workflow.

Policy Was Decided behind Closed Doors

A second theme that emerged was that hospital administration often made policy decisions without consulting other stakeholders in the organization. Surgeons noted that administration frequently changed aspects of their practice without transparency or consideration of the lift that the policy change would require. They

5 Implementing Change in Surgical Culture

indicated that this made them feel powerless as practitioners of their craft and excluded in their work environment, which resulted in resentment and push back against decision making. For nurses caught in the middle between these two management groups, this lack of transparency lead to anxiety and frustration.

"Us" against "Them"

The organizational structure of our surgical ward manifested in a combative environment. Structurally, the lack of clear hierarchy pitted the nurses and OR personnel against the physicians when making policy related decisions. In practice this meant that nurses and administrators managed the OR with very little input from physicians. Adding to this mix was the fact that there were academic as well as private practitioners who inherently had different goals.

Informants identified a general lack of collaboration, where there were no shared aspirations. We also identified a lack of shared knowledge about the way to achieve the ultimate goal of providing efficient and safe care. Some stakeholder groups expressed feelings of isolation and ineffectiveness. We heard anecdotal evidence suggesting that this work environment had caused the hospital to lose high quality staff, a practice that can initiate a vicious cycle of talent drift.

Relational Mapping

Construction of a relational map, displayed in Fig. 5.1, shows that the anesthesia group had the highest RC ratings both between work groups and within their own group. The anesthesia group exhibited the strongest overall RC with other groups.

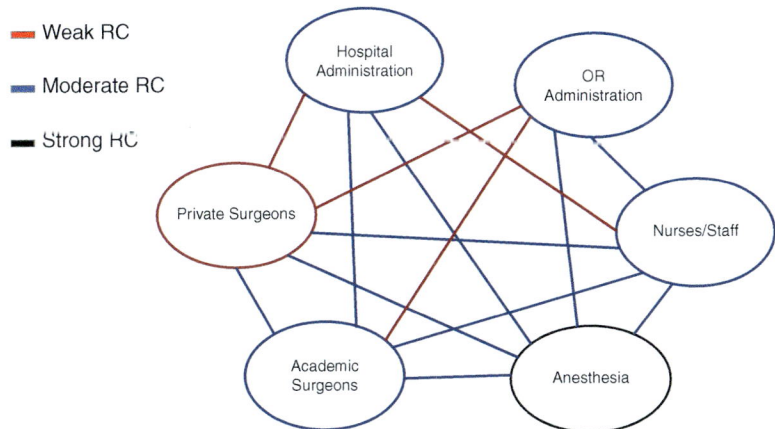

Fig. 5.1 RC Map of the Stakeholders

The RC map also shows that the anesthesia group worked well among themselves. They communicated frequently and timely among themselves sharing high quality information. In contrast the private surgeons were shown to have the lowest internal RC and were tied with the two administrative groups for lowest between group RC. More broadly the RC map pointed to a need for improved communication between surgeons and administration.

Organizational Structures Analysis

Organizational structures analysis, displayed in Table 5.1, demonstrated that Shared Protocols and Shared Information Systems were accessible as platforms to improve processes and provide communication to all stakeholders with the exception of some private surgeons. A conflict resolution process was accessible to all stakeholders in the unit, excluding private surgeons and hospital administration. The two surgery groups were excluded from shared meetings and huddles, making them further isolated from communication.

Breaking these results into the categories of current state and desired state produced the categories displayed in Table 5.2. Broadly the themes of the current state

Table 5.1 Characterisitics of the Stakeholders

	Hosp Admin	OR Admin	Nurse/Staff	Anesthesia	Academic Surgeons	Private surgeons	Support for RC
Selection for teamwork	x		x	x	x		4/6 = 66.7%
Training for teamwork			x	x			2/6 = 33.3%
Shared accountability for outcomes	x	x					2/6 = 33.3%
Shared rewards for outcomes	x			x	x		3/6 = 50%
Shared conflict resolution process		x	x	x	x		4/6 = 66.7%
Relational job design			x	x	x		3/6 = 50%
Relational leadership	x		x		x		3/6 = 50%
Boundary spanner roles		x	x		x		3/6 = 50%
Shared meetings/huddles	x	x	x	x			4/6 = 66.7%
Shared protocols	x	x	x	x	x		5/6 = 83.3%
Shared information systems	x	x	x	x	x		5/6 = 83.3%

Table 5.2 Current vs. Desired States

Current state
- Untimely and infrequent communication; blaming culture
- Nurses are afraid of being in the middle and being blamed for any failure by admin (hospital and OR) and by surgeon groups (academic and private)
- Surgeons and other stakeholders tend to isolate into their silos feel that they lack 'control' and 'autonomy' in the OR

Desired state
- Shared values and mutual respect
- Creation of a system where communication is frequent, accessible, and done in a safe space devoid of harmful power dynamics.
- Creation of boundary spanner role and frequent huddle to help close the relationship gap
- Building trust and breaking down silos

described poor communication and relationships. We crafted the desired state to reflect insight from the theory of Relational Coordination.

We took this information and decided to create a physician of the day (POD) role to serve as boundary spanner. We observed that the POD served as an arbitrator, which buffered nurses and other OR personnel from managing conflict with physicians. The POD further served as boundary spanner between policy makers and physicians, which noticeably relieved nurses from the responsibility of performing this role. Establishing a POD further sent a message to physicians that they would be held accountable for their actions and that they were responsible for participating as part of a larger unit. If the POD was not able to resolve the problem, the issue would be escalated to the division director and subsequently, the surgeon-in-chief.

The quasi-experimental pre/post comparison of on-time start rate and turnover time indicated that the POD intervention was associated with an increase in efficiency. The percentage of on-time starts improved from 78.7% in the 6 months prior to the implementation of the POD to 82.5% a year after the introduction of the POD role. The turnover time similarly improved, with the average time dropping from 29.2 min to 20.5 min. We believe that this was a remarkable improvement.

Discussion

Culture is the labor capital of an organization, something that can predict efficiency and safety. Our surgical culture rose organically without intentional design. Our experience manifested in infrequent and inadequate communication and a lack of clear leadership that resulted in variable accountability. The end result was a battle of wills between physicians, nurses and OR staff that caused frustration and hampered workflow for all parties. The goal of the boundary spanner role was to establish a third-party form of leadership to increase objective accountability. We found this intervention to be highly effective.

Lessons Learned

The first key takeaway from this project was that structure defines function in our organization. Roles that were naturally third-party boundary spanners had good internal and external relational coordination. In this project the Anesthesia group demonstrated highest internal and external RC. This was not surprising considering that they work directly with all other groups providing anesthesia for all surgeries.

It is similarly unsurprising that the private surgeons were the most disparate group. This group consisted of the largest number of physicians who were in multiple private practices. The fact that they did not spend as much time in the hospital as the other groups meant that they had less opportunity for timely and frequent communication. We found that their interactions were generally sporadic. We found that they distrusted the hospital and OR administrators, and that their assumptions about administrative actions often were untested, which further reinforced poor communication. Hospital and OR administrators had weak relational connections with the surgeons and nurses. It was unclear if shared goals existed as they were not clearly articulated.

We also learned how important it is to incorporate workers from the gemba, or the actual workfloor in decision making [9]. Incorporating these front-line workers helped to blend theory with practice and highlight specific barriers to adoption that were crucial to consider during implementation. In our case this was helpful in identifying the problem with asking nurses to manage physicians before taking steps to reduce existing power dynamics which are carried over from the historical toxic hospital hierarchy that puts physicians above nurses.

A predictable takeaway was the importance of soliciting the perspectives of all stakeholders involved in the care process. To do this, leaders must be on the lookout, ready to expand the stakeholder map to include additional stakeholders. Leaders can not presume to have successfully diagnosed the problem before listening to all stakeholders and identifying their assumptions. This helps to identify critical barriers to change implementation. This process also means challenging one's own assumptions about what other people are thinking. Though time consuming and often nuanced, engaging the stakeholders in the change process is vital if one wants the change to be durable. We found that taking the effort to go through this process paid off substantially.

A last takeaway was that change must be meaningful for all stakeholders. The change leader needs to articulate the rationale for the change and why it benefits the stakeholder. Because changing the culture will reshuffle the relationships and potentially change power dynamics, stakeholders must be engaged and regularly reminded about the value of the change.

Reflections on Change Management

At the time of project rollout I knew that details and careful project planning was not one of my strong traits. To successfully place these interventions in the hospital culture I needed to identify collaborators and champions. I was fortunate to have partners in the perioperative services who managed that aspect.

We engaged the Chief Medical Officer (CMO) early in the process regarding the POD role. The CMO was often the 'police' for the organization who had to deal with conflicts. He saw that establishing a POD would provide him with another level of support at the local level. It was an easy concept for him to champion and it was an early win for our project. He communicated this to the Chief Operating Officer and Chief Executive Officer and they were also supportive.

We found the process of changing culture for non-management stakeholder groups to be hard work, requiring a sense of urgency, perseverance, and trust. We found that trust can be earned by staying on message, listening to different perspectives, and questioning one's own assumptions. Our staff greatly benefitted from having a credible champion who showed interest in listening to them about ways that the hospital culture could change to help them do their job better. This came as a surprise considering that no one had previously taken the time to understand their needs. In reflection I found that they had expected the meeting to be another critical assessment of their behavior. This simple action transformed their commitment to culture change.

I was surprised at how much the stakeholders wanted change and embraced my message of enhanced communication, mutual respect, and working towards aligned goals. They wanted everyone to be held accountable to policies and processes that have been vetted and implemented. This partnership meant that we were all in this together, a sentiment that led to improvement in the operation of the ORs. The message that all participants were respected members of the same team translated into vastly improved morale.

In addition to the POD policy we made a decision as a group to no longer implement new policies without physician/stakeholder input. This meant that surgeons would have their perspectives taken into consideration and that implementation would not be the first time that the physicians would hear of the new policy. This further meant that nurses no longer had to play the role of go-between, translating policy into action. This improved morale tremendously among the nursing staff and gave the physician a sense that they had a voice in the change process. Having a fair process was an important step to implement hard changes.

We took special effort to establish a shared understanding of the primary goal, improving care for our surgery patients. That message made all of the difference and helped push all stakeholders to put in the work needed to establish consensus despite our differences in opinions regarding the process. This central mission helped us to win over late adopters and successfully incorporate the new position of POD.

Conclusion

Culture is the soul of an organization. It is the background upon which everything happens. Unfortunately for many organizations, the culture develops organically as a result of misunderstood intentions and assumptions that are not tested. The result is lack of cohesiveness and dysfunction. This case study shows that culture change is possible when all stakeholders are included in decision making and goal setting. One can define a high functioning culture in many ways, but we learned that central themes must include shared knowledge, shared goals, mutual respect, fair process, and effective communication.

References

1. Gittell JH, Fairfield KM, Bierbaum B, Head W, Jackson R, Kelly M, et al. Impact of relational coordination on quality of care, postoperative pain and functioning, and length of stay: a nine-hospital study of surgical patients. Med Care. 2000;38(8):807–19.
2. Gittell JH, Weinberg DB, Bennett AL, Miller JA. Is the doctor in? A relational approach to job design and the coordination of work. Human Resource Manag. 2008;47(4):729–55.
3. Farrell JB. The impact of high quality relationships on proactive behaviour at work: evidence from independently owned hospitals in Ireland [internet] [doctoral]. Dublin City University; 2012 [cited 2020 Jun 5]. Available from: http://doras.dcu.ie/17508/
4. Havens DS, Vasey J, Gittell JH, Lin W-T. Relational coordination among nurses and other providers: impact on the quality of patient care. J Nurs Manag. 2010;18(8):926–37.
5. Newell CL. The relationship between relational coordination, shared mental model, and surgery team effectiveness in preventing wrong site-surgery [Internet] [Ph.D.]. [United States–Minnesota]: Walden University; 2009 [cited 2020 Jun 5]. Available from: https://search.proquest.com/docview/305080399/abstract/D8D772008DE245B2PQ/1
6. Bae S-H, Mark B, Fried B. Impact of nursing unit turnover on patient outcomes in hospitals. J Nurs Scholarsh. 2010 Mar;42(1):40–9.
7. Romanow D, Rai A, Keil M. Cpoe-enabled coordination: appropriation for deep structure use and impacts on patient outcomes. MIS Q. 2018 Mar;42(1):189–A11.
8. Gittell JH. Coordinating mechanisms in care provider groups: relational coordination as a mediator and input uncertainty as a moderator of performance effects. Manag Sci. 2002 Nov;48(11):1408–26.
9. Womack JP, Shook J. Gemba walks. Version 1.0. Cambridge, MA: Lean Enterprise Institute; 2011. p. 348.

Fast Track Approach Following Heart Surgery in Infancy and Early Childhood: Implementation Strategy with Outcome and Cost Analysis

6

Anastasios C. Polimenakos

Key Learning Points
- Research on the outcomes for early extubation in postoperative management in infants and young children/toddlers who have congenital heart surgery vary depending on institutions and philosophy toward ICU management.
- Early extubation in pediatric heart surgery can improve the length of ICU stay and reduce postoperative morbidity.
- The patients in the EE cohort were less likely to develop postoperative complications and had lower complication rates.
- Higher complication/procedure ratio and need for reoperation during the same hospitalization were major determinants for reintubation and failing fast track strategy.
- Early extubation post-operative care strategies save in costs for both the hospital and the patient.
- Fast track strategy is justified during infancy and early childhood following heart surgery but requires team approach and buy-in by all involved caregivers/stakeholders.

Executive Summary

Institutions have varying philosophies toward ICU management, which ultimately impacts the use of early extubation and fast track strategies in infants and young children/toddlers after congenital heart surgery (CHS) and patients with single ventricle. This inconsistency results in scattered series having various outcomes. The purpose of this study was to better describe fast track strategies and associated

A. C. Polimenakos (✉)
Pediatric Cardiothoracic Surgery, Medical College of Georgia, Children's Hospital of Georgia, Augusta, GA, USA
e-mail: apolimenakos@augusta.edu

outcomes in our institution when applied to infants and young children after CHS. The preoperative data and intraoperative factors affecting early extubation in the operating room prior to arrival in the ICU and fasttrack strategies after arrival in the ICU were reviewed. Main goals of the study were not only related to the clinical applicability of such fast track protocol, but also to evaluate the elements of team building and refinements of strategies in order to better serve our patient population and based on individual risk factors to reduce potential morbidity and mortality. Furthermore, through cost analysis and system-based evaluation we intended to help our institution's strategic goal for quality improvement with emphasis on cost-reduction and customized care effectiveness to promote value care.

We performed a retrospective review of prospectively collected data of all patients under 6 years of age with CHD who underwent surgical repair, at Children's Hospital of Georgia. From July 2017 to June 2018 112 consecutive patients who underwent CHS were identified. Patients with Society of Thoracic Surgeons (STS) and European Association of Cardiothoracic Surgery (EACTS) classification for Congenital Heart Surgery Complexity Categories (STAT) 1–5 were followed from the index cardiac operation until hospital discharge and included in the study. Patient groups were evaluated based on: Fast track/EE approach [group A] versus the one that did not [group B].

Through this project we proved feasibility and capacity in the care of a very demanding subset of patients. Key findings highlighted were: (1) Selective deployment of fast track strategy is justified during infancy and early childhood following heart surgery but requires team approach and buy-in by all involved caregivers/stakeholders; (2) Patient specific and modifiable parameters can guide judicious use of fast track protocols; and (3) Proper customization and implementation can have a powerful impact on Institutional strategic goals for quality improvement with emphasis on cost-containment and care value of best practice. This study can be the trigger for future intra-institutional initiatives regarding (1) Synergies/campaign in pursuit of strategic advantage advocacy; (2) Organizational alignment and integration of care protocols with profound impact on quality of care and cost-containment; (3) Initiatives for care path alignment with performance improvement processes (trans-discipline workforce for implementation of metrics and benchmarking expectations); (4) Accountability care intradepartmental initiatives that involve service-specific and provider-specific targets.

Brief Narrative of Key Values to Lead Change

Key values to assess the existing environment prior to engaging into this project, embrace and engage stakeholders, identify key participants, define expectations, build the momentum within the team, create accountability and establish feedback report to navigate through the steps necessary to complete the project:

- Fair processing encouraged all parties' participation and interconnectivity
- Delegation, Feedback and Accountability Without exercising Authority

- Collective intelligence was valued from the initial steps between stakeholders and team project's participants
- Leading by example; going into GEMBA (ICU, OR, Perioperative care)
- Communication: Influence and Persuasion to commit and the importance of the project not only for the Congenital Heart Surgery program, but also, its impact on organizational goals towards cost-containment and care value (quality/cost)
- Core team interconnectivity and integration of goals based on timetable and open communication to solve issues de-novo and proceed to alternate plan or facilitate given plan
- Conflict resolution and difficult conversations core team sessions during the project's evolution targeting clarity of goals and buy-in
- Assessment of the Seven S's to support/constrain capabilities "AS IS" (strategy, structure, skills, systems, staffing, shared values, style)

Introduction

Early extubation in pediatric heart surgery has become an invaluable tool in the postoperative management of children with congenital heart disease (CHD) for improving length of ICU stay and reducing postoperative morbidity [1, 2]. Despite established efficacy in postoperative management in older children and adolescents, early extubation and fast track strategies in infants and young children/toddlers after congenital heart surgery (CHS) and patients with single ventricle varies between different institutions based on philosophy towards ICU management [3, 4]. Therefore, scattered series have reported various outcomes [5, 6].

In this chapter, I will discuss the research my team and I collected on fast track strategies following heart surgery and the associated outcomes in our institution when applied to infants and young children/toddlers. The goal of this study was to review the results of all patients with CHD during infancy and early childhood, as well as, those with single ventricle through staged palliation and assess our strategy for fast track following heart surgery. In addition to analyzing the outcomes associated with fast track strategies after heart surgery, my second goal in this study was to evaluate the elements of team building and refinements of strategies in order to better serve our patient population. Instrumental concepts to lead change, such as (a) fair processing in encouraging all parties' participation and interconnectivity, (b) collective intelligence between stakeholders and team project's participants, (c) communication and persuasion for stakeholders to commit in integration of goals, (d) conflict resolution and targeting clarity of goals and buy-in through difficult conversations of core team, were pursued. Furthermore, through cost analysis and system-based evaluation we intended to help our institution's strategic goal for quality improvement with emphasis on cost-reduction and customized care effectiveness to promote value care. The following section discusses the methodology of the study, followed by the results and lessons learned from the research.

Methodology

We reviewed the pre-operative data and intraoperative factors affecting early extubation in the operating room prior to arrival in ICU and fast track strategies after arrival in the PICU. Our sample included prospectively collected data of all patients under 6 years of age with CHD who underwent surgical repair at Children's Hospital of Georgia. The study was approved by the Institutional Review Board and the need for parental consent was waived.

From July 2017 to June 2018, 112 consecutive patients who underwent CHS were identified. Patients with STS/EACTS STAT classification 1–5 were followed from the index cardiac operation until hospital discharge and included in the study. Patients with tracheostomy needing mechanical ventilation (MV) prior to CHS, pre-operative extracorporeal membrane oxygenation (ECMO) support, non-index STAT case as lone procedure were excluded. Patient groups were evaluated based on: Fast track/EE approach [group A] vs the one that did not [group B].

Fast track strategy was consisted of the following expected required steps:

1. Maximization of cardiopulmonary bypass (CPB) circuit volume reduction (as per protocol)
2. Implementation of blood conservation strategy (as per protocol)
3. Caudal regional anesthesia
4. A-adrenergic agonist receptor management administration when appropriate immediately after weaning off CPB
5. Maintaining bilateral lung parenchyma recruitment with low set of continuous positive airway pressure (CPAP) an inhaled nitric oxide throughout the case
6. Immediate early or secondary early extubation* to a non-invasive airway support without need for reintubation within 48 h from index extubation
7. Aggressive pulmonary toilet strategy in the ICU (as per protocol after extubation)
8. Early mobilization within 12–24 h following arrival in the ICU
9. Removal of Foley (indwelling ureteral) catheter within 24 h from ICU arrival
10. De-escalation of invasive monitoring within 24 h from arrival in the ICU
11. De-lining from invasive monitoring with 72 h from arrival in the ICU
12. Removal of chest drain within 72 h from ICU arrival

*Immediate early extubation (EE) is defined as extubation in the operating room. Secondary EE is defined as extubation within 12 h from admission in the ICU. Delayed extubation is defined as any extubation after 12 h following admission in the ICU. Extubation failure is defined as the need for reintubation within 48 h from initial extubation.

Variables

This study used demographic and pre-operative measures such as age, gender, prematurity, chromosomal anomalies, cardiopulmonary bypass time (CPB), single vs two ventricle anatomy, complication/procedure ratio with reference to EE and ICU length of stay. Pre-operative anatomic and demographic parameters were evaluated, including fetal diagnosis and congenital heart defect diagnosis with stratification for complexity assessment (STS/EACTS STAT classification). From health and operative medical records collection of data included the type of surgical intervention, CPB and cross-clamp times and the timing of postoperative extubation. Postoperative data included early and late post-operative morbidities, total mechanical ventilation (MV) time, need for non-invasive ventilation, ICU length of stay, the need for re-intubation, inotrope support and vasoactive inotropic score (VIS) [7], incidence of renal or hepatic failure, healthcare-associated infections, arrhythmias, neurodevelopmental morbidity and overall mortality.

Statistical Analysis

Initial analyses included frequency distributions and patterns in the data and are presented as frequency, median with range, or mean ± SD as appropriate, with the number of non-missing values indicated. Group comparison (between patients with early extubation versus those without) was performed with ANOVA or Student t-test for continuous variables and χ^2 for categorical data, as appropriate.

Predictors of extubation failure or failure to complete fast track approach at any step of its deployment is identified using multivariable logistic regression analysis. Cox regression is used to determine the independent predictors of early outcomes. Adjusted odds ratios with 95% confidence intervals were estimated for independent variables. The appropriateness of variable transformations will be determined by means of univariate analysis. Variables with a univariate p-value of less than 0.05 or those with known biologic significance but failing to meet this critical χ^2 level will be submitted to multivariable models. Statistical analysis will be performed using p value less than 0.05 as statistically significant.

Lastly, cost analysis between the 2 groups was pursued. We determined the average cost per day in the ICU. Other medical costs included diagnostic imaging (X-ray, CT scan, ultrasound, MRI), special procedures (i.e., cardiac catheterization, etc.), medications, and allied health care (clinical nutrition, physiotherapy, occupational therapy, social work, and child life). Cost Analysis included hospital costs from the index procedure to hospital discharge. Primary cost analysis included (1) total hospitalization cost, (2) direct, and (3) indirect (e.g. overhead) costs. Total costs were calculated from Children's Hospital cost accounting reports using the detail balance of gross patient revenue and expenses. Part of the total cost included devices and associated disposables, equipment and room allocated times, and time-driven activity-based cost (ABC) [8]. As a result, the final formula used for cost analysis is the following:

$$\text{mean total direct cost} = \text{mean LOS in ICU} \times \text{mean daily cost in ICU} + \text{mean daily cost of}\left(\text{imaging} + \text{allied health care} + \text{pharmacy} + \text{blood bank / lab}\right) \times \text{mean LOS} + \text{mean non} - \text{ICU cost} + \text{time} - \text{driven ABC}$$

Direct costs were allocated by the expense of each cost center. Indirect costs were calculated on the cost center's building square footage, equipment depreciation, and number of annual nursing hours. The summation of direct and indirect constituted total cost. Costs were allocated inside each cost center to the charge code level for both hospital and professional fees. Professional and hospital fee schedules were updated annually using the Center for Medicare/Medicaid Services, and the institutional-based cost studies, respectively. ABC methodology addressed the inherent variability associated with cost to charge ratios by using a bottom-up costing methodology mapped directly to the actual patient-specific episode of care. The cost centers, analyzed in our study, included pharmacy, radiology, echocardiography, cardiac catheterization laboratory, intensive care unit, operating room, laboratory and blood bank. The cost data excluded the preoperative workup in both the groups.

Project's Organizational Format/Participants

One goal in this study was to evaluate the elements of team building and refinements of strategies in order to better serve our patient population. The participants in this study included: (1) Team's Participants: Pediatric heart surgery, anesthesia, ICU team, medical school scholars (3rd year medical students assigned, funding); (2) Leadership and/or sponsorship buy-in into your project: Chairman of Surgery, CMO, ICU Director, Chairman of Anesthesia; (3) All stakeholders and team members buy-in was exercised; (4) Collection of relevant data / Children's Hospital of Georgia Clinical Research Ethics Board approved the study and resources were allocated; (5) To address potential obstacles we conducted team meetings biweekly and checked in on the data collection process on a weekly basis in order to meet time targets. The key tasks related to the designed framework are depicted in Fig. 6.1.

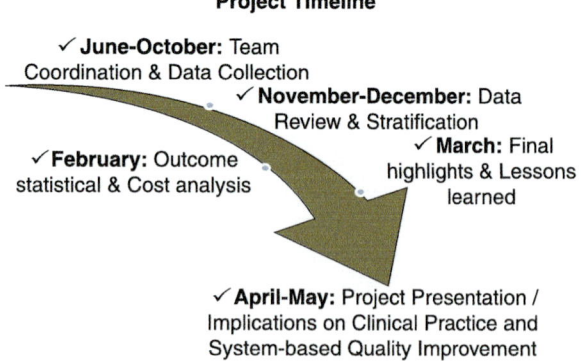

Fig. 6.1 Project Timeline—Key tasks related to the designed framework

Results

Demographics

Our cohort consisted of 112 patients (55% male). Sixteen percent were neonates (age < 30 days old), 47% infants (older than 1 month old) and 37% >12 months old, at the time of CHS. Of the 112 patients, 15 (14%) had chromosomal abnormalities, including trisomy 21. Six neonates (5%) were born prematurely (gestational age < 36 weeks).

Procedural Details

The median patient age at surgery was 9.1 months (IQR, 0.9–47.4). The complexity of each case was assessed using STS/EACTS STAT classification: 17% were assigned to risk category 1; 38% to risk category 2; 32% to risk category 3; 9% to risk category 4; and 4% to risk category 5.

The median CPB and cross-clamp time was 77 min (IQR,47–123) and 43 min (IQR, 21–76), respectively. The CPB (median, 130 vs 64 min; $P < 0.001$) and cross-clamp (median, 77.5 vs 33 min; $P < 0.001$) times were considerably longer for the neonates compared with all other patients.

Complications/Survival

The overall complication rate in our cohort was 4.1 complications per 10 procedures, with 27% of all procedures associated with 1 complication. The patients in the EE cohort were less likely to develop postoperative complications (20% vs 85%; $P < 0.001$) and had lower complication rates (3 vs 22 complications per 10 procedures; $P < 0.001$). Higher complication/procedure ratio and need for reoperation during the same hospitalization were major determinants for reintubation and failing fast track strategy ($p < 0.05$) (Table 6.1). Overall mortality was 1.3% (with lower unadjusted mortality for Group-A; 0.8% vs 6%, $P < 0.05$).

Table 6.1 Determinants of EE failure following Congenital Heart Surgery

Variables	Odds Ratio (95% Confidence interval) Group A (N = 81) Group B (N = 31)	P
Age	1.11 (0.98–1.38)	0.07
(neonates vs infants vs > 1 yr. old*)	1.59 (1.41–1.88)	0.02
Stat (I-III VS IV-V)	0.80 (0.71–.0.89)	0.001
Single Ventricle vs Two-Ventricle Anatomy	1.99 (1.79–2.12)	0.04
Prematurity	2.32 (1.97–2.54)	0.05
Chromosomal Abnormalities/Syndromes	1.76 (1.61–2.01)	0.03
CPB Time	0.81 (0.76–0.91)	0.04
Need for Reoperation/Complication During Same Hospitalization	2.05 (1.89–2.45)	0.03

Early Versus Late Extubation/Determinants of Failure

Fast track/EE was achieved in 81 (72%) patients; of which more than 60% were extubated in the operating room. In patients younger than 1-year old, neonates were less likely to follow the EE path (EE was achieved in 21% of neonates; $P < 0.05$) (Fig. 6.2). Prematurity in neonates had a prohibitive effect on fast-track strategy ($P < 0.001$) (Fig. 6.3). Chromosomal anomalies/syndromes were associated with

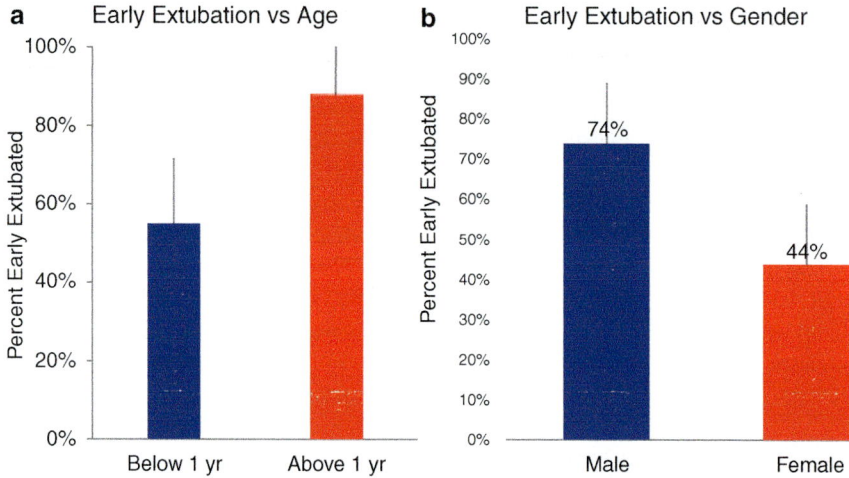

Fig. 6.2 Demographics and Patient-specific Variables for fast track / EE. [**a.** Early extubation vs Age (<1 year old vs >1 year at the time of surgery); **b.** Early extubation vs Gender]

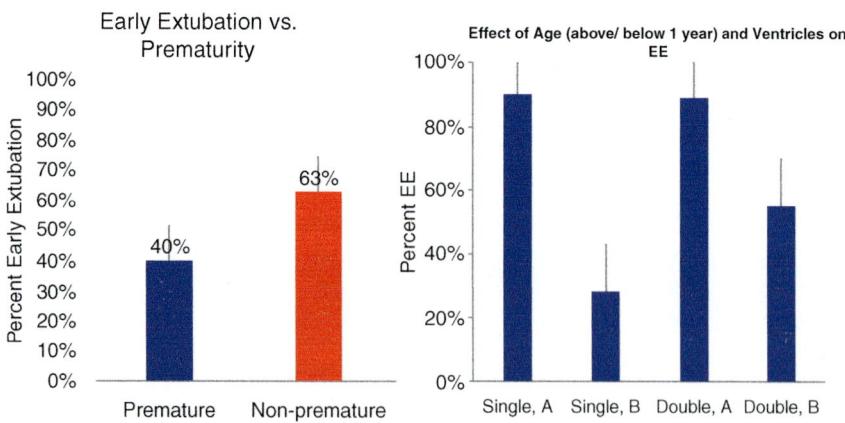

Fig. 6.3 Demographics and Patient-specific Variables for fast track / EE. [Left: Early extubation vs Prematurity; Right: Early extubation vs Age referenced to ventricular anatomy: Single Ventricle (single)—Two ventricle (double)]

early EE failure (P < 0.05). Higher STAT complexity (4 and 5) were associated with unfavorable outcome towards fast track (P < 0.05). Vasoactive-Inotropic score was not statistically different between groups (P > 0.05). The overall reintubation rate was 7%; 92% required reintubation within 24 h and 8% after 24 h. ICU length of stay was directly correlated with EE/Fast track and was longer for single ventricle patients regardless of EE (P < 0.05) (Fig. 6.4). The predictors of EE failure determined by the multivariable logistic regression model are listed in Table 6.1. Significant determinants (modifiable and non-modifiable) of outcome have an independent and cumulative effect on EE failure and the fate of fast track strategy.

Cost Analysis

Daily ICU cost was approximately 4.0-fold greater than daily non-ICU cost ($30,274.77+/−4505.42 vs $110,888.74+/−9857.97; p = 0.005). Average additional direct daily hospital costs, independent of ICU cost reached statistical significance between groups (P < 0.05). Total direct hospital cost in EE-Fast track group remained substantially lower ($50,139.07+/−7714.72 vs 188,061.39+/−19,418.63; p = 0.001) (Fig. 6.5a, b). The breakdown of mean post-operative hospital costs was 68% for the ICU stay (including time-driven ABC), 19% for the non-ICU stay (including time-driven ABC), 6% for imaging, 3% for pharmacy, 2% for allied health, and 2% for blood bank/lab (Fig. 6.6). There was a near three-fold increase in cost for patients failing EE/fast track irrespective of case complexity (Fig. 6.7).

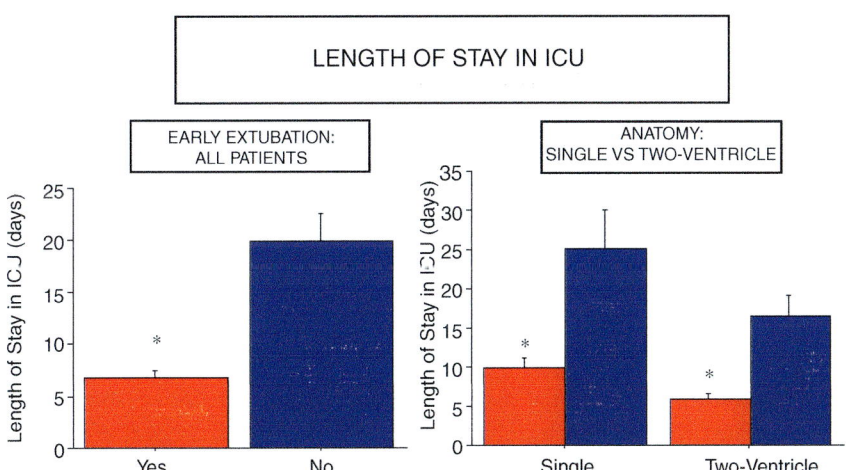

Fig. 6.4 Fast Track /EE and ICU length of stay. [Left: All patients; Right: Referenced to single- vs two- ventricle anatomy Red indicates YES for early extubation; Blue indicates NO for early extubation]

a

Direct Cost ($) mean(SD)	EE-FAST TRACK (N=81)	NON-EE (N=31)	P
ICU	30,274.77±4,505.42	110,888.74±9857.97	0.005
ICU time-driven ABC	3,819.75±983.19	12,352.26±1,353.99	0.02
Ward/Floor (non-ICU)	8,466.73±1077.73	31,551.78±4,492.27	0.003
Non-ICU time-driven ABC	1,059.68±412.53	2,997.52±662.86	0.05
Imaging	3,008.34±707.23	10,874.23±1,102.34	0.004
Pharmacy	1,504.17±466.71	5,437.11±995.42	0.01
Blood bank/Laboratory	1,012.78±382.34	3,601.64±801.31	0.02
Allied Health	992.73±343.42	3,647.83±797.19	0.01

b

Cost ($) mean(SD)	EE-FAST TRACK (N=81)	NON-EE (N=31)	P
Total Hospital	54,200.32± 7,714.72	188,061.39±19,418.63	0.001
-Total Direct	50,139.07±6,804.85	181,237.03±18,331.34	0.005
-Total Indirect	4,061.25±909.87	6,824.36±1,087.29	0.07

Fig. 6.5 Cost Analysis between groups. Sub-analysis of cost (**a**) Direct by segment; (**b**) Total Cumulative

We demonstrated substantial cost savings with relatively narrow credible intervals associated with an early extubation post-operative care strategy that persisted with broad variation of input data. Therefore, there was a consistent relative reduction of costs throughout all cost estimates. The percent cost reduction is perhaps more meaningful than the absolute dollar value for generalizing cost reductions relative to other institutions given the considerable inter-hospital cost variation demonstrated in the literature.

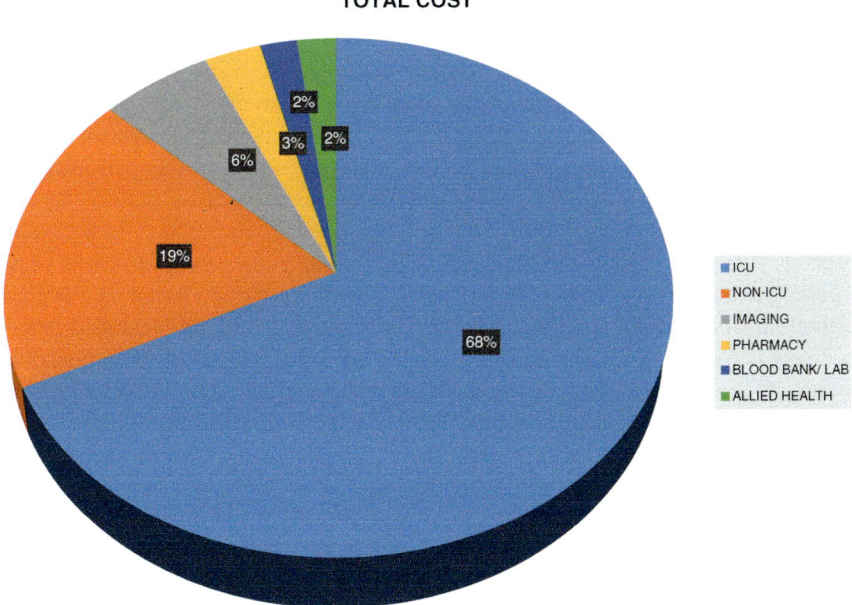

Fig. 6.6 Percentage of cost distribution

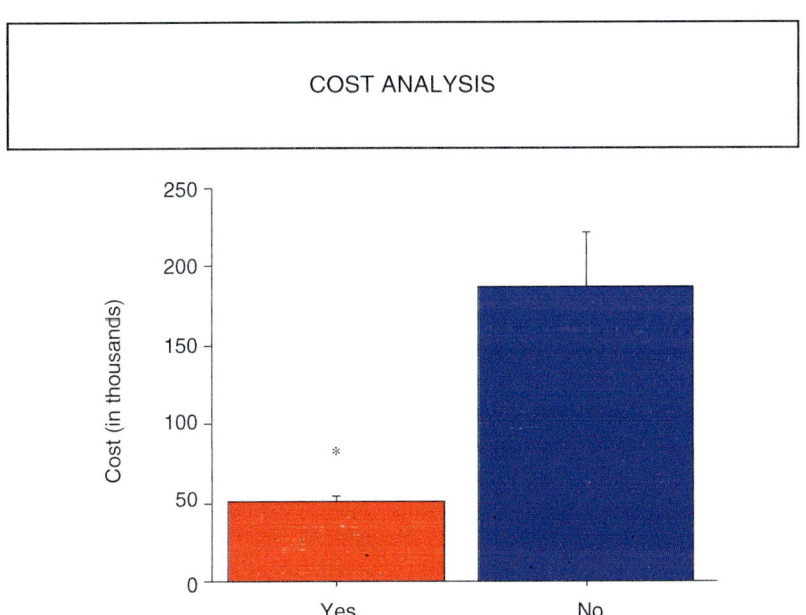

Fig. 6.7 Cost Analysis between groups [*Indicates total direct cost*]. Fast track (YES) vs Non-Fast track (NO)

Limitations

Our study was limited by the retrospective nature of the analysis, although data were prospectively collected. Given that there was a programmatic implementation of early extubation at our institution, we did not have a contemporary control cohort. Nonetheless, comparing our present results with the adoption of this perioperative management strategy with contemporary published benchmarks, it is clear that the outcomes, complication rates, and resource usage compare favorably. Given the differences in case distribution among centers, the results of the present study serve as a demonstration of the feasibility of this approach in the environment fostered within our organization. The lack of a suitable control group has precluded determining whether a causal relationship exists between EE and improved clinical outcomes. Race and ethnicity were not included in the analysis as social determinants of health. Hence, the generalizability of such approach is institution dependent, because it requires broad-based support from cardiac surgery, cardiology, anesthesia, and ICU to be successfully implemented.

Discussion

Implications/Impact on Organization or Clinical Practice

It was demonstrated that selective deployment of fast track strategy is justified during infancy and early childhood following heart surgery but requires team approach and buy-in by all involved caregivers/stakeholders. Patient specific and modifiable parameters can guide judicious use of fast track protocols. Proper customization and implementation can have powerful impact on Institutional strategic goal for quality improvement with emphasis to cost-containment and care value. Fast Track and EE has been shown to be an effective management strategy for improving resource utilization by shortening ICU length of stay [9]. Correspondingly, characterization of the economic impact of implementing an EE/fast track strategy becomes an important indicator of program success in the healthcare setting. Therefore, complex congenital heart surgical care, which has been shown to have the highest healthcare resource utilization in pediatric cardiac surgery may benefit most from implementing an EE/fast track post-operative strategy on a per patient basis. However, since lower complexity congenital heart surgery is more common, and shown to have highest inter-institutional variation, this cohort may generate increased cost savings for an institution dependent on the surgical patient demographics. Improving cost efficiency within a resource limited setting is particularly attractive for health budget allocation. The EE/fast track strategy following CHS offers an opportunity to reduce hospital costs without compromising post-surgical outcomes. Given the marked difference in costs associated with ICU care compared to general floor care, future identification of factors associated with reduced ICU stays may further improve resource utilization in this patient population. We have demonstrated a high rate of EE in many infants undergoing higher risk procedures. One of the key strengths of the present study was that we included all patients in our analysis unless excluded as indicated above based on set criteria. Given the morbidity and known risks associated with intubation and mechanical ventilation, our institution has developed an approach such that EE is the norm, and patients only remain intubated if a compelling cardiorespiratory benefit is present, regardless of age. Reducing the length of ICU stay leads to improved resource utilization. Hence, broad implementation of EE has the potential to reduce the total costs associated with pediatric cardiac surgery and reduce the interinstitutional variability.

The goal of our study was to determine the feasibility and assess the clinical effect of implementing a fast track/EE strategy for all children under 6 years old undergoing CHS, including neonates and infants, irrespective of the complexity of surgical intervention. Our findings further expand the global understanding of prolonged intubation or failing EE after CHS, including identifying potentially modifiable factors. Our data open several avenues for inquiry, including early identification and reintervention for major residual disease and avoidance of postoperative complications. Further research aimed at understanding other potentially modifiable factors affecting EE, including anesthetic strategy and fluid overload, require analysis of multi-institutional databases to determine all relevant covariates. A prospective, multicenter analysis is necessary to confirm these findings and determine the effects of these modifiable factors on fast track/EE strategy.

Based on our current knowledge, as surfaced by the study, we advocate a predetermined fast track/EE protocol to all infants and children under 6 years of age unless the following parameters are met:

Preoperative Parameters
– Extreme low weight (<2.5 kg) at operation
– Prematurity (<36 weeks birth age)
– Associated chromosomal abnormalities
– Requiring immediate MV support prior to index cardiac operation
– Requiring cardiopulmonary resuscitation (including extracorporeal membrane oxygenation support (ECMO) prior to index cardiac operation
– STAT category V complexity for congenital heart surgery

Intraoperative Parameters
– Immediate intraoperative extubation could not be pursue for clinical etiology or surgeon's preference
– New onset arrhythmia requiring MV continuation
– Echocardiography demonstrated residual lesion with hemodynamic significance
– Ongoing coagulopathy

Postoperative Parameters

- New onset arrhythmia requiring MV continuation
- Early assessment in the ICU based on clinical, laboratory and hemodynamic criteria preclude reliable execution of fast track approach
- Echocardiography demonstrated residual lesion with hemodynamic significance
- Ongoing coagulopathy

Proper customization of patients and implementation of such predetermined protocol is aligned with our Institutional strategic goal for quality improvement with emphasis to cost-containment and care value which will be, not only associated with CHS, but also across surgical services at the Children's Hospital of Georgia.

Assessment of Team Performance and Leadership: Lessons Learned

Key values were used to assess the existing environment prior to engaging into this project, embrace and engage stakeholders, identify key participants, define expectations, build the momentum within the team, create accountability and establish feedback report to navigate through the steps necessary to complete the project:

1. Fair processing encouraged all parties' participation and interconnectivity
2. Delegation, Feedback and Accountability Without exercising Authority
3. Collective intelligence was valued from the initial steps between stakeholders and team project's participants
4. Leading by example; going into GEMBA (ICU, OR, Perioperative care)
5. Communication: Influence and Persuasion to commit and the importance of the project not only for the Congenital Heart Surgery program, but also, its impact on organizational goals towards cost-containment and care value (quality/cost)
6. Core team interconnectivity and integration of goals based on timetable and open communication to solve issues de-novo and proceed to alternate plan or facilitate given plan
7. Conflict resolution and difficult conversations core team sessions during the project's evolution targeting clarity of goals and buy-in
8. Assessment of the Seven S's to support/constrain capabilities "AS IS" (strategy, structure, skills, systems, staffing, shared values, style) as shown in Fig. 6.8.

Seven S Factor	Support capabilities	Constrain capabilities
Strategy	Small group with clear values; serves the community and supports Institutional vision for cost containment and quality	Quality management guidelines across services and institution not well defined
Structure	Top-down leadership style; Organization with elite services towards catering patient's expectations	Limited resources to support expanding the concept protocol across all surgical services; need for integration in management expectations and system-based alignment
Skills	Few, but highly qualified providers and personnel in where matters the most	Quick employment turnaround time limits sustainability and commitment to shared goals
Systems	Small core groups is the platform for change	System-based disconnect and quality integration is the predicament
Staffing	Policy driven work standards; benefits and incentives based on RVU and impact within the organization	Cumbersome for staff of different service-lines to engage due to silos; staff retention strategies missing
Shared Values	Quality care close to home vision; Integrity; team-based approach in projects impacting care value and cost-containment	Loyalty of the staff; staff retention to provide continuity and positive feedback towards relational coordination
Style	Leadership driven by financial metrics; theme "quality with cost containment – customer/patient satisfaction geared management"	Not visible; not going to GEMBA; some disconnect with staff and divisions leaders

Fig. 6.8 Assessment of the Seven S's to support/constrain capabilities "AS IS" (strategy, structure, skills, systems, staffing, shared values, style)

Managing Change: Reflections

As the leading figure in the Taskforce for the Conceptualization and Implementation of changes I was able to influence and lead through the process. Being a full-time surgeon carried constraints in time availability, but also, provided opportunities to get involved. As Divisional leader, though, and being in the GEMBA allowed me for being influential within the framework of my care-path (transdisciplinary) and serving as an active advocate of accountability and quality expectations towards patient satisfaction and performance improvement initiatives. Thus, these targeted efforts were instrumental in promoting innovation in clinical and care delivery framework (such as in this project). Furthermore, "islands of excellence" linked to these initiatives in pursuing excellence and value of care. Finally, transdisciplinary initiatives were introduced towards transparency and BEST CARE Value accountable for improving quality/cost ratio (fast track and EE).

Conclusion

In summary, through this project we proved feasibility and capacity in the care of a very demanding subset of patients. Through this process, we highlighted that: (1) Selective deployment of fast track strategy is justified during infancy and early childhood following heart surgery but requires team approach and buy-in by all involved caregivers/stakeholders; (2) Patient specific and modifiable parameters can guide judicious use of fast track protocols; and (3) Proper customization and implementation can have a powerful impact on Institutional strategic goals for quality improvement with emphasis on cost-containment and care value of best practice. Looking into the future the foundation of this work can lead to the following venues:

A. At the Administrative Leadership domain:

It can be the vehicle for joining synergies/campaign for strategic advantage advocacy, fostering active leading role in organizational alignment and integration of care protocols with profound impact on quality of care and cost-containment, and participating in Accountability Care intradepartmental initiatives that involve service-specific and provider-specific targets.

B. At the Clinical Care Path Leadership level:

It can be a stepping stone for Initiatives for care path alignment with performance improvement processes (trans-discipline workforce for implementation of metrics and benchmarking expectations). Feedback looping of transparency with simple self-sustainable communication schemes and accountability reinforcement applications can be supported. Furthermore, it might assist with promoting talent and assign responsibilities towards innovation across service-lines and institution-wide.

Declaration of Conflicting Interests The author(s) declared no potential conflicts of interest with respect to the research, authorship, and/or publication of this article.

Funding The author(s) received no financial support for the research, authorship, and/or publication of this article.

Acknowledgements Many thanks to Raquel Esquivel and Emma Geister (Research scholars), Danielle Crethers (Research Coordinator), Departments of Surgery, Anesthesia and Critical Care, and the Chief's Medical officer collaborators for their contribution and participation.

References

1. Hamilton BCS, Honjo O, Alghamdi AA, Caldarone CA, Schwartz SM, Van Arsdell GS, Holtby H. Efficacy of evolving early-extubation strategy on early postoperative functional recovery in pediatric open-heart surgery: matched case-control study. Semn Cardiothorac Vasc Anesth. 18(3):290–6. https://doi.org/10.1177/1089253213519291.
2. Harris KC, Holowachuk S, Pitfield S, Sanatani S, Froese N, Potts JE, Gandhi SK. Should early extubation be the goal for children after congenital heart surgery? J Thorac Cardiovasc Surg. 2014 Dec;148(6):2642–7. https://doi.org/10.1016/j.jtcvs.2014.06.093.
3. Davis S, Worley S, Mee RBB, Harrison AM. Factors associated with early extubation after cardiac surgery in young children. Pediatr Crit Care Med. 5:83–8. https://doi.org/10.1097/01.PCC.0000102386.96434.46.
4. Polito A, Patorno E, Costello JM, Salvin JW, Emani SM, Rajagopal S, et al. Perioperative risk factors for prolonged mechanical ventilation after complex congenital heart surgery. Pediatr Crit Care Med. 2011 May;12(3):e122–6. https://doi.org/10.1097/PCC.0b013e3181e912bd.

5. Gaies M, Tabbutt S, Schwartz SM, Bird GL, Alten JA, Shekerdemian LS, et al. Clinical epidemiology of extubation failure in the pediatric cardiac ICU: a report from the pediatric cardiac critical care consortium. Pediatr Crit Care Med. 2015 Nov;16(9):837–45. https://doi.org/10.1097/PCC.0000000000000498.
6. Iodice FG, Thomas M, Walker I, Garside V, Elliott MJ. Analgesia in fast-track pediatric cardiac patients. Eur J Cardiothorac Surg. 2011 Sep;40(3):610–3. https://doi.org/10.1016/j.ejcts.2010.12.032.
7. Gaies MG, Gurney JG, Yen AH, Napoli ML, Gajarski RJ, Ohye RG. Vasoactive-inotropic score as a predictor of morbidity and mortality in infants after cardiopulmonary bypass. Pediatr Crit Care Med. 2010 Mar;11(2):234–8. https://doi.org/10.1097/PCC.0b013e3181b806fc.
8. Garrison RH, Noreen EW, Brewer PC. Activity-based costing. In: Managerial accounting. 15th ed. New York, NY: McGraw-Hill; 2015. p. 286–312.
9. Holowachuk S, Zhang W, Gandhi SK, Anis AH, Potts JE, Harris KC. Cost savings analysis of early extubation following congenital heart surgery. Pediatr Cardiol. 2019 Jan;40(1):138–46. https://doi.org/10.1007/s00246-018-1970-0.

7. Decreasing Variance in Care: Implementation of Protocolized Postoperative Feeding as a Proxy for Discharge

Anne C. Fischer

Key Learning Points
- Choose a project strategically to be something that is achievable. Aim for low-lying fruit.
- Your involvement and visibility to the front line is critical. Time spent on the floor to get to know front line workers is instrumental to a project's success. Be a visible hands-on leader, yet avoid micromanaging your team, so empower them to continually move the football down the field.
- Involve stakeholders in all points of decision making so all can participate either actively or passively: bumps in the road inevitably occur.
- Buy-in from leadership is mission critical; keeping them abreast of ongoing positive outcomes is essential for the change leader's success. Promoting your successes, even small wins, is key in managing up positive newsfeeds.
- Pick an inexpensive and noncontroversial project when new to an organization. You will be judged by that success. Failure in a more complex assignment will be viewed negatively and typically bring controversy.
- Professional titles infer accountability but do not guarantee the authority needed.
- Understand the political context of the organization and how tolerant it is to change.
- A project can be viewed as a proxy war for those with seniority in the institution to undermine the process and subsequently the change leader.

A. C. Fischer (✉)
Palm Beach Children's Hospital, West Palm Beach, FL, USA

Charles E. Schmidt College of Medicine, Florida Atlantic University, Boca Raton, FL, USA

- Leadership is about managing people and problems. Managing disputes requires social capital which is limited for a new recruit to an institution.
- The perception of change is negatively inferenced and galvanizes old informal social networks to align against new leadership. The longevity of a CEO in healthcare has shortened to a 3–5 year cycle. This can dramatically disrupt initiative in clinical programs and strategy needing that timeframe at the minimum to take hold: clinical programs need a longer trajectory for longevity and success.

Historically the Chairs, were visionary leaders in medicine with great clinical experience and authority. They had great power over finances, personnel and clinical programmatic development. However, the move to corporate medicine has transitioned chairmen, from the height of clinical leadership, to being middle management in hospital organizational charts. Changes of senior management in the C suite can silence and negatively impact a Chair's capacity for clinical initiatives. The visionary leaders of the past who created entire new fields of clinical care are rarely championed. Instead that type of personae are often being driven out in the newer corporate environment in the clash between excellence of clinical care, strategic clinical development, and fiduciary limitations.

Executive Summary

This chapter studies change management strategies during a time of organizational flux. The team piloted a new policy of standardizing postoperative feeding for pediatric surgical patients in a newly affiliated academic hospital that was in the process of undergoing a merger and management change. Change was ongoing on all levels: system merger, affiliation with a newly minted medical school, and new leadership in many departments, including the division of pediatric surgery. Despite the success of the study and achieving its desired endpoints, the project was unable to reach its full potential since the change leader was not provided with sufficient authority to fully enact the principles. The leader had the titular recognition of authority without the infrastructure and support of the senior leadership needed for sustainability. This paper adds to medical management literature by (1) discussing strategic selection of a change management project and the consequences of so doing, (2) how to identify an environment where change is tolerated and can succeed, and (3) pitfalls and best practices for structuring management to operationalize continuous improvement.

Introduction

A Historical Basis for Stakeholder Perspectives

Opened on Jan. 24, 1955 as a 238-bed community hospital, Beaumont, Royal Oak evolved to become a 1100-bed major academic and referral center with Level I adult and Level II pediatric trauma status. The hospitals and eventual school of medicine were all named for William Beaumont, a U.S. Army surgeon who became known as the "Father of Gastric Physiology" following his research on human digestion started at Fort Mackinac on Mackinac Island, Michigan.

As the flagship hospital, the Royal Oak campus had 55 residency and fellowship programs, something that distinguished it as more 'academic' than its twin campus in Troy, Michigan located 11 miles away. This 2-hospital system thrived by serving a very well insured patient population from the upscale wealthy Oakland County, Michigan. Analysis of CMS data identified Beaumont, Royal Oak as one of the top-grossing hospitals in the country in 2013, with $3.31 billion in in-patient revenues and tremendous profit margins. By 2014 the hospital system became a not-for-profit organization despite having longstanding decades of positive revenue streams, something that reflected its perceived need to actively court the tremendous philanthropic opportunities present in Oakland County. Beaumont's biggest competitors are the University of Michigan and the Henry Ford System associated with Wayne State Medical School, both about an hour drive away. In contrast neither Beaumont campus was affiliated with any medical school. Royal Oak strove to be perceived as "academic" in order to optimize market referrals and public perception. They did this by affiliating with their newly created Oakland University William Beaumont School of Medicine to become the school's only teaching hospital. By 2015 the first medical school class graduated from Oakland University William Beaumont School of Medicine.

Beaumont's two-campus hospital system, Royal Oak and Troy, had attending physicians who were either in private practice or were hospital employed. Historically the staffs originated from private practices growing centrically around either campus. Neither hospital was truly academic in the traditional sense but did have longstanding residency programs. In practice this meant that there was no longstanding academic culture or hierarchy to lean on as an organizational flow chart. Informal networks of old associations and referral patterns were palpable. The Dean, at a site far from the hospital, was not involved in shaping the tone and culture of the institution and was strictly focused on the education of medical students. Since all physicians were employed by the hospital system and not the University, this further reduced the Dean's influence on "faculty" and programs. Further confounding academic pursuits at the hospital campuses was the fact that there was a constant C suite awareness of market penetration into the geographic areas of the wealthy Oakland County by their competitors in the vicinity, including Henry Ford Systems, Detroit Children's, and University of Michigan.

Beaumont health system, like other hospitals in the area, faced a landscape of extraordinary financial and regulatory pressures at the federal and state level. Mergers between regional and national heavyweights were understood at the time to be the way to adjust to the intense need for cost containment and offset infrastructure costs. This strategy might have been far-fetched in the prior decade, but serial partnerships were being actively courted by Beaumont. One anticipated merger between two giants, Beaumont Health System and Henry Ford Health System, based in Detroit, failed in 2013. Henry Ford's board ended talks when Beaumont's physician leadership rejected Henry Ford's proposed terms to have all physicians be employed by the single hospital system as opposed to their private practices. Ultimately the two institutions recognized they had completely different institutional cultures—one based in private practice groups and one with a single employer.

The hospital was in a period of extreme flux. Physician leadership was culled during this period of anticipated mergers, and practically all the Chairs were removed/exited in a clean sweep of clinical leadership. The leadership change, quietly orchestrated, was so opaque that the Chairs just returned to their private practice across town as if nothing happened upon losing their chair leadership position.

By 2014 federal antitrust and tax-exempt status was approved to move forward with the creation of Beaumont Health as a non-profit to cultivate philanthropy more successfully. Beaumont Health System joined with local community hospitals, Botsford Health Care, and Oakwood Healthcare, to become the largest medical system in Southeast Michigan. The merger was promoted as benefiting residents of SE Michigan by providing greater access to care. There were widely anticipated objections to this merger given that at $3.8 billion, this would be the largest hospital system merger in Michigan. However, the Attorney General made no objections and the establishment of the 8-hospital system from the prior 2 hospital system was approved in 2016. Beaumont Health now would control roughly 30 percent of the inpatient market with 3337 beds, 153 outpatient sites, 5000 physicians and 33,093 employees. The anticipated rapid growth of merging 8 hospitals from 2 hospitals into one dominant health care system caused tremendous anxiety in specialty services operationalized to support these hospitals.

A Service Line for Pediatric Surgery

Beaumont Children's Hospital (BCH), located on one floor at Royal Oak, is contained within the adult hospital, with 40 pediatric floor beds, 8 PICU beds, and around 50 NICU beds. Its strategy was to build health services for infants, children and adolescents in nearly every medical and surgical subspecialty with 80 pediatric subspecialists either working in private practice, or for an employed physician model. This expansion of specialty care would allow BCH to compete with the draw of the much larger Detroit Children's comprehensive specialty care. Detroit Children's was actively constructing a comprehensive surgery center on the main artery between the two Beaumont campuses.

The focus on hiring a Surgeon-In-Chief was to bring the Beaumont Children's Hospital to the next level in Children's hospitals and establish programmatic growth and an academic presence. A not-so-minor detail was that Beaumont did not have an existing Surgeon-In-Chief, so there was no template for the relationship that this role had with other departmental chairs and hospital senior leadership. Hired by the Chair of Surgery, this role was then to collaborate with the Chair of Pediatrics who in fact wanted to hire his former associates from another hospital to control the Children's Hospital Surgeon in Chief position.

Recent changes on all levels of institutional leadership were not obvious to any outsider. This milieu of tremendous institutional change was especially precarious for any recruitment, with the on-again and off-again courting of mergers, loss of market share due to competitor penetration, financial pressures, and the clean sweep of departmental chairs being changed out all at once. In this time frame, the institution was contemplating its mission and value to the surrounding public. Its highly successful marketing campaign "Do you have a Beaumont Doctor?" reflected exclusivity for the wealthy in Southeast Michigan. The stated goals for the pediatric surgical service line were to develop and recruit enough pediatric surgical attendings for 24/7 coverage, as well as have sufficient staff for programmatic advancement and to undertake quality initiatives to align with national initiatives meant to designate and 'top tier' children's hospitals.

The availability of a sufficient number of pediatric surgeons is expensive due to a very limited resource pool. When considering the large catchment area, it was going to be quite challenging to ensure access to care and adequacy of coverage. Overcoming the underlying supply-demand mismatch of pediatric surgeons to patients was critical to the bottom line of the children's hospital. Its ability to care for critically ill patients and retain high reimbursement procedures all depended on recruiting and retaining pediatric surgeons. The program's success would insure stabilization of Beaumont Children's Hospital. This would prevent loss of its clinical volume that was previously being sent to nearby independent children's hospitals and help retain the NICU level III status critical for reimbursement levels.

Given the tremendous regional need of pediatric surgical expertise, the new Surgeon in Chief was able to establish an alliance of care delivery at a third nearby hospital which was desperate for pediatric surgical coverage to retain cases locoregionally. They had been in long standing coverage agreements with free-standing children's hospitals that ultimately led to diminution of case volumes by siphoning all pediatric patients and sending them to the freestanding children's hospitals. This led empty pediatric floors in the community hospitals. The transporting out of all pediatric cases led this economically struggling community to be underserved, and the pediatric residency program to be at risk at the hospital. By stepping up to create a geopolitical alliance between two competitive adult hospital systems, the Surgeon in Chief strategically stabilized local regional pediatric surgical care to maintain volumes critical for pediatric specialists. The Surgeon-in-Chief used her much-needed expertise and availability to allow for geographic stabilization for pediatric specialists overlooking any ongoing political infighting along adult service lines between the two hospital systems.

Building a contractual relationship with this adult hospital allowed for the generation of increased surgical case numbers, referrals, and positive revenue stream for coverage to Beaumont's pediatric surgery service line. In any other situation these two hospitals could have competed on a pediatric level as they did on the adult side. Many of the patients were uninsured or Medicaid recipients and the hospitals serving these communities wanted to retain those patients. Beaumont was not anxious to attract poorly insured patients, so this coverage model benefitted both hospitals and communities and still exists today.

Given its history of highly insured patient population, Beaumont still functioned intrinsically as a for-profit entity despite having a not-for-profit designation. A limited coverage model was set up to allow for increased coverage as needed by clinical demand for the participating hospital's staff, ED, and pediatrics programs. The Surgeon-in-Chief forged these partnerships with a trauma activation-like contract for pediatric surgical services. The success of this alliance further proved the feasibility of a multi-site coverage model with the capacity of the current faculty. The Beaumont hospital in Troy likewise had to commit the needed resources for pediatric surgery for the program to be successful there as well. Developing a pediatric surgical program clinically active on two campuses had not been achieved by any other service line in the area: in contrast Beaumont pediatric surgery was functioning at three sites. The expectation was to continue to operationalize this endeavor since it created a positive financial stream and allowed expanded community coverage with improved access to excellent pediatric specialty care and a great deal of institutional "good will".

Piloting a Quality Improvement Project

To successfully develop a multi-hospital program, the Beaumont pediatric surgery program needed to demonstrate that this initiative resulted in improved care and cost. This would be key to get the support of all stakeholders. The strategy was to align this change with cost containment, considering the anticipation of a policy of a single payment per diagnosis. This required that they transform an environment where care was individualized to each attending into one that created uniformity and championed a best clinical pathway. To do this, it was decided to start with a kaizen, focusing on a small change, on a small percentage of patients substantial enough to show feasibility to have positive impact both in cost containment, patient experience, and scalability. This typified the type of low-lying fruit ideal for a pilot.

One problem was that the main hospital had a culture where clinical decisions were set by attendings individually on daily rounds which is perfect for private practice model. Other advances on patient care were held up since nurses were not empowered to move a patient along their trajectory toward meeting discharge criteria. This hospital had surgical residents who also rounded once a day, which was similarly unhelpful and patterned on attending's rounds, considering that there was no way to ensure that care advanced *throughout* the day.

This study was an attempt to demonstrate in a pilot the administrative benefit of a standardized pediatric surgical service line. Pre-intervention envisioned pediatric surgeons only for call coverage instead of how achieving collaboration to institute programmatic delivery of continuity of care. Rollout of this project aligned performance initiatives as embodied in the American College of Surgeon's program for verification for Children's Surgical Services to raise the visibility of our program. This national program was in the initial phased rollout to identify best sites for children's surgery by ensuring sufficient resources dedicated to a level of pediatric surgical care.

To specifically prepare to apply for ACS verification, Beaumont needed senior leadership's commitment to performance improvement. The administration, a major stakeholder, wanted to ensure the pediatric surgical quality designation as well as to participate in the national Pediatric NSQIP database with a full-time administrator, which was another ~$100 K annual commitment.

Everyone recognized that high rankings in quality are critical in ensuring success in this competitive market for pediatric specialty care, particularly with insurers. Already the US News' Hospital report showed solid rankings for adult care at Beaumont. Beaumont Children's Hospital had not completed the questionnaires important to being ranked so remained unranked in current US News Hospital reports [1].

At the time of this study, Beaumont Children's Hospital also had not applied for Level I ACS designation for pediatric trauma despite having an adult Level I ACS designation and sufficient pediatric trauma volume. The absence of these two very normal initiatives, both through the American College of Surgeons, and consistent with a Children's Hospital's growth and reputational value, was striking and stymied their regional reputation as well as allowing further market penetration.

Focus on Procedural or Nonprocedural Component of a Surgery

The goal for the Division of Pediatric Surgery was to build a center of advanced laparoscopy for children, even newborns; thus, a project to highlight the expertise of more novel technology as applied to babies, could demonstrate multidisciplinary collaboration, as well as developing programmatic clinical pathways to drive positive outcomes.

Hypertrophic Pyloric Stenosis (HPS) is one of the most common indications for nonelective surgery in neonates, occurring in 2–3.5 of 1000 live births [2]. Technically a pyloromyotomy can be done laparoscopically or traditionally by an open approach, as in a Ramstedt pyloromyotomy. Despite multiple meta-analyses and randomized trials [3–5], existing literature struggles to substantiate the superiority of a minimally invasive approach. Laparoscopy as the newest approach was presumed to be unnecessarily expensive technology particularly for babies, with only cosmetic benefits, with potentially more risks. Since the benefits for neonates were not initially recognized, the popularization of minimally invasive surgery was presumed to be unnecessary yet highly desirable to the public.

For over a decade the type of procedure (open vs minimally invasive surgery) was presumed to impact the length of stay (LOS) and complication rates. Optimizing nonprocedural parts of care, the postoperative refeeding, has come to light as the primary driver of LOS, extended hospital costs, and patient experience. Since the diagnosis of HPS was not frequent enough to recognize how many different types of refeeding protocols existed, there was a lack of consensus on best practices [6–8]. A meta-analysis on refeeding techniques showed the superiority of ad libitum (unstructured feeding) or early rapid refeeding as the second-best approach [9]. The potential savings associated with a decreased LOS were estimated to range from $392 to $1290 per patient in 2002 which is $557 to $1848 today adjusted for inflation [7, 8].

The Goals and Timing of this Project

The literature has long debated the benefit of *the surgical approach* for HPS - laparoscopic versus open; whereas it is the underappreciated cousin to this debate, *the importance of the nonprocedural aspects of care* that is the actual driver in determining length of stay. Many organizations like to focus on procedural differences between surgeries; any difference is often immediately presumed to be associated with the type of surgery. Identifying low-lying fruits to improve performance is often overlooked since the first focus of surgeons, staff, and administrators is on 'the procedure' as opposed to the 'nonprocedural' aspects of the case. Leinwand et al. first reported in 2000 that a standardized postoperative feeding protocol resulted in a decrease in LOS [2]; however, then subsequent studies have equivocated whether a postoperative protocol can positively impact LOS. Finally, Clayton et al. did show the benefit of implementing a comprehensive postoperative protocol, resulting in a shortened LOS [10, 11]. This study postulated that including even more than one feeding regimen added confusion among front-line nursing staff and could stall feeding advancements [10].

Multiple refeeding methods resulted in confusion and explained the lack of consensus on a single plan. The challenge was to differentiate the signs of emesis routinely seen from perioperative edema as opposed to emesis indicating a complication such as a perforation. Routine emesis can last up to 3 days if not protocolized in a way to manage low level emesis. Given this concern we created a physician-designed protocol that nursing implemented to feed through low level emesis and identify more concerning patterns of emesis. Nursing engagement for feeding advancements throughout the day avoided the constraints of once-a-day advances based on attending rounds. With nursing ownership of this process, we transitioned from a more *hierarchical* decision-making process to one that is *patient-centric*.

Administration stood to benefit from this intervention because it gave them the ability to iterate a cost/benefit ratio for a standardized procedure. Moreover, this was intended to advance other additional quality improvement efforts. Getting positive results from this pilot study, to support our advanced laparoscopy for neonates, was hypothesized to promote the adoption of other expensive programs [12].

Observing the association between national rankings and hospital level innovations takes time and requires hospitals to develop a national reputation at academic meetings. At this hospital, which has a for-profit model as part of its historical DNA, policy makers struggled to appreciate the non-fiscal benefit of doing advanced laparoscopy. The new Surgeon-in-Chief directed their goals toward achieving quality benchmarks to incorporate a larger vision of care.

Proving the feasibility of this project had the potential to positively create (1) a template to implement other ERAS-like (Enhanced Recovery After Surgery) protocols for many more diagnoses avoiding narcotics and strategies for earlier discharge, (2) allow the option to promote a noncontroversial topic as a newly hired manager, (3) build a prototypic multidisciplinary team, that relationally can bridge the divide from residents to nursing-directed care, (4) empower nurses to take the lead on implementing and standardizing order sets to minimize care variation, (5) improve

LOS and thus cost containment over time. This cost containment could further validate our service line's approach, a 'programmatic approach', to improve expected timing of discharge. This was a dramatic change from having individual attendings functioning as private practitioners in implementing care. This project further had the potential to improve patient experience by being more patient-centric, by avoiding the waiting for the attending surgeon to advance feeding protocols. This last point enabled nurses to better time patients' discharges, which was important to patient and family satisfaction.

Methods

The plan was to initiate a single postoperative pathway. Implementation required a protocol, designed by physicians, to move a postoperative child along a pathway to advance feeding by nurses. The nurses were instructed to use a decision tree for management of emesis, which allowed them to overcome the bottleneck created by being tethered to the once daily physician rounds. Successful collaboration in this team-building approach required a culture of teamwork across groups to remove the existing gap in communication between nurses and surgical residents.

The impact of this intervention was measured using metrics including length of stay, compliance to the HPS pathway, and patient satisfaction with the delivery of care (access to sequentially advancing feedings and to be able to expect the timing of discharge). The latter two measures were both important to gaining support of the hospital's Family Counsel. They also tracked the variance in feeding pre- and post-intervention, as well as readmission rates within the first week postoperatively. The tested hypotheses were that structured feeding would improve measures of efficiency including LOS, as well as nursing and parental satisfaction. An untested hypothesis is that a decreased LOS would improve utilization of hospital resources which would increase net profit given the prohibitively limited number of pediatric beds.

The problem with the postoperative reintroduction of feeding is that the feedings can be reintroduced either early or late, and feedings could ramp up quickly or slowly. A third variation is structured vs. ad libitum feeding regimens recommended by physicians. A fourth variation comes from the dilutions of formula that was fed to children. Anyone can see the confusion caused by this paradigm. The researchers found that choosing regimens at the time of implementation was confusing and negatively impacted nursing adherence. They needed to do this comparison in a deliberate way in a central location rather than ad hoc in the ward.

Focusing on the introduction of only one regimen that was tracked by a decision tree that was available to all bedside nurses, shown in Fig. 7.1, allowed the implementation of advancing feeding, and further facilitated order sets, and provided charts and other information that could be used for nursing and resident education.

Although the literature advocates for ad libitum feedings as the best strategy for decreasing LOS [9], the team chose a structured feeding strategy with a midpoint NPO (nil per os, or nothing by mouth) time of 4 h. They chose to do this because the physicians were most comfortable with a structured reintroduction of feedings and

Protocol with Shared ERAS Elements

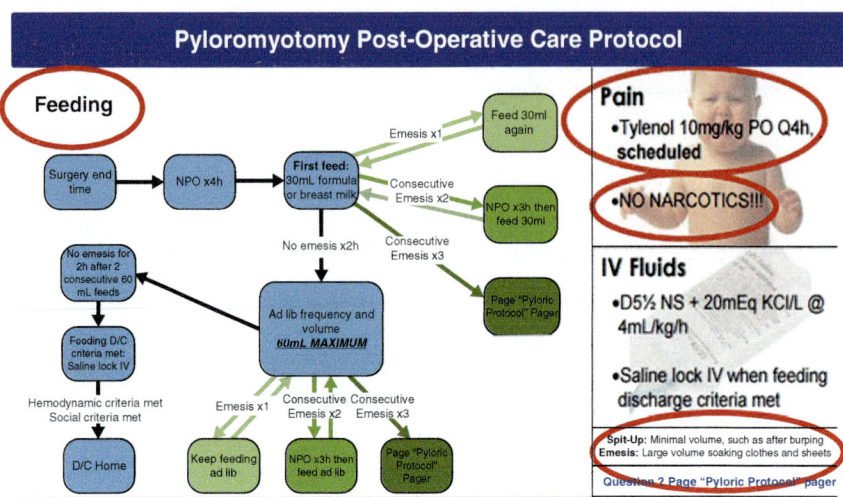

Fig. 7.1 Red circles represent measures consistent with principles of ERAS (enhanced recovery after anesthesia) such as early reintroduction of feeding, non-narcotic pain measures and management of emesis [10]. Reprinted from Clayton JT, Reisch JS, Sanchez PJ, Fickes JL, Portillo CM, Chen LE. Postoperative Regimentation of Treatment Optimizes Care and Optimizes Length of Stay (PROTOCOL) after pyloromyotomy in Journal of Pediatric Surgery, Vol. 50/Issue 9, pgs. 1540–3, ©2015, with permission from Elsevier Science and Technology Journals, W. B. Saunders

were not comfortable with the ongoing emesis with ad libitum feedings. It was decided to not provide any narcotics, a quality measure that was consistent with ERAS protocols. Scheduled Tylenol dosing was used to ensure consistent pain control after intraoperative local was given to avoid the typical sine wave of postoperative pain management.

The goals of this project were to minimize the variability of care, prove feasibility and improve outcomes (decreased LOS and patient/family satisfaction). This project shared elements with a larger project the Surgeon-in-Chief wanted eventually to implement, an ERAS-type of protocol for improved outcomes without narcotics. ERAS regimens have been the go-to strategy for allowing protocolization of surgical care from pre- operation to post- operation. Setting the stage with a prototypic study to address low lying fruit allowed for a demonstration of feasibility, making the case for a for a larger initiative, like ERAS, which needed a longer timeframe to enact larger programmatic change.

Assembling a Policy Team

They identified the relevant stakeholder groups to be the nurses, physicians (attendings and residents), mid-level providers, the Family Counsel Group, and 'hyper users" for IT order sets. The researchers started team building right at the outset of the project, involving stakeholders from each of these groups. A second move was to establish content experts by initiating a comprehensive review of the literature to decide what would be applicable in our institution.

The intervention was adapted to reflect the communication needs in the organization. The physicians and nurses seemed to round in parallel and did not interact. This meant that each group needed to be involved in designing the order sets. At the outset of the project the order sets were rolled out in the following way: Advanced nurse practitioners were responsible for initiating the order sets, the surgical residents approached the attendings to sign off on the order sets, and the surgical residents would then implement the order sets for the attendings.

The intervention changed this process by empowering nurses, using the decision tree poster, to implement the HPS protocol by managing the frequency and volume of emesis. Since these variables became so important in the decision-tree, they were tracked better by nurses. Such tracking had a secondary benefit of documenting these nurses' adherence to the protocol. When emesis did not resolve by the third time, nurses were instructed to page the surgical team, which included attendings, residents, and midlevel providers. Dedicated information technology (IT) resources were critical for implementing order set design, observing compliance, tracking nursing documentation for adherence to the protocol, and identifying deviations.

Analysis

The team used retrospective chart data for analysis. As previously discussed, clinical variables of interest in the data included length of stay (LOS), time to feeds, feeds to discharge (DC), amount of emesis, as well as qualitative nursing documentation. The sample consisted of all pediatric patients with HPS who did not experience surgical complications, which would have skewed the expected LOS. A sample size of 70 allowed for 80% of power to detect a 50% reduction in proportion of patients with prolonged LOS ($\alpha = 0.05$) given how spread out the LOS was. They analyzed the difference in these measures using a quasi-experimental pre/post design without a control group. As an implementation of a clinical guideline for our practice, this work constituted a shift in clinical management, and not a research study. This means that this study did not meet requirements for IRB approval.

Results

The retrospective chart review indicated that that prolonged length of stay (LOS) hovered around 45% for infants without surgical complications. The research team then rolled out the decision-tree and pager system using change management strategies. Implementation of their study was associated with a 50% decrease in LOS of those staying over 1 day (i.e. 2 days or ≥ 3 days), as well as a greater than a two-fold

Table 7.1 Metrics

Metric	Measure used	Baseline	Results	Impact Assessment
1	Decrease pLOS (in hours)	35% had pLOS	50% reduction of pLOS Reduced to 15% of pts. with pLOS of more than 1 MN	• 50% reduction • Fewer pts. spending >1MN post-operation
2	Decrease time to first feed	362 min	248 min	• Approximates protocol
3	Recorded #feeds to DC	Up to 33 feeds	Reduced to 6 feedings	• Narrowed variance
4	Recorded # emesis	Variable 0–21 emesis	Reduced to 0–6 emesis	• Narrowed variance
5	Nursing adherence to ordered feeding	41%	55%	• Less confusion on stepwise advancement • Improved documentation

pLOS = postop LOS > 1 or more MNs, i.e. 1MN, 2MN, or 3MN and greater

increase in cases that were discharged within the first day. They similarly observed time to first feed decrease from 362 minutes to 241 minutes. They also noticed that the spread of data decreased. The number of feeds to DC was reduced to 6, and the variance in postoperative emesis was reduced from 0–21 to 0–8 episodes. Also observed was that documentation regarding the amount and frequency of emesis and inputs and outputs improved substantially, 41% to ~55% of total time. Additionally, they noticed that nursing compliance improved regarding the correct type of feed that was ordered. Table 7.1 summarizes the change in metrics that were tracked in this study.

Patient surveys, conducted by patient care coordinators, indicated an improvement in patient reported outcomes. Testimonials from families were generally positive regarding the reduction in length of time and improvements in the ability to anticipate discharge. Generally, testimonials indicated that we had addressed the concerns of the Family Counsel.

Discussion

Change Management

Before embarking on a change implementation project, one needs to weigh the cost-benefit ratio of attempting to lead change at Beaumont Health by initiating this type of performance improvement process. The Mckinsey 7S Framework [13] and Porter's 5 Competitive Forces that Shape Strategy were used to align the Surgeon-in Chief with the institution's strategy [14].

Being a change agent or program builder can be associated with a shorter institutional life span and is not something for the faint of heart. To preserve one's ability to make change, a watchful eye on one's degree of institutional support is key.

Social capital in any institution is limited and waxes and wanes with early wins. This was especially true in the case of a change leader, where it is even more important to be strategic with this capital.

It was also necessary to identify and understand the underlying organizational structure of the old guard. These informal relationships could work around any explicit hierarchy by using their "buddy" network. Titles add responsibility and accountability, but authority is not guaranteed by senior leadership who maybe giving titles on one side and 'a nod and a wink' on the other side. Authority can be earned over time and be supported or undermined by these informal networks. Tacit approval by these informal clubs is important to have resilience. This buddy network ultimately represented the greatest challenge to lasting change in this program and this change implementation project evolved into one of many proxy wars for who actually ran the division.

The first management tactic that the new Chief employed was to generate a strategic plan regarding the type and scope of the project. Considering that change can be potentially threatening, the plan was to choose a nonthreatening topic that could be changed without too much impact to other areas of the hospital. There could not be a more boring project to surgical attendings than refeeding. This meant that the senior partner, with a history of 40 years at the hospital, would not be tremendously interested, which would mitigate his scrutiny. However, his insecurity on not being able to do laparoscopic surgery may have added to his anxiety regarding all the other changes in the program, and its new leadership as well as new affiliations with other hospitals in the practice.

Once the topic was chosen, steps were taken to justify the project into the organization by aligning the project with goals that benefit stakeholders. Consideration of stakeholders that were not involved in the project but were tangentially affected by the outcome was key. Messaging to other quality improvement managers was that any positive outcomes from any study would highlight the benefit and value of a dedicated service line/program. Building a program is fundamentally easily aligned with the interests of all quality initiatives. Tying the project to tangential initiatives and stakeholders in this way created a mutually enforcing network of like-minded practitioners.

The team was chosen to be a multi-disciplinary change team. Team building was organized using the relational aspect of the Relational Coordination framework that emphasized shared goals, shared knowledge, and mutual respect [15]. They achieved shared knowledge by discussing literature reviews bi-weekly, and then used the knowledge to identify potential projects, which allowed them to establish shared goals. These components were co-reinforcing with mutual respect.

While the majority of the team were adopters of the change initiative, a senior partner stood in stark resistance. He was concerned that the project would focus on technical differences in approaches surgically for pyloromyotomies rather than feeding regimens, despite being told that this was not the aim of the project. This partner's concern arose from the fact that he only did open surgery over laparoscopic pyloromyotomies. That obviously dated him surgically. He feared his preeminence as the senior partner and that he may lose his ability to use his preferred method. After a long period of dissent, they were able to work around this adversarial team member by giving them power in the project. An advanced registered nurse practitioner, someone who the senior partner respected, ran the drafted order set by him to get his approval in concept. This consideration made it possible to avoid some of his interest in blocking the project.

This exercise brought up the point that, in many cases, late adopters/resistors are threatened by false assumptions about the project. In this case the partner, threatened that this project was really about surgical approaches, did not want to budge. It took lengthy communication to bring this to the surface and reassure them that their interests would be protected. Advertising the positives of a protocol and how it can benefit the attendings by decreasing floor calls with a well-designed decision-tree protocol is important to remind every stakeholder of the benefits of change.

Convincing nurses about the benefits of the change project was more straightforward. Something that they could refer to if they had a question or disagreement with the way that protocol was managed as shown in Fig. 7.1. The nurses had a 'pyloric pager' that they could use for cases of emesis that required the attention of physicians to have an early way to recognize those patients falling off the clinical pathway and an early marker for postoperative issue. These tools allowed them to better advocate for care and prepare the patients' families for anticipated discharge.

Lessons in Management

Lesson 1 *Choose the project strategically* to be both feasible and have observable impact. This allowed for positive managing up, where the 'C' Suite was rewarded for their investment in the initiative. A 'win' could be perceived by senior leadership in the institutional dedication to laparoscopic build for neonates and toddlers and the 'buy in' for investing in components of the ACS Children's Verification of Surgery program. It also helped that our project scored high patient satisfaction scores, which were previously immobile and in need of attention.

Choosing a project that did not introduce controversy in the institution was also key to strategy. Unfortunately, not enough attention was paid to this last point, and small controversies pushed by the nonadopters/resisters ultimately made the project less effective than it could have been, given a senior partner's insecurities once he was passed over for leadership.

Lesson 2 A key to project success was *'Walking the Gemba'* and understanding the issues involved so key to do for the first year in any leadership role [16]. One can understand the many levels and drivers of involvement and become a visible and hands-on leader by participating with the delivery of care at the front line. Front line support however does not compensate for any pushback from the informal networks unaligned with the change leadership. Informal networks can use constant negative commentary politically to erode decisions by senior leadership to implement change.

Lesson 3 *Involving stakeholders at all points of decision making regarding the care process* helped the Surgeon-in Chief to bring key stakeholders along in the decision-making journey. This started with the literature review process, which gave a forum to study perspectives on each point of care in open meetings and make decisions collectively. Stakeholders were encouraged to participate in the process of policy development rather than chastised for breaking protocol once policy was established. We exposed these stakeholders to AIDET sessions (Acknowledge, Introduce, Duration, Expectation, and Thank you) as well as role playing to brainstorm the best way to improve clinical quality measures and patient satisfaction. *The success of improving patient satisfaction* was key to the positive impact and mutual reinforcement of *AIDET training* [17]. This built strong group dynamics. Moreover, the fact that feedings were about post-surgery care rather than about surgery created a new dynamic where nurses felt that they could contribute and be empowered regardless of their position in the hospital.

This new dynamic helped to expose a lack of consensus regarding rounding times, which resulted in the fact that physicians rounded independently from the nurses. We were able to use this feedback to craft a new regimen that allowed these team members to coordinate their rounding times to work together.

Lesson 4 Obtaining '*buy-in*' and involvement from the surgical attendings is mission critical. In some cases, resistance can be avoided by bringing these stakeholders in and finding a project that does not threaten their ability to do their job as they see fit. Getting buy-in requires understanding and addressing the work that you are asking people to do. One senior partner that did not buy into the project or into the program and he had a substantial impact on the project's success. He certainly slowed every step to try to have the study not advance. He may have best understood that early successes from a project ensures positive newsworthy program and that would ensure longevity. He opposed change and change leadership so he would obstruct any forward progress. There are multitude of reasons he functioned as an obstructionist- being passed over in leadership, perceived loss of administrative control, possible future revenue loss, and diminution in his roles and relevancy. Never underestimate the power and influence of any non-adopter, potentially an obstructionist, particularly if he/she is one with decades of institutional history and can mobilizing informal networks against the change leader in an effort to ensure his/her own influence.

Lesson 5 *Pick an inexpensive project (low lying fruit) when you're new to the organization.* This project did not require substantial resources, which made the process of getting support of senior administration much less complicated. Achieving buy-in requires understanding the risks that you are asking people to take. Picking a low-cost project requires less risk and therefore inherently removes barriers to buy-in particularly in traditionally non-academic environments.

Lesson 6 *Titles yield accountability, but do not guarantee authority.* In this case, the institution was not aligned to support the role of Surgeon-In- Chief in the Children's Hospital which was a new role to the institution. It took applying the *Seven S's* to this institution [13, 18] to identify the depth of disconnect between shared values, style, and staffing, which together constrained and stymied the capabilities of programmatic growth. No wonder Beaumont could not merge with Henry Ford since the power of informal networks of the private practices could not be removed for a system approach, such as transitioning into being all employed by one employer. This realization highlighted the depth of disconnect between C suite and clinical thought leaders regarding their appetite for change. Understanding that authority is gained over time helps to explain why hiring outside of the organization for senior management proves so often to be unsuccessful for the recruitment in the long term but it is used to initiate a change, nonetheless. This explains why these managers often leave after a short period of time but the institution is positively impacted by having an impetus to change; that leader recruited as a change leader may not have longevity.

Lesson 7 *Recognize the importance of political context within the organization.* Merger and changes in leadership can dramatically unravel a new program or unintentionally strip resources and handicap a program overnight. The mission appeared to be aligned with the vision of 2 campuses, where pediatric surgical specialty care was a priority. The eventual expansion of the health system to potentially 8 hospitals sent reverberations throughout our health group. They had to juggle the competing interests of the children's hospital with the merger, which ultimately proved to be very difficult since any change caused the senior partner to create a perception of a crisis. The perception of a limited resource specialty accommodating an 8-hospital merger as opposed to the 2–3 campuses became the destabilizing issue to the faculty.

Lesson 8 *The role of proxy wars to challenge a change leader.* There were so many elements of change- a new medical school, the firing of a whole group of Chairs, the mergers considered and hospital acquisition and now the concept of system coverage not just hospital coverage were all threatening issues. Change on other fronts in the division (such as this study) easily could become the *proxy wars* for a much larger destabilizing factors--the potential 8 hospital system expansion that could make surgeons cover other hospitals, reignited the controversy over currently covering 3 hospitals. Before all these change elements for system expansion, the surgeons could focus and cover only one campus but that was not a competitive strategy with all other systems vying for market share and congenital cases. Recognize and identify all the change elements to recognize which one is the most disruptive to the change leader.

Lesson 9 *Managing leadership disputes requires social capital.* This is how managing leadership on every front is a cost to a leader's social capital: recognize any decision can be a potential dispute, so choose them carefully. A nonadopter to a study may reveal an obstructionist whose strategy is to ensure that the change leader runs out of social capital so he can continually rehash negative comments to informal networks to undermine the program's change leader. Given the degree of change and uncertainty in the institution, the reins of power were always in motion and lacked stability as a result. As a new member of senior management, the change leader was given little ability to assert authority, easily challenged by the senior partner pushing informal networks to use to his advantage. The C suite does not manage a power struggle such as this, since it can be a politically expensive cost and the longevity in healthcare is now short-lived to 2–5-year cycles. If an obstructionist is not appropriately managed, then he can stymie or undermine organizational change. Accountability is often promised but often not delivered if authority of the change leader is not actively supported. Implicit tacit support is not sufficient.

Lesson 10 The perception of change is seen as threatening to entrenched faculty or staff. The 'deep institutional history' that entrenched faculty or staff share then galvanizes old informal social networks to align against the change leader. There is a precarious balance of a reporting clinical hierarchy and the informal social networks that undermine such a reporting structure. These informal social networks align unlikely non-adopters to strategically align to undermine the newly appointed leadership. This can ultimately destabilize the program as it was envisioned by the change leader. The project succeeded and showed the benefit of a program focused service line. The paradigm of covering 3 hospitals in a collaborative mission all succeeded to this day as envisioned. The change was fiscally good as designed for the institution and its regional influence as a children's hospital.

There are many cultural issues when a younger surgeon, trained in the era of multidisciplinary teams, works with older private practitioners trained in the pyramidal system of residency at the time of an 'eat what you kill' paradigm. Surgeons trained in this style of practice, typified in private practice, learned to make money on individual cases rather than through programatic driven outcomes. Because of this training, they fail to see the value in developing a collaborative comprehensive program for full coverage, whether it is the benefits of performance improvement or the benefit of a comprehensive group model to manage surgical specialty care in local regional hospital system. While implementation was possible on a small scale, the program never realized its full potential without the blessing of one of these senior surgeons.

The longevity of a CEO in healthcare is often in a 3–5-year cycle which can dramatically disrupt clinical programs and strategy. Historically the Chairs, were visionary leaders in medicine, and they had great power over finances, personnel and clinical program development; however, the move to corporate medicine has transitioned chairmen to being middle management who are greatly impacted and silenced by the changes of senior management. As healthcare has become corporate, clinical leaders (department chairs and divisional chiefs) are now considered to be only middle managers without the control of the resources to implement and underwrite programmatic growth. Successful programmatic growth requires a continuity and stability in leadership with a trajectory longer than a 3–5 year cycle.

Implementation of the Project

The team did a great job of implementing this project by the end, but it was a slow process to groom. Since this was a first project of its type, it was difficult to get different stakeholder groups to participate. This type of quality improvement project would be much easier in a hospital that has a high absorptive capacity for change management initiatives.

One of the largest contributors to the success of the project was the team nature of the work. We delegated components of the project to each person, which caused everyone to be involved in the journey of implementation. At first it was difficult to get the nurses to feel empowered to share their thoughts. Communication was key in overcoming this hierarchy. Giving people a platform to discuss their position and creating a space to discuss problems allowed everyone to appreciate the struggles and share their experiences, which generated a shared sense of reciprocity [19]. Some examples of what we found from these open discussions were that (1) having multiple feeding regimens confused everyone, (2) keeping babies endlessly NPO when the literature showed we could feed so much earlier put stress on patient's families, (3) there was a need to educate clinical staff regarding the difference between emesis and small emesis or spit up. Going through each step of the patients' journey together allowed us to collectively understand stakeholder's perspectives and identify pain points.

One consideration is to be a more passive member of the team, one who lets the team be empowered to move forward without a change leader seen as its figurehead. Had I championed the project harder it would have only further enraged the senior partner and other non-adopters. Strategically to be under the radar is ultimately helpful in managing non-adopters and ideally encourages the team to take the reins as an empowered group. Nurses were empowered to protocolize the management, and the residents worked to get the appropriate IT power plans on the chart to ensure the attendings' approval. There is a healthy balance that needs to be struck between being under the radar as a leader to empower one's team and as a change leader managing up and advocating 'good news' regarding the program. Change requires balancing the championing the project to the C suite as a 'early win' for the program, while making the project quietly succeed.

Any larger project such as a larger ERAS project would not have been easily implemented in this timeframe. Ultimately this fact emphasizes the point that strategic project selection is vital for project completion, especially when the change leader is new to an organization and early wins and positive press are the coin of the realm.

Conclusion

This project took place in a hospital that was in flux, where leadership and resource allocation were constantly changing. The rapid merger magnified the degree of resource constraints we faced for a program in its infancy. Pediatric surgery was

Beaumont's second program to build and first as a multi-hospital coverage model. The rapid growth of the hospital system to 8 hospitals with a whole new clinical leadership created an all-too-common backdrop of change.

This paper looked at the strategy and development of change in this organization-in-flux. How key it is to recognize all levels of change. By building a prototype to study a policy shift we were able observe the capacity of an organization to accept a nuanced change in care paradigm, and the ensuing outcomes that are brought about by that change. Even at the moderate levels of adoption described in this paper we were able to observe substantial change to measured outcomes, including length of stay and patient reported satisfaction with earlier discharges.

This project found that empowering nurses made it possible to standardize and champion feeding routines and advancing a patient toward discharge at all hours of the day. In operationalizing refeeding postoperatively, we were in effect implementing protocolized discharge timing. We were able to design order sets upfront with physician input, and then implement protocolized postoperative care via computerized order sets from the PACU. This stepwise process of up-front design of the order sets by physicians and residents ensured the buy-in for a consistent comprehensive plan for postoperative management. While this project certainly showed proof of concept and was an early win for the program, and the institutional investment in the program, as an early pilot project it was not sufficiently endowed for the proxy wars it came to symbolize. This process reaffirmed the need for the change leader to be supported in a way that provides authority and resiliency. All logistical changes at the time in the project, the program, and coverage models of care still exist today in the way they were fiscally envisioned by the change leader, despite another round of leadership changes that ensured.

References

1. U.S. News & World Report. How Does Beaumont Children's Hospital Rank Among America's Best Hospitals? [Cited 2020 Jun 5]. https://health.usnews.com/best-hospitals/area/mi/beaumont-childrens-hospital-PA6442245
2. Leinwand MJ, Shaul DB, Anderson KD. A standardized feeding regimen for hypertrophic pyloric stenosis decreases length of hospitalization and hospital costs. J Pediatr Surg. 2000;35(7):1063–5.
3. Hall NJ, Pacilli M, Eaton S, Reblock K, Gaines BA, Pastor A, et al. Recovery after open versus laparoscopic pyloromyotomy for pyloric stenosis: a double-blind multicentre randomised controlled trial. Lancet. 2009;373(9661):390–8.
4. Sola JE, Neville HL. Laparoscopic vs open pyloromyotomy: a systematic review and meta-analysis. J Pediatr Surg. 2009;44(8):1631–7.
5. Oomen MWN, Hoekstra LT, Bakx R, Ubbink DT, Heij HA. Open versus laparoscopic pyloromyotomy for hypertrophic pyloric stenosis: a systematic review and meta-analysis focusing on major complications. Surg Endosc. 2012;26(8):2104–10.
6. Adibe OO, Nichol PF, Lim F-Y, Mattei P. Ad libitum feeds after laparoscopic pyloromyotomy: a retrospective comparison with a standardized feeding regimen in 227 infants. J Laparoendosc Adv Surg Tech A. 2007;17(2):235–7.
7. Garza JJ, Morash D, Dzakovic A, Mondschein JK, Jaksic T. Ad libitum feeding decreases hospital stay for neonates after pyloromyotomy. J Pediatr Surg. 2002;37(3):493–5.

8. Puapong D, Kahng D, Ko A, Applebaum H. Ad libitum feeding: safely improving the cost-effectiveness of pyloromyotomy. J Pediatr Surg. 2002;37(12):1667–8.
9. Sullivan KJ, Chan E, Vincent J, Iqbal M, Wayne C, Nasr A, et al. Feeding post-pyloromyotomy: a meta-analysis. Pediatrics. 2016;137:1.
10. Clayton JT, Reisch JS, Sanchez PJ, Fickes JL, Portillo CM, Chen LE. Postoperative regimentation of treatment optimizes care and optimizes length of stay (PROTOCOL) after pyloromyotomy. J Pediatr Surg. 2015;50(9):1540–3.
11. Costanzo CM, Vinocur C, Berman L. Postoperative outcomes of open versus laparoscopic pyloromyotomy for hypertrophic pyloric stenosis. J Surg Res. 2018;224:240–4.
12. Miles JA. Absorptive capacity theory. In: Management and organization theory: a Jossey-Bass reader. 1. ed. San Francisco, CA: Jossey-Bass; 2012. p. 17–23. (The Jossey-Bass business & management reader series).
13. The McKinsey 7-S Framework: - Making every part of your organization work in harmony. [cited 2020 Jul 6]. http://www.mindtools.com/pages/article/newSTR_91.htm
14. Porter ME. The five competitive forces that shape strategy. Harv Bus Rev. 2008:1–18.
15. Gittell JH. New directions for relational coordination theory. The Oxford Handbook of Positive Organizational Scholarship. 2011 [cited 2020 Jul 6]. https://www.oxfordhandbooks.com/view/10.1093/oxfordhb/9780199734610.001.0001/oxfordhb-9780199734610-e-030
16. Womack JP, Shook J. Gemba walks. Version 1.0. Cambridge, MA: Lean Enterprise Institute; 2011. p. 348.
17. Braverman AM, Kunkel EJ, Katz L, Katona A, Heavens T, Miller A, Arfaa JJ. Do I buy it? How AIDET™ training changes residents' values about patient care. J Patient Exp. 2015;2(1):13–20.
18. Waterman RH Jr, Peters TJ, Phillips JR. Structure is not organization. Bus Horiz. 1980;23(3):14.
19. Cialdini RB. Harnessing the science of persuasion. Harvard Business Review. 2001 Oct 1 [cited 2020 Jul 6];(October 2001). https://hbr.org/2001/10/harnessing-the-science-of-persuasion

8. Institutional and Professional Transition: The Foundations of Business Management in the First 100 Days of a Chief Medical Officer

Thomas F. Tracy

Key Learning Points
- Physician executives must understand how to analyze leadership structure and activate networks in order to build lasting partnerships.
- Building a team of direct reports is a useful mechanism for establishing leaders of cross-functional teams that will be required for achieving an organizational transformation.
- Establishing clarity in goal setting and design is a critical stage in the transformation process and a key management foundation for the individual to be successful.
- In the face of uncertainty, learning how to communicate effectively and setting expectations with the best immediate understanding and situational awareness up through management and down through responsible teams is critical for bridging knowledge and action.
- Positively positioning critical teams of influence and engaging stakeholders in operational processes, both under and outside the purview of the executive, is a key strategy for success.
- Taking efforts to mend or remove broken relationships is essential for proper coordination within the organization.

Introduction

The transitional steps and experience required for physician executives to advance or take on new roles is poorly documented. The vast majority of physicians that transition to administrative roles, such as the Chief Quality Officer (CQO), Vice President

T. F. Tracy (✉)
The American Pediatric Surgical Association,
East Dundee, IL, USA

Adjunct Professor of Surgery and Pediatrics, Brown University, Providence, RI, USA

of Medical affairs (VPMA), or Chief Medical Officer (CMO) arrive at the opportunity through their local accomplishments, reputation, and respect. In academic institutions, these physician leaders have generally demonstrated high degrees of individual accomplishment across the patient care, teaching, and research missions of the institution or health system in which they are working. They have also achieved an even greater understanding of the interdependencies among cross-functional teams that are needed in order to unify and coordinate efforts between administrations and their physician leadership partners. This is generally also true for physicians at other large hospitals, ambulatory centers, and community institutions delivering healthcare.

In both worlds of healthcare delivery and business management, the increasing complexity of the positions that these physician executives hold has often led to the use of specialized search firms and committees for their recruitment and selection [1]. Through my experience in these roles, I have observed how physician leader's roles in a hospital or health system administration have evolved well beyond the more limited scope of medical staff oversight, as was the former limited purview of the Vice President of Medical Affairs [2]. These positions now include responsibilities to provide complex understanding, counselling, and execution in the areas of clinical quality, finance, legal, strategy, operations, and health systems engineering, that all business administrators must address and collaborate on [2, 3]. Table 8.1

Table 8.1 Three major challenges for Chief Medical Officers

Challenge	Skills and resources	Examples
1. *Managing the economic or policy disruption and uncertainty while leading innovation in patient centered quality and value*	Human Behavior and Engineering	1. Understand the entire patient care continuum 2. Eliminate variability in care and outcomes 3. Balance clinical research and innovation vs. core measures. 4. Align system initiatives and evidence based best practices. 5. Facilitate translational and patient centered outcomes research
2. *Finding the best way to express our medical message and common purpose*	Enterprise, Marketing and Learning Community	1. Develop mechanisms to partner with patients and caregivers 2. Develop centers that study, develop and report clinical excellence 3. Introduce and implement business intelligence software for medical insight 4. Provide responsible feedback systems and meaningful measurements for genuine transparency
3. *How to take advantage of population, community, and diversity to deliver health and wellness.*	Public Health and Economics	1. Ensure access for all patients 2. Develop fluid, transparent delivery networks 3. Reinforce clinical effectiveness and facilitate patient navigation 4. Participate in value-based organization or specialty unit demonstration projects 5. Demonstrate and coordinate community partnerships for population health 6. Tackle the coordination required for the transitions in chronic disease

categorizes these expanded roles as viewed by the author within three main challenges for the CMO, proposing the necessary skills and resources needed to address these challenges, and examples of possible solutions.

With this understanding, many physicians now find that the role of CMO at the corporate level achieves parity with other senior leadership roles, including reporting to both physician and non-physician Presidents or Chief Executive Officers as well as their institutional boards. Although there is no available data on the numbers of physicians that obtain these positions or the ideal path to selecting these individuals for their roles [3], there is better understanding of the necessary competencies and executive practice track records for those that have joined a healthcare executive administration in these roles [2]. Furthermore, and perhaps equally important for those preparing for this direction in their professional development, is having the necessary tools, experience, and insight to choose the type of position and institution that would be the best fit for the individual and their potential for success [1].

Similar to professional progression in any field, the applicant's breadth and depth of successful past experience is the best indicator of suitability for the position and pre-requisite to compete for the job. However, even so, there are no guarantees for either the institution or the incumbent of the success that both anticipate through the recruitment process. The transition into an executive role presents a very different course from the professional progression at an academic or professional physician practice, usually demonstrated by advancement in successful group practices, clinical units, divisional, departmental or institute leadership [2]. As such, failures in executive recruitment and transitions occur when either the applicants have incomplete individual capacity to achieve all of the responsibilities of the roles as described above or, they are unable to address the magnitude of the collective challenges facing the institution and its leadership team. Selecting the right candidate and choosing the ideal institution requires extreme diligence for both parties.

In this chapter, I will take the position that the first introductory observations and insights for a new CMO, translated into positive contributions, will not guarantee, but may afford a positive start. The business and management elements that translate to the bedside need to be constantly implemented during care delivery to not only achieve the patients' best outcomes but also assure the financial and operational long-term growth and development of the institution. The observations that form this chapter are personal and should be considered as unique, as no two institutions or roles for CMOs are the same. While the findings presented in this paper may, therefore, not be able to be generalized to every other setting, this chapter will cover some common general business approaches that were used in this case and the transition of a physician leader within an academic medical center and health system.

Role of the Chief Medical Officer

In my transition to become a new CMO at a major university medical center in 2016, I had the opportunity to apply my experience and knowledge of business management to designing a strategy for my first 100 days in the position. The first 100 days in a position is a well-known critical time in management for confirming the observations made during applicant recruitment and provides the chance to reevaluate any prior perceptions and correct course on behalf of the institution and the executive leadership [4]. With both myself and the leadership of the Medical Center having the same goal for a successful start, this time frame offered me the opportunity to work toward achieving an orderly transition into my role and early success.

The role of CMO was a newly designed position at the Medical Center and was within the context of a relatively nascent health system, being less than 2 years old. As articulated through the recruitment process, the stated expectation of the role by the Medical Center leadership was to begin to extend the mandate of the Medical Center's leadership team to cover an expanding outpatient network across the continuum of acute care and to expand the responsibility of these centers by partnering with academic physicians in primary and specialty care. As expressed during the interview process, the overarching goal was to have the CMO take on a broad leadership function and to work as an integral part of the strategic vison of the health system, which would serve a growing regional population. The Medical Center, along with the adjoining College of Medicine, were both relatively young. While the institutions were founded in 1963 [5]; with over five decades of past clinical care, research and teaching experience, the institutions had become highly respected tertiary and quaternary academic medical enterprises [6]. When I assumed the role of CMO, the leadership of these institutions were seeking to merge the Medical Center with another regional system or either acquire or build new institutions on a larger regional footprint in order to create a larger and more boldly designed system [7].

Prior to my recruitment, the previous CMO was positioned largely as a leader for the medical staff. It was only with the recent reimagination of the Medical Center into a larger health system that the CMO role was reconceptualized as ideally able to share the responsibilities for the broader outpatient network with the responsibilities to operate across the entire continuum of care. As explained during my recruitment process, this would allow strategic and operational integration of roles, to include responsibilities for inpatient services as well as services at ambulatory and other new hospital sites. Administratively, the position reported to the Executive Director of the Medical Center and the Executive Vice Dean the Faculty for the College of Medicine, who served as the Chief Operating Officer (COO) of the Faculty Medical Group (Fig. 8.1).

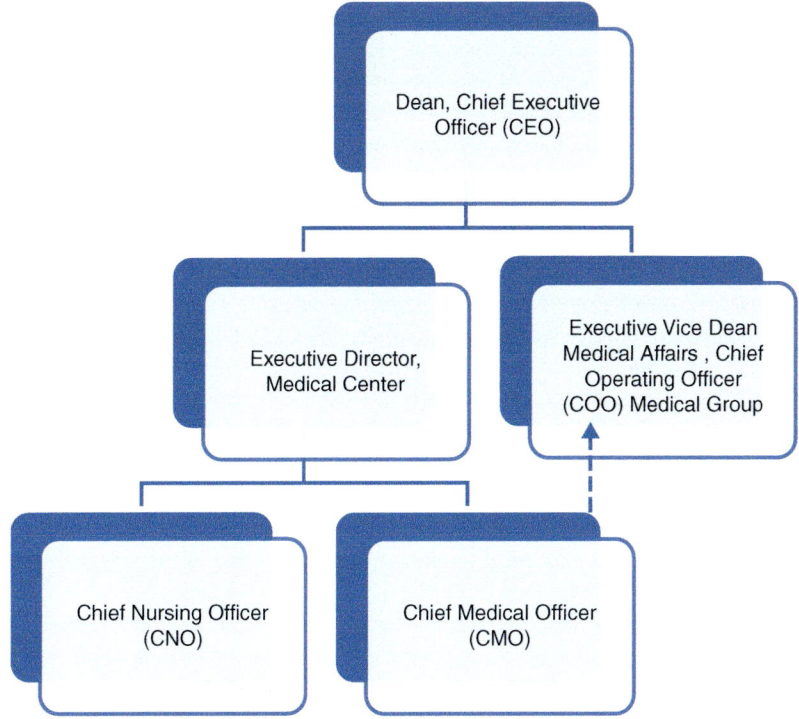

Fig. 8.1 Diagram of CMO reporting structure*. *Solid lines represent direct reporting responsibilities and dotted lines represent indirect reporting responsibilities

Defining the Problem

The operational status for the academic and clinical administration at the Medical Center was based on a traditional academic structure, where the Dean is the Chief Executive Officer (CEO) of the entire system and College of Medicine [8, 9]. Under the past leadership, this framework for operation naturally promoted a siloed environment, largely directed by Chairs of departments to achieve clinical and academic success [10]. As such, programmatic or management support from a partner CMO was not seen by most of the leadership team to be necessary, but rather, an interesting idea in the face of required growth and perhaps cultural change.

The region had an established favorable payment environment, consisting of a persistent fee for service reimbursement. This important economic reality could theoretically limit the success of attempts to rationally distribute services and faculty practitioners throughout a larger healthcare system, without a strong focus on value of care as in value-based payment models [11]. Additionally, while major strides in quality and patient safety had been made and recognized through improved national rankings–including being ranked amongst the top ten organizations in the rigorous Vizient Quality and Accountability Study and earning a Leapfrog Hospital Safety Grade of A, there was an urgent need to establish pathways for capital acquisition, resource development, process design, and care integration that would anticipate the healthcare policy changes toward alternative, value-based payment models, and focus on durable clinical outcomes and enhanced efficiency [1].

A key issue for me to consider, as the new CMO, was whether the new organizational structure could be designed to achieve partnership with and deployment of specialty and primary care resources across a large region, without sacrificing the research and teaching mission that was so much a part of the clinical environment. Additionally, lurking in the background was the proposition of a merger with a local health system and the urgent need to expand current in- and outpatient facilities to accommodate growth in the face of near universal 100% capacity [12].

When beginning my new position, I was advised by the Dean that a thoughtful and collaborative redesign of clinical care models and redistribution of services would allow for greater patient access to leading specialty care and primary care providers. There were three primary benefits that could be derived if that proved true. The first and most essential benefit was that the quality and value provided to the population served would be enhanced, as measured by key risk-adjusted outcome metrics, such as the Vizient rankings. Secondly, resource use in key high-level care areas, such as the emergency department and surgical services, would benefit through enhanced patient flow and enhanced physician-supported and evidence-based value analysis of the clinical supply chain [13, 14]. Finally, by careful analysis and measurement of both the healthcare market needs and barriers to healthcare access for patients, the necessary investments in infrastructure would become more apparent and realized sooner. It was expected that significant improvements in efficiency would be achieved through the redesign processes, leading to greater provider satisfaction, improved and innovative patient-care models, a lower cost of care, and measurable increases in meaningful access to care for patients across a region.

Creating a Plan

The analysis, understanding, and action plans that I derived during my first 100 days in the position, together with measures of success from targeted projects, determined the overall acceptance of the new CMO position and its role in leadership. I identified three elements that were critical to this process and provided sequential areas of focus in the proposed timeline of the first 100 days, including: **(1) building**

foundations of leadership and organizational structure, (2) providing clarity in terms of goal-setting and design, and (3) ensuring communication with the best immediate understanding. These drew from the key pillars of fair process work, which link work processes, staff attitudes, and staff behaviors together with the aim of achieving staff trust and commitment to leadership goals, and ultimately, active cooperation in change [15]. These pillars, including adequate stakeholder engagement, clear explanation of goals and the processes to achieve those goals, and clarity around expectations were essential in quickly building partnerships, a team of direct reports, and positively positioning critical teams of influence. Building the individual capabilities within the existing organizational structure helped to reaffirm not only my personal fidelity to the institutional mission as a trusted member of the team, but also provided the foundation for me to appreciate challenges to the status quo and initiate solutions. Within the organizational structure, communication and clear transparency from my side allowed for the best efforts of those setting and following the direction of the business at the multiple points of care. Finally, as in any new or dynamic situation, together with other leaders, I had to be willing and able to accept the best evidence upon which to base my decision making.

With my position start date in mid-August, I was able to plan a visit to the Medical Center in late June to begin to define the current leadership situation by meeting with direct supervisors. During this time, I was also able to clarify and refine the proposed role of the CMO with respect to responsible areas and direct reports. This allowed me to consider the best prospects for team formation and the optimal and preferred communication, goal setting, and progress measurement mechanisms through the summer, before the formal start of the position. I hoped to achieve clarity and consensus on the immediate needs of the institution to be addressed by the CMO with the leadership of the Medical Center, which would allow me to prioritize my initial exposure and introductions across the institution and begin to consider the steps to propose for action and resolution.

From the initial visit and the subsequent early conversations, I gained enough familiarity with the leadership, people, team, and culture of the Medical Center to have the ability to build an initial team that upheld the pillars of robust quality, safety, and patient experience that CMOs are responsible for and require passionate and expert leadership to carry out [2, 10]. Highlighting the recognized achievements in those areas was a way to gain insight into the successful ways in which the team currently worked together across the organization and the networks that already existed within the institution and supported the positive work— structures that together have been termed "relational coordination" [16]. By first focusing on the previous successes of the team, I was able to cultivate an understanding of the institutional, financial, information technology (IT), and other support systems that existed before I joined and would be necessary to ensure that all facets of those systems were well-established and optimally measured and reported.

During my initial visit, I spent considerable time observing and listening to Department Chairs and institute Directors in order to identify and analyze the organizational structure, interpersonal relationships, and critical social networks within the administration and physician leadership. This required travel to all outpatient sites and inpatient clinical units to make direct introductions and gain a situational understanding of the patients' needs and the system capabilities. I found it absolutely necessary to develop relationships with the Department Chairs and their clinical division leaders to determine their priorities, current limitations, and future aspirations. They perhaps best defined the "Gemba"—or the key place of value for both assessing and creating opportunities and resistance within departments [17–20].

Building on this foundation, the next phase of my work included designing and offering new or modified care delivery models to be presented to the relevant Chairs, Institute Directors, and the leadership group. It was clear that the ability to build and deploy cross-functional teams was going to be the most effective tool to break any detrimental patterns or broken processes. Consensus across the stakeholders could only result from clarity of communication and well-coordinated systems in order to see any direct financial benefits and achieve diminished institutional and departmental stress [15]. I felt hopeful that smaller, initial tests of implementing these models would achieve wins that would encourage increased engagement, enthusiasm, and trust amongst the team.

As expected, later in the 100 days, the coordination and collaboration between team members emerged that, after a fair examination, needed to be addressed and celebrated. The strength of my role and my ability to build the trust required from the team for the long- term success of the position was based upon my ability to work with new colleagues and to protect the interests of the institution, the staff, and the patients that they serve. The use of an action plan proved essential in allowing me to identify the best resources for resolving conflicts and to solidify plans for better coaching of staff to ensure continued progression toward leadership roles and career development [21].

Finally, it was evident that my ability to plan and execute change management and other initiatives would rise from the personal vision that I would put together in the first 100 days and ensuring that this resonated within the leadership team. At the time I took my position, the team was trying to transition its image from that of an isolated academic medical center, focused solely on serving its immediate population, to a true regional contributor, as a health system with a credible approach to population health. Considering the medical center as a broader health system would only be achievable if we were ultimately able to demonstrate partnership with new affiliates and successfully integrate our strengths in order to overcome our weaknesses. It was foreseen that other specific outcomes would come from consistent delivery of leading clinical outcomes or research that yielded growing national recognition and advanced our tripartite mission of providing excellent clinical care, research, and training of the next generation of clinicians on behalf of our patients.

Getting to Work

Upon my recruitment, I was immediately faced with the realities of a new physician leader in a new position for the institution. The prior CMO had developed as a long-standing member of the Department of Medicine, where there had been positive elements of relational coordination, especially in terms of the relationship and communication with a strong Chief Quality Officer (CQO). There was an ongoing search for a new Chief Nursing Officer (CNO) that offered the opportunity for a dyad partnership that could examine together the needs for interdisciplinary work, support, and integration.

Through my first introductory meetings with the CEO, I expressed my desire to work only in a dyad model of leadership, uniting the roles of CNO and CMO to demonstrate to both clinical and administrative units that unity and collaboration in our work together could be modelled at any point of care [22]. I was asked to join the search committee for the new CNO and help influence the Medical Center's choice for a leader that would be able to reverse the prior setbacks and vacancy gaps that they were experiencing, as highlighted by internal staff survey results.

Similarly, according to discussions with executive leaders, the prior CQO had a close relationship with and was highly respected by the Dean as a result of projects that had impacted the College of Medicine. However, this individual had very weak coordination with the external systems of care. In an effort to repair that deficiency, I was able to launch an immediate search for a new CQO who would report directly to me, and to whom I could provide clear direction to establish a broader focus on patients, rather than attention to just a limited set of goals and tactics that were pertinent to the institutional ranking. The new CQO was hired after having served in an accomplished quality role in a large academic children's hospital and was able to coordinate her reporting teams to have more expanded responsibilities and influence for both inpatient and outpatient care. This enabled the new CQO to extend the accomplishments in quality projects well beyond those for standard reporting and value-based payment.

Within the first 60 days of the plan, there was also the opportunity to transfer the Chief Medical Information Officer (CMIO) from the IT department to my team. The institution had committed to a major revision of the electronic medical record system due to sunsetting revenue cycle software and other data and informatics platforms that needed replacement or growth. These two institutional changes allowed me to gain insight into both finance and IT services, which were rapidly moving into system support structures, under a corporate services model. Understanding the strengths and weaknesses of each service would give me a greater credibility when responding to the needs of the clinical models of care that we might propose. With the CMIO as a part of my team, we were poised to be able to respond to several institutional process changes, including addressing issues that could potentially alter provider and nursing workflows, establishing much needed decision support to providers, providing meaningful data through informatics to both providers and leadership, and helping to reduce the time and documentation burdens that are a major source of staff burnout that plague all clinical providers and cripple productivity [23].

Furthermore, with the Dean's interest in Lean methods of business management and drive to continuously improve work processes, purposes, and people [18, 24, 25], a unit known as "Operational Excellence" had been developed in recent years to provide project management oversight. As I began to learn about that team, I found that they were largely poorly understood with variable connections and involvement with the major clinical units or the operational managers for the departments and clinical institutes. Drawing from my past experiences and my familiarity with Lean practices from working at a former institution, I requested a transfer of the small group to my team and rapidly established a senior management Steering Committee that could bring the capabilities and capacity to increase their exposure in the Medical Center and create buy-in for their engagement in a growing set of projects directly to them. This included projects such as cutting waiting times in the cancer center to reducing costs in the supply chain.

I insisted that we present the return on investment for each proposed project by the unit and then held monthly reviews with my co-leaders on the progress of each initiative and the financial results accomplished. We took advantage of every chance we had to present the successes of the unit to the medical staff and clinical leadership. Through these demonstrations of every tool that the team had, including the 5-S tool for Lean management [26] to full value stream mapping [27], we rapidly expanded the demand for all levels of Lean management education at the Medical Center, which was evidenced by the inclusion of Lean management education as a part of the health systems studies and required medical students and residents to have quality project portfolios.

However, along with the quick wins achieved through the few tactics outlined above, the best work emerged with the highest coordination between quality teams and Operational Excellence—a unit which was placed as a potential barrier to project engagement and initial consideration of projects. On the other hand, there were strong individual relationships between the Dean, Medical Group Chief Operating Officer (COO) (who also was a long-standing Chair), and the Hospital Executive Director, that provided a strong triangle of coordination in the Medical Center leadership that could be useful in opening doors to these teams.

Several discussions and observations with the Medical Group illuminated the relational barriers and distinctions between different units within the organization that they wanted to overcome and redesign. However, despite these relational and leadership challenges, cultural change in the organization was still possible. Through continued discussions and growing relationships between a group of four Medical Group Associate CMOs, the sources of the limited collaboration between units and an understanding of the potential of those opportunities emerged in the period after the first 100 days, opening new doors for change and perspective on the part of the Medical Group.

As CEO of the Medical Center, the Dean recognized that opportunities for the Medical Center to engage in mergers and acquisitions with other hospitals or healthcare systems were emerging, which would broaden the scope of the institution. His solution was to form a cross-functional group with a weekly round-table with the legal, finance, strategy, clinical, and operational leaders where he would be able to provide direction and receive advice. I was invited and encouraged by the CEO to become part of that roughly 9-member group, which gave me essential exposure to the decision-making mechanisms and divisions of power and responsibilities that were established between leadership units. This advisory board would become the key platform used by the leadership team for managing the advanced health system challenges faced by the institution and to build mergers and acquisitions, as this group was presented with the financial opportunities or implications for all these critical decisions. Robust market analyses were provided to the advisory board and strategic plans were then generated by the group, to be used as constant references for opportunities for growth and other regional partnerships with payors or provider groups and institutions. Although it might have initially been perceived to be well above the level of operations that the CMO would directly impact, being a part of this board offered me immediate insights into the executive culture, tolerance, and capabilities that formed the framework within which we needed to plan, execute and grow.

For the large groups of concerns that were within my individual responsibilities, such as institutional capacity and patient flow, discussions within my team and our first proposals for action were quickly launched and implemented. These quick transitions were made following a few key steps: for each key observation, solutions were proposed to provide structural support for the new recruitment or action in question and presented to relevant teams clearly and in relation to the highest goals of clinical processes. Ultimately, the work process to be considered was clearly articulated based on the best immediate understanding and the benefits that could be gained for the institution.

Reflections and Results

The success of my transition into the role of CMO within the context of cultural and institutional changes within the Health Center was based on the application of clear behavioral and management tactics and an understanding of good business foundations. Upon my entry into the position, it was necessary to move rapidly to initiate the three elements of fair process work, including engaging stakeholders, offering clear explanations of processes and goals, and setting clear expectations [15], in order to achieve my goals of finding and creating partnerships, building a team of direct reports, and positively positioning critical teams of influence [28]. These steps are summarized in Table 8.2, which outlines the main tactics that I used by the key elements of the first 100-day plan, along with the specific actions that I took to guide these processes.

Table 8.2 Tactics used in implementation of 100-day plan

Formal business foundations for understanding	Tactics used	Specific elements of this transition
1. Leadership foundations and organizational structure	• Build partnerships through engagement	• Joined search for Chief Nursing Officer (CNO) and CEO's health system roundtable • Acquired Chief Medical Information Officer (CMIO)
2. Expectation clarity in goal-setting and design	• Build a team of direct reports	• Recruited Chief Quality Officer (CQO), Vice President Of Operational Excellence, and Director of Care Transitions
3. Communication and explanation with the best immediate situational assesment and understanding	• Positively position critical teams of influence	• Elevated the presence and impact of Operational Excellence

Along with the introduction of a new CMO, the institution accepted the opportunity to recruit new executive leadership and other central roles for administrative coordination. A new Chief Quality officer and the acquisition of the employees in Operational Excellence brought a fresh start and alignment from which other collaborations and networks developed and were energized. With an new structure and leadership in Care Transitions there was an immediate connection into the traditional framework of hospital and nursing operations that brought not only a new model of care to support the clinical practitioners, but also it gave a dramatic financial advantage to Utilization management and patient flow throughout the acute and chronic care settings.

In addition to these structural enhancements, there was a better understanding of the positive new work processes and relationships between individuals and teams. My engagement with the various Medical Center leaders and teams through frequent communication for collective problem-solving and the exploration of ideas that took place in the first 100 Days of my new role as CMO narrowed the gaps that had developed in the past and were potentially detrimental to future programs. The application of this relational coordination was essential to augment or alter the paths of communication and coordination within the organization that mirrored those of traditional siloed healthcare environments. This also placed relationships at the center of our immediate and future communication strategies in ensuring that communication took place with the appropriate frequency, accuracy, timeliness, and problem-solving value [16].

The work to reinforce relationships not only helped to remove relational barriers between units, but also helped allow for mutually agreed upon performance outcomes. This permitted a better collective identity that enabled work to be coordinated more effectively. Additionally, by recognizing spaces for conflict between individuals and groups early on, and by applying relevant action plans to remedy these conflicts in a timely manner, my team was able to avoid the potential creation of damaging animosity within the team.

The creation and positioning of the Operational Excellence team also proved to be an essential step in establishing leadership and creating structures for sustaining the positive changes. The Operational Excellence unit became one of the central elements of the Medical Center leadership. After the first 100 days in my position, Operational Excellence became seen as the core of the cross-functional teams that brought even more relevance to our dyad, presented new paths for collaboration, and provided evidence for the necessary efficiencies that would need to be implemented.

Together, these steps also positively contributed to the Medical Center's focus on quality and innovation. According to internal survey results of staff within department units, quality and innovation are now thriving and dyad models for leadership have been applied to all of the major operational units.

Conclusion

In the fields of business or medicine, the primary measurements of success for a new hire at the end of the l00 days period will always be the degree of successful engagement between that individual and the team, how effective they are able to perform internally with leadership, and how they are viewed externally to patients, providers and in terms of overall performance [29]. Changing the personality or structure to a certain position is simply not enough [30, 31]; the application of fair process pillars and attention to relational coordination are essential managerial and business tools for success. Building on this initial 100-day period, the successes and failures of the transition of a new CMO will largely be based on the ability to extend visible and tangible connections that reach out to the system leadership. Using this case based on my own experiences of transitioning into a CMO role at a hospital undergoing considerable organizational and structural change, this paper highlights how positive relationships within organizational units and leadership can be built through three key elements, including (1) creating strong foundations for leadership and structure, (2) providing clarity in terms of goal-setting and design, and (3) ensuring communication with the best immediate understanding within the first 100 days. These relationships and foundations of trust will hopefully take important shape in time beyond the critical impressions made in the first 100 days.

References

1. Greenspun H, Rowe C. The next generation of healthcare leadership: new demands in the shift to value-based care. Korn Ferry Institute; 2017. https://www.kornferry.com/content/dam/kornferry/docs/article-migration//HealthcareVBC_Summer17.pdf [Accessed 25 January 2021].
2. Angood P, Birk S. The value of physician leadership. Physician Exec. 2014;68(6):152.
3. Schreiber L. Leading from the top—Chief Medical Officers and Their Leadership Styles. In: Leadership in Healthcare and Public Health. The Ohio State University Pressbooks; 2018. https://ohiostate.pressbooks.pub/pubhhmp6615/chapter/leading-from-the-top-chief-medical-officers-and-their-leadership-styles/ [Accessed 25 January 2021].
4. Hargrove R. Your first 100 days in a new executive job: powerful first steps on the path to greatness. 4/20/11 edition. Boston, MA: CreateSpace Independent Publishing Platform; 2011.
5. History. Penn State College of Medicine. https://med.psu.edu/history [Accessed 25 January 2021].
6. Healthcare. Penn State University. https://www.psu.edu/healthcare [Accessed 25 January 2021].
7. Federal Trade Commission and Commonwealth of Pennsylvania, Plaintiffs-Appellants v. Penn State Hershey Medical Center and PinnacleHealth System, Defendants-Appellees. 2016. https://www.ftc.gov/enforcement/cases-proceedings/141-0191-d09368/penn-state-hershey-medical-center-ftc-commonwealth [Accessed 25 January 2021].
8. Schieffler DA, Farrell PM, Kahn MJ, Culbertson RA. The evolution of the medical school deanship: from patriarch to CEO to system dean. Perm J. 2017;21:16–069. https://doi.org/10.7812/TPP/16-069.
9. College of Medicine Dean and Penn State Health CEO Craig Hillemeier to retire. Penn State News. 2019 Feb 2; https://news.psu.edu/story/560230/2019/02/21/administration/college-medicine-dean-and-penn-state-health-ceo-craig. [Accessed 25 January 2021].

10. Longnecker DE, Patton M, Dickler RM. Roles and responsibilities of chief medical officers in member organizations of the Association of American Medical Colleges. Acad Med. 2007;82(3):258–63. https://doi.org/10.1097/ACM.0b013e31803072fb.
11. Burwell SM. Setting value-based payment goals—HHS efforts to improve U.S. Health Care. N Engl J Med. 2015;372(10):897–9. https://doi.org/10.1056/NEJMp1500445.
12. Change and dynamic growth marks fiscal year at Hershey Medical Center campus. Penn State News. 2018. https://news.psu.edu/story/535938/2018/09/11/impact/change-and-dynamic-growth-marks-fiscal-year-hershey-medical-center. [Accessed 25 January 2021].
13. Lakdawalla DN, Doshi JA, Garrison LP, Phelps CE, Basu A, Danzon PM. Defining elements of value in health care-a health economics approach: an ISPOR special task force report. Value Health. 2018;21(2):131–9. https://doi.org/10.1016/j.jval.2017.12.007.
14. Silbaugh BR, Leider HL. Physician leadership is key to creating a safer, more reliable health care system. Physician Exec. 2009;35(5):12–6.
15. Chan Kim W, Mauborgne R. Fair process: managing in the knowledge economy. Harv Bus Rev. 2003; https://hbr.org/2003/01/fair-process-managing-in-the-knowledge-economy. [Accessed 25 January 2021]
16. Gittell JH. Transforming relationships for high performance: the power of relational coordination. Palo Alto, CA: Stanford University Press; 2016.
17. Chilingerian JA. Teaching surgeons how to Lead. In: Köhler TS, Schwartz B, editors. Surgeons as educators : a guide for academic development and teaching excellence. Cham: Springer International Publishing; 2018. p. 341–75. https://doi.org/10.1007/978-3-319-64728-9_20.
18. Toussaint J, MD. In: Womack J, editor. Management on the mend. 1st ed. Appleton, WI: ThedaCare Center for Healthcare Value; 2015.
19. What is a Gemba Walk and Why is it Important?. Six Sigma Daily. 2018. https://www.sixsigmadaily.com/what-is-a-gemba-walk/. [Accessed 25 January 2021].
20. About Catalysis. Catalysis. https://createvalue.org/what-we-do/about/. [Accessed 25 January 2021].
21. Patterson K, Grenny J, McMillan R, Switzler A, Maxfield D. Crucial accountability: tools for resolving violated expectations, broken commitments, and bad behavior, second edition. 2nd ed. New York: McGraw-Hill Education; 2013.
22. Baldwin KS, Dimunation N, Alexander J. Health care leadership and the dyad model. Physician Exec. 2011;37(4):66–70. http://www.lucereleadership.com/wp-content/uploads/2013/07/Healthcare-Leadership-Dyad-Model.pdf. [Accessed 25 January 2021]
23. West CP, Dyrbye LN, Erwin PJ, Shanafelt TD. Interventions to prevent and reduce physician burnout: a systematic review and meta-analysis. Lancet (London, England). Lancet. 2016;388(10057):2272–81. https://doi.org/10.1016/S0140-6736(16)31279-X.
24. Earley J. The lean book of lean: a concise guide to lean management for life and business. 1st ed. Chichester, West Sussex: Wiley; 2016.
25. George ML, Maxey J, Rowlands D, Price M. The lean six sigma pocket toolbook: a quick reference guide to 100 tools for improving quality and speed. 1st ed. McGraw-Hill; 2004.
26. ASQ. What are The Five S's of Lean?. Five S Tutorial. 2020. https://asq.org/quality-resources/lean/five-s-tutorial. [Accessed 25 January 2021].
27. ASQ. What is value stream mapping?. Value Stream Mapping. 2020. https://asq.org/quality-resources/lean/value-stream-mapping. [Accessed 25 January 2021].
28. Chappell RW. Secrets of a chief medical officer: what they didn't teach you in medical school but you wish they had. Physician Exec. 2004:30.
29. Stoller JK. Developing physician-leaders: a call to action. J Gen Intern Med. 2009;24(7):876–8. https://doi.org/10.1007/s11606-009-1007-8.
30. Kirschman D. Leadership is the key to chief medical officer success. Physician Exec. 1999;25(5):36. 39
31. Cors WK. The chief medical officer: a critical success factor. Physician Exec. 2009;35(5):60–2.

Part III

Value Creation in Health Care I: Improving Technical Outcomes and Patient Experience

National Surgical Quality Improvement Program (NSQIP) Improvements: A Case Study

9

Mark A. Talamini and Apostolos Tassiopoulos

Key Learning Points
- NSQIP results measure the surgical system, not the surgeons in the system.
- Key stakeholders range in authority from hospital leadership to frontline workers.
- Multidisciplinary change teams are needed for large policy shifts in matrix organizations.
- Quality of documentation determines NSQIP results
- Choose case sets to avoid risk when ramping up NSQIP.
- Invest time and resources into information technology services.
- Policy has unintended consequences.

Executive Summary

The national surgical quality improvement program (NSQIP) measures risk adjusted surgical outcomes at 30 days on a hospital basis. This chapter discusses an academic medical center in New York that elected to execute a broad strategy to improve NSQIP results. We established standardized reporting procedures aimed at aligning workflow to maximize NSQIP results for four surgical events: catheter associated urinary tract infections, prolonged intubation, surgical site infection, and perioperative myocardial events. This chapter further discusses the management strategies

---

M. A. Talamini
Northwell Health Physician Partners, Manhasset, NY, USA

Northwell Health, Manhasset, NY, USA

Zucker School of Medicine at Hofstra/Northwell, Manhasset, NY, USA

A. Tassiopoulos (✉)
Division of Vascular and Endovascular Surgery, Department of Surgery, Stony Brook University Hospital, Stony Brook, NY, USA
e-mail: apostolos.tassiopoulos@stonybrook.edu

that we used to operationalize these changes in the hospital. This study found that outcomes were not significantly improved after 1 year despite substantial support from leadership. To course correct, we instituted a dashboard analytic system that allowed us to iterate according to real time results.

Introduction

New focus and attention has been paid to surgical quality. Led by government, payers are shifting reimbursement models, both for hospitals and doctors, from fee for service or bundled payments, to payment for quality [1]. The big question is how quality will be defined moving forward. The American College of Surgeons judged that defining quality and being the steward of surgical quality measurement in the US is vital to the successful management of patients by surgeons in America [2]. Who better to define surgical quality and outcomes than the national leaders of Surgery [3]?

The National Surgical Quality Improvement Program (NSQIP) is a risk adjusted outcomes method offered by the American College of Surgeons with a subscription framework financial mode [4]. Participating hospitals must meet a set of criteria, including hiring RN's who abstract charts according to strict protocols and who contact patients for quality improvement surveys by phone at 30 days for an independent assessment. Hospitals are measured against one another, creating one source of potential error bias. Interestingly, preliminary results indicate that there is no difference between hospitals that choose to participate in NSQIP and hospitals that do not participate [5, 6].

NSQIP uses risk adjusted data to create an observed to expected (O/E) ratio for each risk category. Then for each category the program orders all participating hospitals into deciles of performance as compared to the total group of participating hospitals. If a hospital's performance is considered to be statistically better or worse than the mean of hospitals for that measure, that difference is indicated. The comparative and risk adjusted data is not available for 6 months because all data sets must be submitted before this detailed analysis is complete. Data is further delayed by the fact that the quality measurement program requires each unit of analysis to have thirty consecutive days of data.

Our hospital had been a participant with NSQIP for about 10 years upon the initiation of this project. For us, participating meant hiring nurses and other personnel to abstract data from charts according to specific criteria, working the sampling methods, obtaining patient follow-up data, and interfacing with the American college NSQIP organization. Over those 10 years, and particularly in recent years, the results have been unimpressive. Among other reasons, this posed a problem for our hospital because; (1) The department's slogan is "innovation and excellence", (2) As payment shifts towards outcomes, these results become a financial liability for the organization in contract negotiations, and (3) Public reporting of NSQIP results was imminent. Poor results were slated to become a public relations issue. It was this project's goal to improve the NSQIP outcomes measures for the Hospital. This objective was, and still is, important to the strategic goals of the Medical Center, the School of Medicine, and the Department.

We sought to address the unimpressive surgical outcomes as measured by NSQIP for the hospital. The quality of care issue negatively affected patients, providers and support staff in many ways. It directly affected the morale of the workforce, particularly the surgeons, as many assumed that they were the "problem". Addressing and fixing this problem required resources. The financial aspects of the problem loomed large, as all contract negotiations on both the professional and medical center sides included quality measures as a part of the reimbursement scheme. To the extent that improving NSQIP results required less variability, some efficiency could be improved. However, quality improvement was sometimes at odds with efficiency and time considerations, as is the case in operating room turnover or start times. These cases of competing interests posed a problem for getting approval from management.

Conceptual Framework

The hospital invested significant resources and over a year of time to understand the NSQIP results and the issues that make improving these results challenging. Poor NSQIP results have a number of possible components. Since it is a risk adjustment, data collection methods and the specific phrasing used is critical to maximize results. The outcomes data obtained does not measure surgical skill alone, or even necessarily in large part. It measures the effectiveness of the whole system. We categorized issues into surgical practice state, and risk adjustment data collection and assessment goals, shown in Fig. 9.1. Items in the surgical practice state are hypothesized to predict meeting the NSQIP data collection and assessment goals.

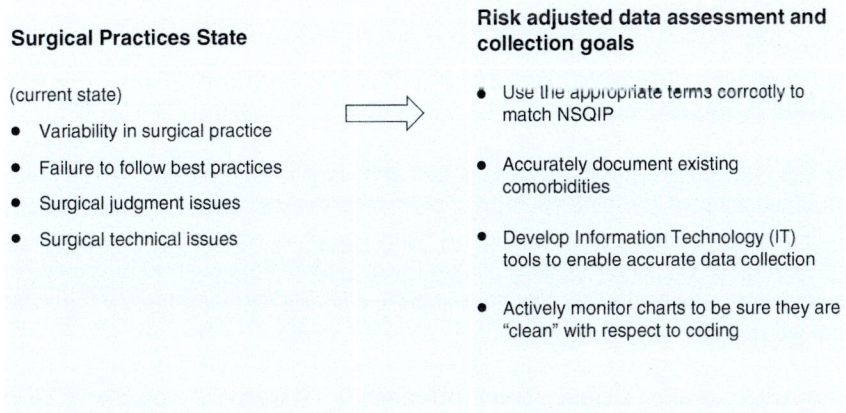

Fig. 9.1 Surgical practices state and data collection and assessment goals

As we analyzed this data, we found that a small set of poor patient outcomes disproportionately impacted our results. In other words, patients with very high risk were often flagged for multiple events, such as peri-operative myocardial events, prolonged intubation, surgical site infection, catheter associated urinary tract infections (since they have catheters for a long time), and mortality. This dramatically impacted the outcomes numbers in many categories. We also realized that attempting to directly impact overall mortality or morbidity (both measures in NSQIP) would be nebulous and difficult. On the other hand, directly affecting specific flags, such as surgical site infection or prolonged ventilation, was a strategy that was actionable. Patients at high risk for morbidity and mortality tended to also be most vulnerable to problems with these "sub-categories" of outcomes. This led to the hypothesis that Impacting a focused set of NSQIP outcomes elements that are actionable and achievable will improve all NSQIP results.

The hypothesized benefits of improvements in these discrete categories are many, and include; (1) Demonstration to the surgeons that if they focused on specific goals they would succeed (something that sets them up for further quality achievements); (2) Improving other surgical outcomes; (3) Providing an opportunity to understand the details of data elements, collection systems using information technology, and our early warning system. Considering ways to design the delivery system to address these elements provided the opportunity to build a system to continuously improve the NSQIP outcomes.

Methods

We started by taking the time to understand how NSQIP actually worked. This helped us to identify factors that negatively affected our current results. We then developed a five step plan to improve results: (1) choose areas of focus, (2) determine steps to address each area of focus, (3) put information technology mechanisms in place to enable change, (4) align incentives with stakeholders, (5) Put tools in place for real time and mid-term monitoring.

Outlier Analysis

We used outlier analysis to determine our strategy for this program. We carefully examined each of the patients with a poor outcome and found critical patterns. Outlier analysis led us to our strategy of focusing upon four areas that would make a difference in the larger general outcomes categories. This method informed our intervention, which addressed the four identified clinical events using the following strategies:

Catheter Associated Urinary Tract Infection [7] (1) Reduce the number of Foley catheters placed in the operating room; (2) Create an automatic Foley catheter removal order for all patients at 48 h; (3) Educate nursing floors on the correct management of Foley catheters (collection bag not placed on the floor, not hung from the top of a wheelchair, etc.); (4) Minimize placement variation by mandating placement by OR nurses in pairs following training.

Prolonged Intubation/re-Intubation (1) Create a mandatory electronic medical record data entry for every re-intubation following surgery to increase awareness and gather data; (2) Communicate to surgical faculty to not push for extubation in the operating room when Anesthesia advises otherwise; (3) Move away from a culture of waiting until the following morning to extubate rather than at night; (4) Provide a dedicated set of respiratory therapists in the surgical intensive care unit to develop unified protocols; (5) Encourage anesthesia to limit fluids and use twitch monitors to titrate paralytics.

Surgical Site Infections [8] (1) Ensure correct wound classification at the OR debrief time out; (2) Establish wound infection protocols for all bowel surgery cases (double gloving, wound protectors, changing instruments at closure, etc.); (3) Establish departmental wound management policy; (4) Have all patients undergo Hibiclens washing/showering preoperatively.

Peri-Operative Myocardial Events [9] (1) Establish heart associated risk screening tool to be used for adult pre-operative patients; (2) Patients who screen positive are assessed by appropriate cardiologists for risk mitigation; (3) Establish Information technology tools to enable application of established protocols for DVT/PE prophylaxis and management of anticoagulants (aspirin, Plavix, etc.) prior to surgery.

Change Management

We formed an initial team that included a surgeon champion, NSQIP nurses, IT specialists and the existing quality management structure. This set the course for a new quality management structure that focussed on improved NSQIP outcomes. A smaller executive steering team was also put in place consisting of the department chair, the physician team leader, a surgical quality improvement nurse, and a NSQIP/decision support nurse. These were representatives of all relevant stakeholder groups.

The hospital agreed to support the department financially for quality outcomes. They committed to a 20% improvement in NSQIP results. The departmental meeting structure included a three-hour faculty retreat to focus on NSQIP results and plans, as well as numerous grand rounds and shorter faculty meetings that were designed to get the faculty to provide ideas and build buy-in.

Stakeholder awareness was established through frequent communication. Three brief conceptual messages from the chairman were effectively delivered. In the first person, they were as follows:

1. "I don't know about you, but I have no interest in working in a center with poor quality surgical outcomes"
2. "I know the surgery world. You guys are not poor performing surgeons"
3. "No one wants to bring their relative to a hospital for surgery with nationally benchmarked poor outcomes"

We established two full time nurse equivalents (FTE) dedicated to independent data collection that can be audited by the American college of surgeons. Additionally we recruited a nurse to identify cases and act in real time to fix documentation or care issues, establishing an early warning system.

NSQIP results are reported on a semi-annual and annual basis depending on the clinical metric. This study compared baseline results to the results 1 year after the start of the project using a quasi-experimental pre/post study without a control group.

Results

With the support of leadership we were able to dedicate the resources needed to implement the three new nursing positions. This made it possible to successfully ramp up NSQIP documentation.

Changing the institutional culture, however, proved much more difficult. We observed that many staff members were dug in, and unwilling to adopt the new strategies for familiar procedures. We experienced difficulty reducing variation in methods used for the procedures in question, which was reflected in the NSQIP ratings.

NSQIP ratings after the first year were not significantly improved from baseline. The second round of NSQIP results were not yet available at the time this study was published.

Discussion

The lack of positive results after the first year was frustrating, demoralizing, and strategically risky. A lot of investment by the department and the organization in terms of both time and resource had been poured into NSQIP, and it didn't appear to be working. We regrouped, dug deeper, and examined the factors that inhibited programmatic success.

Lessons for Changing NSQIP Ratings

Balanced Feedback Loop A huge challenge in this program was the disconnect between actual practices and results both in terms of time and transparency. This was true for three reasons; (1) The nationally risk-adjusted data was not available until 6–12 months after the actual cases have taken place; (2) When caring for a patient it was not known whether the patient would be included in sample that is observed for NSQIP; (3) Lack of pre-intervention data meant that we had no idea how the program nurses were evaluating charts and grading them prior to lock down and submission.

Based upon these facts, we knew we needed to create a system to understand in real-time which patients were at risk of being poor outcomes from a NSQIP Point of view. With the identity of these patients in hand, we needed a system to take immediate action either to alter care plans and/or maximize the effectiveness of documentation to bring about the best NSQIP results. We employed a dashboard analytic tool that gave us feedback in real time.

Importance of Information Technology The most critical resource we harnessed after receiving poor results was the full attention of our information technology specialist on a weekly basis in the "war room". This is where the dashboard application was conceived, designed, and implemented. Absent this bespoke information technology that fed back results, or something like it, we would have had no chance of iterating for success because of the excessively long lag time between key surgical events and the downstream outcome metrics.

Choose Case Sets to Avoid Risk when Ramping up NSQIP This was more complicated. Beyond the required small set of sampled cases, each institution was instructed to choose a set of case types to focus upon. At initiation (prior to my arrival) the institution had chosen a set of cases that have frequent complications (colorectal, pancreatic, esophageal). NSQIP is officially a risk adjustment methodology, so strictly speaking it should not have mattered. But the risk adjustment was not sufficient to manage this case load. Realizing this, we readjusted our sampling methodology. We would not see the results of these two actions for another 6 months, but we believed these changes would make a huge difference.

Quality of Documentation Determines NSQIP Results Initial investigations into why results were less than desirable quickly taught us that record keeping was the main issue. In order for NSQIP to be reliable, the rules regarding documentation must be strict. It is the only program in the surgical world that insists upon 30 day follow-up with patients, either via a clinic visit or a phone call. It has a rigorous and complex sampling methodology. The NSQIP data collection nurses are paid by the hospital, but they are very clearly instructed to not be influenced by the local surgeons, and to exhaustively follow the NSQIP rules. If "demand ischemia" is written in the chart, the patient will be scored with a perioperative myocardial event, whether or not they were eventually shown to have had a myocardial infarction or not. In academic medical centers, where a lot of people write in the chart (medical students, residents, nursing students, etc.) there is a greater chance of someone using such a phrase than a private hospital where all of the notes are confined to fewer caregivers. This is one reason that non-academic smaller hospitals can do better with NSQIP.

NSQIP Results Measure the Surgical System, Not the Surgeons in the System A false assumption is that the National Surgical Quality Improvement Program (NSQIP) measures what surgeons do in the operating room. The assumption is that surgeons who cut and sew well will have good NSQIP numbers and those who don't cut and sew well won't. Nothing could be further from the truth. Cutting and sewing well in the operating room is certainly necessary for good results, but unrelated to the surgical structure imposed by the NSQIP framework.

NSQIP Was Not the Only Quality Improvement Project An obstacle that is generalizable to all quality improvement efforts at our hospital came from the competition within the department for quality improvement resources. In our hospital there was an alphabet soup of quality programs all vying for resource and leadership attention. This was true at baseline, but was particularly true when a new quality initiative was proposed. Ultimately this taught us to be discerning about rollout of the quality improvement initiative.

Tackling a Large Policy Shift in a Matrix Organization Means Building Consensus and a Multidisciplinary Change Team The chairman of the department of surgery and chief of surgical services for the hospital does not have authority and control over all of the formal and informal networks in the organization. For example, floor nurses, and even the OR nurses, would not say that they work for the chief of surgical services, but rather for their nursing supervisors and head nurses. A big accomplishment such as improving NSQIP outcomes can only happen by building consensus that the goal is worth pursuing, and by creating a team with influence among all these groups.

Stakeholders important to adoption of NSQIP at the institution included surgeons, anesthesiologists, OR nurses, recovery room nurses, floor nurses, and information technology personnel. It was further beneficial to get buy in from respiratory therapy, transport, and data analysis personnel.

Policy Has Unintended Consequences Every major policy shift brought unintended consequences. A morbid example of policy not matching reality occurred when policy directed providers to not operate upon very high-risk patients who had no chance of survival. This strategy might have yielded higher NSQIP scores and potentially even been the more efficient action, but in some cases following this policy meant directly contradicting the expectations of the patient and their family which did not sit well with our staff.

Lessons for Leadership

Team Management and Physician Bias I would rather avoid conflict, but have learned that when it is necessary to confront a problem it is best done early rather than late. We discovered a strange dynamic where the hospital-based personnel seemed reluctant to share data with the surgeon leader and myself. Upon investigation, I learned that this was not a new phenomenon in the organization. A decade ago, an incident occurred where we believed that physicians were inappropriately impacting outcomes data. As a result, the hospital created a system in which quality data was collected, interpreted, and reported by the hospital without input from physicians or physician leadership. As a result, the NSQIP data was being "locked down" and submitted without the opportunity for review by the NSQIP surgeon team. This was clearly a major problem. We worked with hospital leadership to convince them that we would not see success without altering this dynamic with the establishment of effective, trusting team relations between hospital quality functionaries and physicians. We had a number of team meetings in which we worked out protocols that would both protect the integrity of the data and allow informed surgical input prior to submission. Some members of the team were replaced. Other established team members were led to understand the importance of transparent teamwork for success.

Motivation and Getting Results Motivation and vision casting are necessary to generate faculty "buy in". Many surgical faculty in our hospital had become numb and willing to accept marginal results. They had been in the program for many years with such results. Others were unaware of the poor ratings.

Motivation began with joint surgery and anesthesia grand rounds in which the results were clearly presented. The communication, in paraphrase, was as follows: "I don't want to work in a place with less than ideal NSQIP surgical results, and I don't think you want to either. I don't believe the numbers reflect who we are. I work in the operating room with all of you, And I know this to be true. In fact I believe we have one of the best surgical faculty groups in the country, but we currently are unable to prove it with our NSQIP outcomes measures. Very soon these outcome measures will be publicly reported. We must band together and create a plan to fix this." This was the theme of our communication strategy, which was supported by continually feeding back results.

Project Management A project management structure was necessary to initiate a culture of continuous improvement. An institution-wide quality meeting structure already existed that was co-opted to be the main vehicle for project management. All of the key stakeholder groups were part of this quality meeting structure (surgeons, nurses, anesthesiologists, administration). To maximize the effectiveness of this monthly meeting, we established an executive planning meeting 1 week prior to the main meeting to maximize the effectiveness of the main meeting. In this preplanning meeting, we established goals, timelines, and previewed results. This drove continuous progress for our overall effort.

Managing Interpersonal Dynamics A dynamic quickly emerged in which our surgeon leader felt some of the other team members were not giving sufficient priority to the program. This likely was true, as these other team members had multiple responsibilities and in general were overloaded by other projects. The hospital team members countered that the surgeon leader was not sufficiently available for successful team functioning. This established a culture of finger pointing without addressing the underlying issue of time constraint. I worked with hospital management to ensure sufficient attention from hospital team members. We then had several team meetings in which we discussed the issue and developed time management strategies.

Leadership Alignment The organization needed to be convinced that surgical outcomes were worth additional investment. Leaders wanted information about why this project needed to stand apart from the sea of shifting quality priorities. During this time frame the organization was assailed (along with all New York hospitals) with regulatory visits for all sorts of issues. It was the "summer of regulatory storm". At this time the contracting team was being asked by third-party insurers how the organization could demonstrate Quality outcomes. Aligning this project with external pressures helped to convince the administration that improving these results was beneficial to leadership.

Communication Focused and sustained communication, both in terms of scope and audience, was critical to success. Communication was the oil that kept the change machine from seizing. Success depended upon continued multichannel communication. This was particularly difficult in a large matrix organization that tends to promote the "the issue of the month". For instance, in the middle of the NSQIP initiative, the organization began to emphasize, "Just culture", a critically important but distracting issue. We argued that the surgical faculty had only so much attention bandwidth to apply to performance improvement programs during any given season, particularly with their already-too-busy surgical practices. We found that persistent structured communication was a way to cut through the distraction. Communication flowed through several domains; (1) NSQIP issues were included in our morbidity and mortality conferences, (2) NSQIP results were published and posted every 6 months, (3) individual NSQIP results were fed back to the surgeons every 6 months, and (4) updates on the multichannel initiatives were presented at faculty meetings. Together these initiatives helped to communicate the goals and progress of the project to our team and the wider hospital community.

Conclusion

This chapter discussed strategies for diagnosing and improving specific NSQIP quality ratings for catheter associated urinary tract infections, prolonged intubations, surgical site infections, and perioperative myocardial events at a hospital in New York. Also included is a discussion of the management steps that were taken to shift hospital culture to adopt the new strategy to improve the NSQIP rankings.

This study found that NSQIP ratings did not improve after 1 year despite successful change management, substantial investment, and high levels of institutional support. In part these low scores were due to the fact that we were focusing on a set of cases that were prone to poor scoring even after adjusting for risk. A second factor that contributed to our poor performance was that we were unable to see the effect of our interventions on NSQIP ratings for 6 months or longer after the implementation of new policy. The delayed results from NSQIP made it difficult to iterate our strategies in a timely manner. We ultimately developed a dashboard application that helped us to track our results in real time. A last observation is that quality improvement ratings, like those found in NSQIP, measure the surgical system, which is slower to change than individual techniques or practices. We were asking our organization to perform a systemic shift, rather than change piece by piece. This effort took time and resources. A project like the one presented in this chapter should only be attempted by managers with high levels of patience and institutional support.

References

1. Linking quality to payment [Internet]. [Accessed 2020 Jul 7]. https://www.medicare.gov/hospitalcompare/linking-quality-to-payment.html.
2. Yount KW, Turrentine FE, Lau CL, Jones RS. Putting the value framework to work in surgery. J Am Coll Surg. 2015;220(4):596–604.
3. Ko CY, Hall BL, Hart AJ, Cohen ME, Hoyt DB. The American College of Surgeons National Surgical Quality Improvement Program: achieving better and safer surgery. Jt Comm J Qual Patient Saf. 2015;41(5):199-AP1.
4. ACS National Surgical Quality Improvement Program. American College of Surgeons. [Accessed 2020 Jul 7]. https://www.facs.org/quality-programs/acs-nsqip
5. Dahlke AR, Chung JW, Holl JL, Ko CY, Rajaram R, Modla L, et al. Evaluation of initial participation in public reporting of American College of Surgeons NSQIP surgical outcomes on Medicare's Hospital Compare Website. J Am Coll Surg. 2014;218(3):374–380.e5.
6. Etzioni DA, Wasif N, Dueck AC, Cima RR, Hohmann SF, Naessens JM, et al. Association of hospital participation in a surgical outcomes monitoring program with inpatient complications and mortality. JAMA. 2015;313(5):505–11.
7. Durant DJ. Nurse-driven protocols and the prevention of catheter-associated urinary tract infections: a systematic review. Am J Infect Control. 2017;45(12):1331–41.
8. Ban KA, Minei JP, Laronga C, Harbrecht BG, Jensen EH, Fry DE, et al. American College of Surgeons and Surgical Infection Society: surgical site infection guidelines, 2016 update. J Am Coll Surg. 2017;224(1):59–74.
9. Smilowitz NR, Gupta N, Ramakrishna H, Guo Y, Berger JS, Bangalore S. Perioperative major adverse cardiovascular and cerebrovascular events associated with noncardiac surgery. JAMA Cardiol. 2017;2(2):181–7.

Addressing America's Opioid Crisis through Community-Based Primary Care

Heidi M. Larson and Priya Agarwal-Harding

Key Learning Points
- Rates of overdose attributed to opioids climbed more rapidly in rural counties from 1999 to 2014.
- Since 2015, drug overdose rates have been climbing more rapidly in urban areas due to the presence of Fentanyl in the illicit drug supply.
- Deaths due to overdose continue to increase at a steady rate throughout the United States, posing a formidable threat to public health and safety.
- COVID-19 worsened social isolation and limited access to treatment, resulting in alarming increases in death from overdose, and reversing earlier gains that brought favorable trends in harm reduction.
- Community-based resources that address a wide range of public health crises—including food insecurity, lack of stable housing, poor access to health care, and weak educational support—can be leveraged to support efforts to reduce rates of drug overdose.
- Strong, community-based primary care networks serve as hubs for collaboration with all available resources within a given community.
- Successful communities will demonstrate tight networks of support that are centered on the needs of individual patients and their families.
- Funding that is specifically directed to support the development of collaborative networks will be necessary to change the course of the opioid epidemic.

H. M. Larson (✉)
Cape Elizabeth, ME, USA

P. Agarwal-Harding
The Heller School for Social Policy and Management, Brandeis University, Waltham, MA, USA

Background

America's opioid epidemic continues to spread across geographic and demographic boundaries [1]. One of the biggest health crises ever to strike our country, opioid abuse and its deadly consequences transcend all categories of geography, age, race, ethnicity, and socioeconomic class [2]. After achieving some degree of success in the treatment of overdoses with the widespread availability and use of Naloxone—a drug used to counter and reverse the effects of opioid overdose—in 2020 and 2021, death rates from overdoses are again spiraling out of control with the use of synthetic opioids such as Fentanyl [3]. Death from overdose is now the leading cause of death for American adults under age 50 [4, 5].

In 2021 there were 106,699 overdose deaths in the United States [5]. Rates of overdose due to Fentanyl roughly doubled year over year from 2013 to 2016, and since 2016 they continue to mount exponentially [6, 7]. The impact of the national opioid epidemic is felt equally in rural and urban settings. While rates of death from opioid overdose increased from 2007–2015 in rural areas, more recently, sharp increases in overdose deaths in urban areas have been seen due to more widespread availability of heroin and synthetic opioids [7, 8].

There is a strong link between opioid use disorders and poverty, inadequate insurance coverage, and transportation issues [9]. These social and economic stressors tend to be more prevalent in rural areas, leaving these communities more susceptible to opioid abuse and its devastating consequences [9]. Additionally, the existence of strong, broad social networks in small towns gives those in rural areas more opportunities to access drugs, including opioids [10].

Data from 2020 and 2021 suggest a surge in overdose deaths in the context of the COVID-19 pandemic [11]. Reported increases in overdose deaths in more than 35 states implicate social isolation, decreased access to treatment, economic devastation, and loss of health care coverage associated with COVID-19 [12]. COVID-19 related social distancing guidelines and reduced opportunities for treatment led many county Emergency Medical Services (EMS), hospitals, and police responders to predict overdose rates that surpassed those of 2019 by more than 30% [11, 13].

Many people who suffer from addiction acknowledge a first exposure to opioids through prescriptions provided to themselves or those close to them [14]. Approximately ten percent of patients who are prescribed opioids for pain management are considered to be at risk for addiction [15]. In many cases, people misuse prescription painkillers by taking the medications in ways they were not prescribed, or by taking medications prescribed for another person [16].

Figure 10.1 shows the total number of U.S. overdose deaths involving prescription opioids from 1999–2021, including those from Methadone [7]. Although rates of overdose from prescription opioids have begun to level off since 2016, those who abuse prescription painkillers are at risk for using heroin due to its relatively low cost and high availability [17]. Additionally, due to the low cost of synthetic narcotic production, such as Fentanyl, these drugs are often added to heroin—many times without the consumer's knowledge [17]. As shown in Fig. 10.2, even a small amount of Fentanyl, when consumed, can be lethal [18]. Consequently, recent

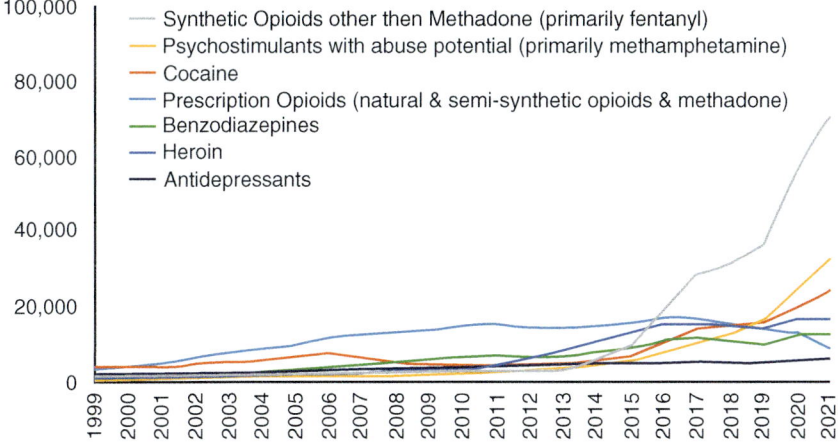

Fig. 10.1 Total Deaths in USA involving prescription opioids (1999–2021) [7]. Reprinted from National Institute on Drug Abuse. Overdose Death Rates. Trends & Statistics. 2023. Available from: https://www.drugabuse.gov/drug-topics/trends-statistics/overdose-death-rates. Originally from CDC/NCHS, National Vital Statistics System, Mortality. CDC Wonder. Available from: https://wonder.cdc.gov/ [19, 20]

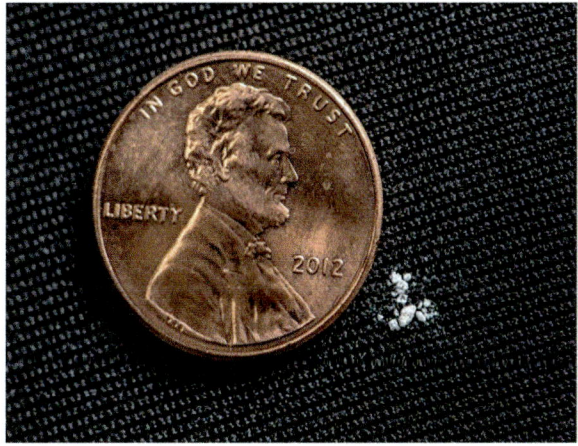

Fig. 10.2 Photograph Illustration of two milligrams of Fentanyl, a lethal dose in most people. Reprinted from PRISM, National Defense University. Comparison of a U.S. penny to a potentially lethal dose of fentanyl. (U.S. Drug Enforcement Administration). Available from: https://cco.ndu.edu/Media/Images/igphoto/2002090915/ [18]

increases in drug overdose deaths are driven by synthetic opioids, such as Fentanyl [7, 19].

A major barrier to the effective treatment of opioid use disorder in the U. S. is the high cost of treatment, especially emergency treatment. From 2001–2018, health care expenses linked to the opioid crisis exceeded $215 billion and continue to climb due to the cost of emergency treatment, including the widespread distribution and use of Naloxone, and inpatient hospital stays [21].

It is clear that what is required is a more comprehensive and community-based response to the crisis, focusing on prevention as a key strategy for avoiding opioid-related morbidity and mortality. Developing strong links between education, healthcare, community services, transportation infrastructure, first responder programs, mobile treatment centers, telemedicine support, law enforcement, and treatment centers is critical to the success of any opioid prevention and treatment program.

The United States Centers for Disease Control and Prevention (CDC) and other federal agencies have outlined a five-point strategy for coordinating efforts to fight the opioid epidemic [22]. The strategy brings together representatives from law enforcement, health care, public health agencies, and community partners to accomplish the following:

1. Improve access to treatment and recovery services
2. Promote use of overdose-reversing drugs
3. Strengthen our understanding of the epidemic through better public health surveillance
4. Provide support for cutting-edge research on pain and addiction
5. Advance better practices for pain management

Community-based primary care practices are uniquely suited to develop and sustain the collaborative approaches that are needed to deploy this strategy at the local level.

Approach

Synthetic opioids are now responsible for the majority of drug overdose deaths in the U.S.A [20, 23]. The convergence of the steady rise in drug overdose deaths due to synthetic opioids and the alarming increase in overdose deaths associated with the COVID-19 epidemic [12, 13] serve as a loud call to action for community-based resources to strengthen collaborative efforts to fight this crisis. A plan that is rooted in a well-organized primary care infrastructure will depend on strong team-based care principles and effective relationships between patients, families, and communities at large. Federal and state funding must be increased to support these efforts and identify creative new ways to collaborate and connect [12].

Community-Based Prevention Programs

The most effective means to address the opioid crisis begins with the development of a comprehensive, community-based prevention program [24]. These programs should aim to provide primary care that is patient-centered—care that is comprehensive, continuous, coordinated, connected and accessible [24]. Strong, community-based primary care enhances clinical quality through the delivery of coordinated, longitudinal care, and uses the approach to improve patient outcomes and reduce health care spending. The hallmark of effective primary care is the presence of close, trusting relationships with patients and their families [24]. Knitting together strong connections between primary care teams and their local resources allows communities to get at the heart of the problem and begin to solve the opioid crisis in a way that relies on evidence-based population health models [25].

Community outreach and education that supports families in understanding the impact of opioid misuse before it becomes a problem is critical to addressing the dangerous consequences of illicit drug use. Capitalizing on opportunities for community education by engaging children and families in places where they gather, such as schools, barbershops, bodegas, churches, Little League fields, dance recitals, rodeos, and county fairs, and soup kitchens is a particularly effective strategy [26, 27]. Working with trusted community partners has been proven to be especially effective for targeting treatment and outreach to communities of color and economically disadvantaged communities and addressing disparities in treatment and access to services [27]. Programs that engage workers in agricultural and industrial settings may be effective models for prevention, as well [28].

Widespread and comprehensive collaboration with stakeholders that are involved in combatting opioid use disorder—both within and outside of the health care delivery system – is an acknowledgement that opioid abuse is more than a health issue; it is a matter of economic opportunity and prosperity. Research has found associations between community prevalence of opioid use disorder and markers of economic opportunity, with those under the poverty line more than twice as likely to have an OUD than those over 200 percent of the poverty line [10]. This relationship likely worsens disparities in access to health care and treatment options in economically disadvantaged communities [10]. As such, collaboration requires the development of community-based monitoring, mental/behavioral health support, and medication-assisted treatment (MAT) programs [24]. Easily accessible prescription take-back and needle exchange programs, as well as first responder training programs that include education and support for Naloxone administration in the community, should be considered as part of a broader effort to support drug task-force and tactical response teams that operate within a broader public health perspective. Recruiting and training providers who are experienced in Buprenorphine/MAT and Naloxone administration is a priority [29].

Organizational leadership has a key role to play in the development of such programs and policies. For example, in some cases leadership may conduct annual substance abuse training on-site and require attendance as a condition of credentialing. In addition, institutions can develop policies and essential education and training programs for staff and providers. Medical staff meetings present opportunities to educate providers and encourage thoughtful discussion. Finally, primary care leaders can help build strong community partnerships that leverage a team-based approach to care that emphasizes prevention while determining appropriate treatment and monitoring options (see Chap. 11).

Pain Management Model

The development of comprehensive pain management programs that are geared toward entire communities should ensure that programs operate within the context of an efficient and effective primary care infrastructure. Proper stewardship of resources that are newly available to combat the opioid epidemic should be geared toward strengthening the primary care platform as a foundation, with the development and integration of a pain management program as a secondary strategy. This approach not only responds to the immediate crisis but provides for a more stable, integrated, and agile primary care delivery system in the long term– a cornerstone for preserving safety-net services to vulnerable and at-risk populations.

The administrative burdens of chronic pain management often become the responsibility of the primary care practice team [30]. Combatting this epidemic requires a team-based approach to providing efficient and effective care, including carefully-designed clinical protocols for the evaluation and management of chronic pain to be treated with opioid medications (see Chap. 11). Safe and effective opioid management requires that the following systems be put into place. Recommendations encompass four key components, including (1) prevention of substance abuse, (2) appropriate treatment options, (3) effective aftercare, and (4) long-term recovery management:

- Clear documentation of the need for pain management with opioids must include a thorough history and physical exam and regular follow-up assessments of pain status along with documentation of other treatment modalities being employed, such as physical therapy, acupuncture, massage, etc. [31].
- Factors potentially contributing to pain and imaging or other diagnostic testing should be addressed and reviewed from time-to-time as part of an ongoing evaluation of patient symptoms [32].
- Specialty consultation to assist in the evaluation and management of pain should be regularly considered by the care team [31].
- Enhanced screening tools such as the Opioid Risk Tool [14] should be utilized to assess risk for substance misuse or addiction.
- Prior to consideration of initiating opioid therapy, patients should be assessed carefully, and a policy of a 7-day maximum prescription of opioids should be adhered to for the treatment of acute injury/pain [33].
- Controlled substance contracts that clearly outline the indications for treatment as well as risks and benefits of opioid use, including but not limited to risk of misuse, addiction, and overdose should be used by providers [34].
- State Prescription Monitoring Programs should be verified regularly to ensure the patient's adherence to the controlled substance contract and to confirm that controlled substances are not being prescribed by multiple providers [35].
- Urine drug screening and pill counts should be carried out regularly to monitor patients for potential diversion or misuse [36].
- Common red flags of concerning behaviors for those patients of long-term opioid therapy must be addressed [37].

- Tapering protocols should be initiated, where applicable, to ensure the lowest effective dose of pain medication is utilized [38].
- Relationships should be cultivated between primary care practices and referral sources for the treatment of substance abuse, including MAT services for people with opioid use disorder and experts for behavioral health support (See Chap. 11).
- Access to training and support for primary care providers on prescribing MAT in their practices should be encouraged [39].
- Chronic care management protocols in critical access hospitals (CAHs), hospital-based practices, and community primary care clinics, including the application of enhanced communication techniques between different care settings and the use of warm hand-offs during transitions of care, can carry many positive benefits for patients and surround those with addiction with strong multidisciplinary supports on a regular and ongoing basis [40].
- Managing depression and anxiety among patients, where applicable, in the context of post-rehabilitative maintenance care is critical [39].
- Regular data monitoring and statistical analyses that ensure patient privacy are critical to better understand the patterns of substance abuse so that data can be funneled back into resources to further inform prevention strategies [22].

There are many programs that have been developed to educate prescribers around pain management and substance use disorders as well as safe prescribing and monitoring practices, which are largely responsible for the leveling off deaths from overdose around 2016–2017, as seen in Figure 10.1. Many states mandate prescriber education as a condition of licensure and work with the boards of registration and licensure to enforce continuing education requirements related to effective pain management; identification of patients at risk for substance use disorder; and counseling patients on the side effects, addictive nature, and proper storage and disposal of prescription medications [41]. These requirements are often promoted in the context of mandatory participation in prescription monitoring programs (PMPs) that are established by individual states [42].

Reducing Barriers to Care

Addressing social factors that create barriers to effective prevention and treatment programs for opioid misuse is a critical component of any program that seeks to engage communities around combatting the opioid epidemic. These barriers, such as stigma and lack of access and affordability of care contribute to underuse of treatment of OUD, with less than one-third of the approximately 1.7 million people with an OUD in 2019 reporting having received any treatment for substance abuse in the previous year [43, 44]. Poverty, transportation, poor or nonexistent insurance coverage, lack of access to primary care providers, low levels of education, a lack of safe and affordable housing, and food insecurity all hinder efforts toward effective education, prevention, and treatment for opioid use disorder [39]. As such, a review of collaborative efforts around the country reveals the following examples of how such barriers can be addressed successfully:

- Chicago-based Advocate Health Care developed a program aimed at reducing the burden of patient malnutrition, saving over $4 million in costs to the system by cutting readmission rates and shortening inpatient stays [45].
- Better Health Through Housing provides stability for chronically homeless individuals by moving them directly from hospital emergency departments in to stable, supportive housing with intensive care management [46].
- The National Farmers Union and the American Farm Bureau Federation teamed up to form the Farm Town Strong campaign to reduce the impact of the opioid epidemic in rural farming communities through advocacy, information, and resources [47].
- Transportation issues are being addressed by many organizations around the country by engaging ride-sharing services such as Lyft and Uber to ensure patients are able to attend appointments [48].
- Massachusetts pairs recovery coaches—people who have completed treatment for addiction themselves—with patients to support them through treatment programs [49].
- Many states have upgraded their PMPs to assist physicians with prescribing opioids and have restricted new opioid prescriptions to just 7 days [50]. Massachusetts reported a 30% drop in the number of opioid prescriptions after requiring doctors to participate in the state PMP in 2016 [50].
- Rhode Island expanded access to treatment for opioid addiction in state prisons [51]; other states such as Maine are leveraging expanded Medicaid funding to maintain treatment during periods of incarceration [52].
- Many states are funding programs based in the emergency department to allow immediate patient access to treatment with Buprenorphine to alleviate symptoms of acute opioid withdrawal [53].
- City health workers in San Francisco are offering MAT to individuals with opioid addictions who are homeless [54].
- Rhode Island integrated their PMP into a population health dashboard with predictive analytics tools to alert practice teams and allow them to gain more visibility into opioid use and potential misuse of prescription drugs [55].
- The Maine Diversion Alert Program (MDAP) mission is to address Maine's prescription drug abuse problem by providing access to drug arrest data for health care providers so they can identify and respond to patients engaged in illegal drug activities [56].
- Through the Consolidated Appropriations Act of 2023, passed by Congress in December of 2022, the Federal Government has removed the requirement for qualified care providers to have special waivers (X-waivers) for the prescription of medications to treat OUD, enhancing the ability of primary care to deliver MAT and facilitating access to treatment for those struggling with opioid addiction [57, 58].

It is unreasonable to expect that an individual community would have access to every type of program. However, community-based primary care teams can lead coalitions that identify local resources as they become available. Local stakeholders can collaborate to develop individualized patient treatment plans that lead to effective treatment and sustained recovery.

Discussion

As the examples of best practices above suggest, multidisciplinary approaches to the safe and effective treatment of chronic pain with opioids will assist in fighting opioid abuse, addiction, and diversion. Close collaboration with those involved in law enforcement, health policy, education, behavioral health, primary care, community services, and other leadership is necessary to reduce the impact of the opioid crisis across the United States.

Federal funding of $41 billion was appropriated to curb the opioid crisis in 2022 [59]. In implementing policies and programs with these funds, it will be critical to identify and connect local stakeholders in resource-starved areas. Although there may be a different mix of personnel available in a certain area from what is available in another, it will be important to leverage the passion and commitment of all available parties to achieve success.

Initial efforts to address the opioid crisis at the community level must involve developing and strengthening a consortium of stakeholders to address education, prevention, treatment, and/or recovery needs. As a first step, performing a thorough inventory of available resources in a given area will be crucial to reveal gaps that need to be addressed in order to optimize current strengths and identify vulnerabilities in existing service area resources. Studying successful models from around the country and adapting concepts to match local available resources is an important step in creating context-specific and comprehensive strategic plans and will allow community teams to add their own innovative approaches around education, prevention, treatment (including MAT), recovery services, and access to care identified in the analysis. Monitoring available data from prescribers, law enforcement, and emergency response personnel helps identify sources of diversion and misuse at a local level to build effective prevention strategies.

A strong primary care infrastructure is central to coordinating efforts around prevention, treatment, and recovery needs. Team-based models of care that incorporate care management functions from a wide range of providers that supply comprehensive and continuous care to populations of patients create sustainability for the consortium and its efforts (See Chap. 11). The core principles of team-based primary care can be adapted to suit the needs of the practice setting and, in turn, leveraged to address myriad social, public health, and chronic medical issues in the community. In this model, special attention to managing transitions of care across multiple settings, such as between primary care offices, addiction treatment programs, hospitals and emergency departments, schools, prisons, and other settings, will also be essential to the sustainability of the consortium's activities (See Chap. 11). Implementation of team-based primary care models that effectively manage such transitions across care settings may also help address issues of workforce shortages in the prevention and treatment of OUD [60].

Recent data has challenged traditional thinking about the duration of treatment for substance use disorder [61]. Those remaining in treatment programs for 6 months or longer, and sometimes even indefinitely, have a much better chance of complete recovery that those whose treatment is limited to 60–90 days [62]. States that have expanded Medicaid coverage have more resources to provide access to and financial support for sustained treatment programs [63]. Primary care teams that nurture trusting relationships with patients, families, and community stakeholders have a strong opportunity to provide the longitudinal support that is required for treatment and recovery efforts to be sustained.

In order to assess the impact of activities and help to direct further efforts, several quantifiable metrics can be employed. Beyond measuring the prevalence of opioid use disorders, the incidence of overdose, and the overdose mortality rate in designated areas, it is also suggested to study measures of economic growth and prosperity. Reduced rates of poverty, joblessness, and unemployment in communities, as well as reduced costs of treating newborn babies with withdrawal symptoms and/or those with Hepatitis C or HIV, are among some of the metrics that should be included in regular data monitoring, as part of a broader system built by a coalition focused on health equity-producing social policy.

Conclusion

The opioid crisis should be addressed in the context of a proactive, comprehensive, community-focused pain management program that is integrated seamlessly within the primary care delivery system. That delivery system must operate with optimal efficiency to create opportunities for high-functioning clinical teams to address the needs of the community. Collaboration across all treatment settings and disciplines, including health care, law enforcement, community-based programs, and public health, is especially important in addressing the rising economic and human costs of the opioid epidemic in America.

References

1. Hedegaard H, Miniño AM, Warner M. Urban–rural differences in drug overdose death rates, by sex, age, and type of drugs involved, 2017. National Center for Health Statistics; 2019. https://www.cdc.gov/nchs/products/databriefs/db345.htm. Accessed 7 Feb 2021.
2. Hampton C, Buckley J, Auld EM, Drewiske K. A nation in crisis: a health education approach to preventing opioid misuse and addiction (Policy Brief). Society for Public Health Education, Inc.; 2019. https://3gceqpmsn92j96fs3py0oq1b-wpengine.netdna-ssl.com/wp-content/uploads/2019/03/Policy-Brief-Heealth-education-and-opioids.pdf. Accessed 7 Feb 2021.

3. Wilson N, Kariisa M, Seth P, Smith IV H, Davis N. Drug and opioid-involved overdose deaths—United States, 2017–2018. Morb Mortal Wkly Rep. 2020;69(11):290–7. https://doi.org/10.15585/mmwr.mm6911a4.
4. Centers for Disease Control and Prevention. CDC's response to the opioid overdose epidemic. 2019. https://www.cdc.gov/opioids/strategy.html. Accessed 7 Feb 2021.
5. Underlying cause of death, 2018-2021. Centers for Disease Control and Prevention/National Center for Health Statistics; 2023. https://wonder.cdc.gov/wonder/help/mcd.html. Accessed 4 Mar 2023.
6. Hedegaard H, Bastian BA, Tinidad J, Spencer M, Warner M. Drugs most frequently involved in drug overdose deaths: United States, 2011–2016. Natl Vital Stat Rep. 2018; 67(9):1–14. https://stacks.cdc.gov/view/cdc/61308. Accessed 7 Feb 2021.
7. National Institute on Drug Abuse. Drug overdose death rates. 2023. https://nida.nih.gov/research-topics/trends-statistics/overdose-death-rates. Accessed 4 Mar 2023.
8. Murphy SL, Xu J, Kochanek KD, Arias E. Mortality in the United States, 2017. Centers for Disease Control and Prevention National Center for Health Statistics; 2018. Report No.: 328. https://www.cdc.gov/nchs/data/databriefs/db328-h.pdf. Accessed 7 Feb 2021.
9. Rigg KK, Monnat SM, Chavez MN. Opioid-related mortality in rural America: geographic heterogeneity and intervention strategies. Int J Drug Policy. 2018;57:119–29. https://doi.org/10.1016/j.drugpo.2018.04.011.
10. Ghertner R, Groves L. The opioid crisis and economic opportunity: geographic and economic trend. US Department of Health and Human Resources Office of the Assistant Secretary for Planning and Evaluation; 2018. (ASPE Research Brief). https://aspe.hhs.gov/system/files/pdf/259261/ASPEEconomicOpportunityOpioidCrisis.pdf. Accessed 7 Feb 2021.
11. Overdose Detection Mapping Application Program. 2021. http://www.odmap.org/. Accessed 7 Feb 2021.
12. Silva MJ, Kelly Z. The escalation of the opioid epidemic due to COVID-19 and resulting lessons about treatment alternatives. AJMC. 2020;26(7):e202–4. https://doi.org/10.37765/ajmc.2020.43386.
13. Hedegaard H, Miniño AM, Spencer MR, Warner M. Drug overdose deaths in the United States, 1999–2020. NCHS Data Brief, no 428. Hyattsville, MD: National Center for Health Statistics; 2021. https://doi.org/10.15620/cdc:112340.
14. Webster LR, Webster RM. Predicting aberrant behaviors in opioid-treated patients: preliminary validation of the opioid risk tool. Pain Med. 2005;6(6):432–42. https://doi.org/10.1111/j.1526-4637.2005.00072.x.
15. Carlson RG, Nahhas RW, Martins SS, Daniulaityte R. Predictors of transition to heroin use among initially non-opioid dependent illicit pharmaceutical opioid users: a natural history study. Drug Alcohol Depend. 2016;160:127–34. https://doi.org/10.1016/j.drugalcdep.2015.12.026.
16. Mars SG, Bourgois P, Karandinos G, Montero F, Ciccarone D. "Every 'never' I ever said came true": transitions from opioid pills to heroin injecting. Int J Drug Policy. 2014;25(2):257–66. https://doi.org/10.1016/j.drugpo.2013.10.004.
17. Cicero TJ, Ellis MS, Surratt HL, Kurtz SP. The changing face of heroin use in the United States: a retrospective analysis of the past 50 years. JAMA Psychiatry. 2014; https://doi.org/10.1001/jamapsychiatry.2014.366.
18. U.S. Drug Enforcement Agency. Comparison of a U.S. penny to a potentially lethal dose of fentanyl. https://cco.ndu.edu/Media/Images/igphoto/2002090915/. Accessed 7 Feb 2021.
19. Multiple Cause of Death 1999-2021. Centers for Disease Control and Prevention/National Center for Health Statistics; 2023. https://wonder.cdc.gov/wonder/help/mcd.html. Accessed 4 Mar 2023.
20. Centers for Disease Control and Prevention/National Center for Health Statistics. National vital statistics system, mortality. CDC WONDER, Atlanta, GA: US Department of Health and Human Services, CDC; 2023. https://wonder.cdc.gov/. Accessed 4 Mar 2023.

21. Altarum. Economic toll of opioid crisis in U.S. Exceeded $1 trillion since 2001. 2018. https://altarum.org/news/economic-toll-opioid-crisis-us-exceeded-1-trillion-2001. Accessed 7 Feb 2021
22. US Department of Health and Human Services. Strategy to combat opioid abuse, misuse, and overdose: a framework based on the five point strategy. 2018. https://www.hhs.gov/opioids/sites/default/files/2018-09/opioid-fivepoint-strategy-20180917-508compliant.pdf. Accessed 7 Feb 2021.
23. Centers for Disease Control and Prevention. New data show significant changes in drug overdose deaths. CDC Newsroom Releases. 2020. https://www.cdc.gov/media/releases/2020/p0318-data-show-changes-overdose-deaths.html. Accessed 7 Feb 2021.
24. National Institute on Drug Abuse (NIDA). Principles of effective treatment. National Institute on Drug Abuse. 2018. https://www.drugabuse.gov/publications/principles-drug-addiction-treatment-research-based-guide-third-edition/principles-effective-treatment. Accessed 7 Feb 2021.
25. American Academy of Family Physicians. Advanced primary care: a foundational alternative payment model (APC-APM) for delivering patient-centered, longitudinal, and coordinated care. 2017. https://aspe.hhs.gov/system/files/pdf/255906/AAFP.pdf. Accessed 7 Feb 2021.
26. Kasworm CE, Rose AD, Ross-Gordon JM, editors. Diversity of adult learning venues and collective endeavors, community health learning. In: Handbook of adult and continuing education. 2010th ed. Los Angeles: SAGE Publications, Inc; 2010. p. 300.
27. Substance Abuse and Mental Health Services Administration: the opioid crisis and the Black/African American population: an urgent issue. PEP20-05-02-001. Office of Behavioral Health Equity. Substance Abuse and Mental Health Services Administration, 2020. https://store.samhsa.gov/product/The-Opioid-Crisis-and-the-Black-African-American-Population-An-Urgent-Issue/PEP20-05-02-001. Accessed 6 Mar 2023.
28. Johns Hopkins Bloomberg School of Public Health. Making workplace health promotion (wellness) programs "work". Johns Hopkins Bloomberg School of Public Health. 2015. https://www.jhsph.edu/research/centers-and-institutes/institute-for-health-and-productivity-studies/ihps-blog/making-workplace-health-promotion-wellness-programs-work. Accessed 7 Feb 2021.
29. Ducharme LJ, Abraham AJ. State policy influence on the early diffusion of buprenorphine in community treatment programs. Subst Abuse Treat Prev Policy. 2008;3:17. https://doi.org/10.1186/1747-597X-3-17.
30. Polydorou S, Gunderson EW, Levin FR. Training physicians to treat substance use disorders. Curr Psychiatry Rep. 2008;10(5):399–404. https://doi.org/10.1007/s11920-008-0064-8.
31. Dansie EJ, Turk DC. Assessment of patients with chronic pain. Br J Anaesth. 2013;111(1):19–25. https://doi.org/10.1093/bja/aet124.
32. Turk D, Robinson J. Assessment of patients with chronic pain—a comprehensive approach. In: Handbook of pain assessment. 3rd ed. New York: The Guilford Press; 2010. p. 188–210.
33. Mundkur ML, Franklin JM, Abdia Y, Huybrechts KF, Oatorno E, Gagne JJ, et al. Days' supply of initial opioid analgesic prescriptions and additional fills for acute pain conditions treated in the primary care setting—United States, 2014. Morb Mortal Wkly Rep. 2018;68(6):140–3. https://doi.org/10.15585/mmwr.mm6806a3.
34. Deep K. Use of narcotics contracts. AMA J Ethics. 2013;15(5):416–20. https://doi.org/10.1001/virtualmentor.2013.15.5.ecas3-1305.
35. Green TC, Mann MR, Bowman SE, Zaller N, Soto X, Gadea J, et al. How does use of a prescription monitoring program change medical practice? Pain Med. 2012;13(10):1314–23. https://doi.org/10.1111/j.1526-4637.2012.01452.x.
36. Florete OG Jr. Urinary drug testing in pain management. Pract Pain Manag. 2018;5(3). https://www.practicalpainmanagement.com/resources/diagnostic-tests/urinary-drug-testing-pain-management. Accessed 7 Feb 2021.
37. Merlin JS, Young SR, Starrels JL, Azari S, Edelman EJ, Pomeranz J, et al. Managing concerning behaviors in patients prescribed opioids for chronic pain: a Delphi study. J Gen Intern Med. 2018;33(2):166–76. https://doi.org/10.1007/s11606-017-4211-y.

38. Murphy L, Babaei-Rad R, Buna D, Isaac P, Murphy A, Ng K, et al. Guidance on opioid tapering in the context of chronic pain: evidence, practical advice and frequently asked questions. Can Pharm J. 2018;151(2):114–20. https://doi.org/10.1177/1715163518754918.
39. Substance Abuse and Mental Health Services Administration (SAMHSA). Evidence-based Practices Resource Center. https://www.samhsa.gov/resource-search/ebp. Accessed 7 Feb 2021.
40. McLellan AT, Weinstein RL, Shen Q, Kendig C, Levine M. Improving continuity of care in a public addiction treatment system with clinical case management. Am J Addict. 2005;14(5):426–40. https://doi.org/10.1080/10550490500247099.
41. Wen H, Schackman BR, Aden B, Bao Y. States with prescription drug monitoring mandates saw a reduction in opioids prescribed to Medicaid enrollees. Health Aff (Millwood). 2017;36(4):733–41. https://doi.org/10.1377/hlthaff.2016.1141.
42. Federation of State Medical Boards. Continuing medical education board-by-board overview. 2020. https://www.fsmb.org/siteassets/advocacy/key-issues/continuing-medical-education-by-state.pdf. Accessed 7 Feb 2021.
43. Congressional Budget Office. The opioid crisis and recent federal policy responses. 2022. https://www.cbo.gov/publication/58532. Accessed 6 Mar 2023.
44. Novak P, Feder KA, Ali MM, Chen J. Behavioral health treatment utilization among individuals with co-occurring opioid use disorder and mental illness: evidence from a national survey. J Subst Abuse Treat. 2019;98:47–52. https://doi.org/10.1016/j.jsat.2018.12.006.
45. Sriram K, Sulo S, VanDerBosch G, Partridge J, Feldstein J, Hegazi RA, et al. A comprehensive nutrition-focused quality improvement program reduces 30-day readmissions and length of stay in hospitalized patients. J Parenter Enteral Nutr. 2017;41(3):384–91. https://doi.org/10.1177/0148607116681468.
46. University of Illinois Health. Better health through housing: improving the health of our community through housing and support. https://hospital.uillinois.edu/about-ui-health/community-commitment/better-health-through-housing. Accessed 7 Feb 2021.
47. Jerome A. Farm groups launch "farm town strong" campaign to address rural opioid epidemic. Farm Town Strong. 2017. https://farmtownstrong.org/2018/01/03/farm-groups-launch-farm-town-strong-campaign-to-address-rural-opioid-epidemic/. Accessed 7 Feb 2021.
48. Coutré L. Uber could improve access for addiction recovery. Modern Healthcare. 2017. https://www.modernhealthcare.com/article/20170726/NEWS/170729934/uber-could-improve-access-for-addiction-recovery. Accessed 7 Feb 2021.
49. Department of Public Health, Department of Mental Health. Bringing Massachusetts' recovery supports to scale moving towards a recovery-oriented system. 2013. https://www.umassmed.edu/globalassets/center-for-mental-health-services-research/documents/brss-tacs-.pdf. Accessed 7 Feb 2021.
50. Massachusetts Department of Public Health. MA prescription monitoring program county-level data measures (2017 Quarter 3). 2017. https://www.mass.gov/doc/prescription-monitoring-program-pmp-data-county-overview november 2017/download. Accessed 7 Feb 2021.
51. Green TC, Clarke J, Brinkley-Rubinstein L, Marshall BDL, Alexander-Scott N, Boss R, et al. Postincarceration fatal overdoses after implementing medications for addiction treatment in a statewide correctional system. JAMA Psychiatry. 2018;75(4):405–7. https://doi.org/10.1001/jamapsychiatry.2017.4614.
52. Russell E. "Time for our state to recover": Mills signs order to combat opioid crisis. Press Herald. 2019. https://www.pressherald.com/2019/02/06/mills-signs-executive-order-to-combat-opioid-crisis/. Accessed 7 Feb 2021.
53. Goodnough A. This E.R. treats opioid addiction on demand. That's very rare. (Published 2018). The New York Times. 2018. https://www.nytimes.com/2018/08/18/health/opioid-addiction-treatment.html. Accessed 7 Feb 2021.
54. Goodnough A. In San Francisco, opioid addiction treatment offered on the streets (Published 2018). The New York Times. 2018. https://www.nytimes.com/2018/08/18/health/san-francisco-opioid-addiction.html. Accessed 7 Feb 2021.

55. Bresnick J. Real-time ADT, PDMP alerts support population health in Rhode Island. HealthITAnalytics. 2018. https://healthitanalytics.com/news/real-time-adt-pdmp-alerts-support-population-health-in-rhode-island. Accessed 7 Feb 2021.
56. Piper BJ, Desrosiers CE, Fisher HC, McCall KL, Nichols SD. A new tool to tackle the opioid epidemic: description, utility, and results from the Maine Diversion Alert Program. Pharmacotherapy. 2017;37(7):791–8. https://doi.org/10.1002/phar.1952.
57. Rep. Connolly GE [D V 11]. H.R.2617-Consolidated Appropriations Act, 2023. 117–328 Dec 29, 2022. http://www.congress.gov/. Accessed 6 Mar 2023.
58. The White House. Dr. Gupta applauds omnibus appropriations bill that will expand access to treatment for substance use disorder. Office of National Drug Control Policy; 2022. https://www.whitehouse.gov/ondcp/briefing-room/2022/12/23/dr-gupta-applauds-omnibus-appropriations-bill-that-will-expand-access-to-treatment-for-substance-use-disorder/. Accessed 6 Mar 2023.
59. The White House. Biden-Harris Administration calls for historic levels of funding to prevent and treat addiction and overdose. Office of National Drug Control Policy; 2021. https://www.whitehouse.gov/ondcp/briefing-room/2021/05/28/biden-harris-administration-calls-for-historic-levels-of-funding-to-prevent-and-treat-addiction-and-overdose/. Accessed 6 Mar 2023.
60. McNeely J, Schatz D, Olfson M, Appleton N, Williams AR. How physician workforce shortages are hampering the response to the opioid crisis. Psychiatr Serv. 2022;73(5):547–54. https://doi.org/10.1176/appi.ps.202000565.
61. Fiellin DA, Schottenfeld RS, Cutter CJ, Moore BA, Barry DT, O'Connor PG. Primary care-based buprenorphine taper vs maintenance therapy for prescription opioid dependence: a randomized clinical trial. JAMA Intern Med. 2014;174(12):1947–54. https://doi.org/10.1001/jamainternmed.2014.5302.
62. Eastwood B, Strang J, Marsden J. Effectiveness of treatment for opioid use disorder: a national, five-year, prospective, observational study in England. Drug Alcohol Depend. 2017;176:139–47. https://doi.org/10.1016/j.drugalcdep.2017.03.013.
63. Sandoe E, Fry CE, Frank RG. Policy levers that states can use to improve opioid addiction treatment and address the opioid epidemic. Health Affairs Blog. https://www.healthaffairs.org/do/10.1377/hblog20180927.51221/full/. Accessed 7 Feb 2021.

Team-Based Care: A Foundation for Success in Value-Based Payment Models

11

Heidi M. Larson

Key Learning Points and Critical Milestones
- **Establish a culture that embraces change.** It is important for an organization to remain nimble and embrace new routines and iterations.
- **Co-location**. Temporary flow stations allow for enhanced communication and collaboration.
- **Pre-visit planning.** Proactive work allows patient visits to be more directed and efficient.
- **Morning huddle.** Identifying bottlenecks and slack points in the schedule helps the front desk to manage workflows.
- **Four stage office visit.** Reorganizing the workflow between physicians and nurses/MA's for the office visit facilitates a new structure that supports team-based care.
- **Utilize resources to troubleshoot.** Having personnel available from IT, Quality, Education, and Administration supports the team in its transition to the new model.
- **Flexible talent.** Emphasize hiring for attitude over aptitude, and recruit people who are interested in iterating workflow. Set the stage for exponential growth by developing team members that are able to mentor others and become team-based care champions for the organization.
- **Empower team members**. Solicit and incorporate regular feedback from practice leadership, providers, staff, patients, and families. Weekly team meetings, if not already established, present excellent opportunities for teambuilding and sharing. The most successful teams will encourage equal participation from all members of the team.

H. M. Larson (✉)
Cape Elizabeth, ME, USA

The Heller School for Social Policy and Management, Brandeis University, Waltham, USA

- **Humble inquiry.** Asking provocative questions like, "What's the rock in your shoe?" helps draw out reluctant players and empowers people to bring up concerns and propose solutions to common problems. Humble inquiry, where management is curious and asks staff questions about their work, breaks down power dynamics and allows the organization to function based on collective intelligence.

Executive Summary

Team based care is a novel approach to workflow optimization in health care delivery. This paper presents strategies for aligning the policy structure of an organization with team-based care in the primary care setting. Team based care requires changing four key components of the primary care practice. (1) Establishing a "flow station" on the floor that allows several providers and staff to meet away from patient waiting rooms and care areas, (2) allocating time to meet before each day to plan for care activities delivered in the visit, (3) having a huddle at the beginning of each day to identify bottlenecks and gaps in providers' schedules, and (4) implementing the four staged office visit that splits activities between the nurse or medical assistant and the provider, and engages the patient in medical decision making and education. We found that these changes, in conjunction with adjustment of existing policy measures surrounding workflow, have been shown to increase staff engagement, patient experience, and practice capacity.

Background

Healthcare spending in the United States continues to grow at an unsustainable trajectory. The United States spends more on health care than any other developed country [1]. Total Medicare costs are expected to grow from 3.9% of gross domestic product in 2020 to 6.0% by 2044 [2]. A recent report from the Medicare Trustees projects that the hospital insurance portion of Medicare will be depleted by 2026 [3].

Unfortunately, our health care investment is not paying off for us. Compared to other wealthy nations, the United States has higher rates of all-cause mortality and preventable death [4]. Our chronic disease burden is high, and our rates of hospitalizations for preventable causes surpasses that of other countries. We have lower life expectancies compared to our peers [1].

Patients in the United States have less access to primary care than many of the other OECD countries [4, 5]. Our support of a strong primary care infrastructure that is focused on prevention and effective chronic disease management is lagging. As a generation of baby boomers ages, further pressures on our already-strained delivery system emerge [6]. The critical shortage of primary care physicians will be amplified by increasing demands for cost-effective care. Fewer graduating students are choosing to enter primary care, opting instead for more lucrative careers in subspecialty care [7].

Currently, our investment in primary care practitioners is less than the mean of OECD countries [5]. Spending for primary care is 6–7% of the US spending on health care, much lower than the average of 14% for other wealthy nations [8–10]. Research has indicated a large return on investment when primary care investment is doubled from less than 5% to approximately 10–12% of total health care spending [9, 11]. Developing primary care delivery is on target with health care's triple aim [12].

Value-based payment models have been proposed to transform the payment and delivery system in this country using a market-based approach to efficiency [13, 14]. Reimbursement models that move away from fee for services, and towards a single capitated payment for a diagnosis incentivize the reduction of total cost of care through more thoughtful and judicious use of resources. We need to conserve the use of hospitals, which generate more cost in the United States as compared to other countries [15]. Primary care is one way to keep patients out of hospitals [16].

Increased investment in changing the payment structure of primary care can reduce overall health care costs [16, 10]. Commercial payers have established programs to incentivize quality and reward reduced costs in primary care [17]. The federal government introduced The Centers for Medicare & Medicaid Services (CMS) Primary Cares Initiative in April 2019 to drive value and results in primary care [16]. Direct Primary Care practices in New England are focusing on strong relationships with patients and families in order to deliver superior value [18, 19].

Team-based primary care, though not a new concept, involves building trusting relationships with patients, families, and communities at large to provide more comprehensive and efficient care that increases provider engagement and reduces burnout [20]. Care coordination is a key foundation for success in realizing the full potential of primary care [5].

The Role of Team-Based Care

A team-based model of care helps to shift responsibilities to make value-based care more efficient using several formulaic components [21]. Team based care makes it possible to shift activities like entering data into the electronic medical record or filling out forms that do not require medical expertise from physician's workload to other clinical staff, which can help to reduce burnout and decrease the cost of labor [22]. Registered nurses (RN), licensed practical nurses (LPN), and medical assistants (MA) share responsibilities of gathering data, reviewing approaching health maintenance due, and updating medication lists. This shifting of responsibilities has been shown to help providers to increase their patient panel size [23].

Physician-led team-based care engages all members of staff in direct patient care, affording providers (physicians, nurse practitioners, physician assistants) the time they need to listen, think deeply, and develop healing relationships with patients [20]. This strategy of emphasizing the physician-patient relationship has been associated with enhanced patient engagement, improved clinical outcomes and increased efficiency [16, 23].

By definition, a team-based model of care involves a high-functioning primary care practice whereby providers, support staff, patients, and caregivers work together to improve the health and well-being of a panel or population of patients while reducing reliance on sick or episodic care [24]. In the clinic, this involves co-location of the core team including physicians, RNs, and MAs, in a single place, what we call the "flow station", where patient requests are addressed directly and in real-time through verbal messaging and desktop management [24]. Innovations in workflow involve the whole team by embracing a proactive model of care, with pre-visit planning and the use of daily huddles. Support staff are empowered through the use of standing orders and expanded clinical protocols for panel management. Shared collaborative documentation, non-physician order entry, and streamlined prescription management have the potential to increase efficiency and help restore joy to the practice of medicine for the entire team.

In a team-based care model, patient service representatives (front office staff) are empowered to schedule patients directly and immediately. They are included in daily huddles and weekly team meetings, and they communicate directly with the care team at the flow station. Practice redesign does not usually require investment in more staff. Instead, changes in workflow and a strategic redistribution of work occur within the constructs of the established team. Starting with the end in mind and including the entire team in the redesign process contributes to the sense of empowerment as the team is able to solve problems together in real time.

Management Methods

Four Core Principles for Team-Based Care

Four core principles are fundamental to the team-based model of care: co-location, pre-visit planning, the daily huddle, and the four-stage office visit [21]. Although these principles seem formulaic, they can be adapted over time to suit the needs of a particular practice. It is important to remember that this is an iterative process. Success depends on team members' ability to remain nimble and engaged. This allows the model to be fine-tuned on a regular basis.

Co-Location

Workspace redesign helps to accommodate changes in workflow associated with team-based care. A flow station must incorporate adequate space for each team member in a way that encourages direct collaboration throughout the day. The flow station space needs to be separated from patient waiting rooms and care areas to protect patient privacy. Designing a space that promotes collaboration while allowing for flexibility in personnel and workflows is essential as teams grow and adapt over time. Desks may be positioned at different heights and in various configurations to avoid a sense of crowding. Care teams have a greater chance of success if their space is designed to support frequent and timely communication according to the design elements laid out by McGough et al. [25].

Co-location allows the team to address the needs of patients and families in real time. Requests for prescription refills, referrals, same-day appointments, and routine paperwork can be handled by any member of the support staff, with provider input batched in between patient visits. This configuration lends itself to a flexible approach where feedback is exchanged regularly. The use of standardized protocols assists with efficient chronic disease management including organizing labs that are due, providing phone calls to check in, ordering medication refills, and disease-specific protocols for medication management by the RN in between office visits [26].

Pre-Visit Planning

Pre-visit planning supports a proactive model of care. Prior to the clinic session, usually the afternoon before, the team reviews the list of patients coming in to identify issues to be addressed in the course of the visit. These might include closing care gaps, such as colonoscopies, mammograms, and immunizations that are due. Whenever possible, orders are prepared and placed in a "pended" status in the electronic health record so they are ready for submission if the patient is amenable. Documentation received from other care providers is reviewed, and treatment recommendations placed in the electronic health record. Likewise, medication refills may be ordered during pre-visit planning sessions. All orders are placed by support staff using standardized clinical protocols and listed in a "pending status", ready for review and signature by the physician at the end of the office visit. This process helps the staff to ensure nothing is forgotten in preparing for the patient's visit and allows more time to listen to the patient's concerns at the time of the visit.

The Morning Huddle

Consistently holding a 5-min daily morning huddle with the entire care team, including front-desk staff, provides an opportunity for the team to check in with each other and make any necessary adjustments for the day. During this time, staff are asked to identify potential bottlenecks in the schedule, and 2–4 spots for same-day visits are communicated to the front desk staff in the morning huddle. This allows the front desk staff to assist with managing the schedule throughout the day without running back and forth to the flow station and distracting the clinical team.

The Four-Stage Office Visit

The office visit is divided into four stages [23]. In *stage 1*, the nurse or medical assistant documents the patient's concerns and uses standardized templates to record additional details through questioning. Next, they update medical, surgical, family and social histories. Health maintenance updates are reviewed, and immunizations administered and documented according to office protocols. Orders for any testing that were placed in the course of pre-visit planning are reviewed with the patient. Medications that are due for refill are highlighted for the provider to sign. The patient is given information about advance care planning, including how to name a health care proxy if one is not listed already in the record.

The nurse/MA steps out into the hallway to brief the provider before they re-enter the room together. For *stage 2*, the nurse/MA remains in the exam room during the visit, sitting at the computer and documenting findings in real time. The provider verifies the accuracy of the information collected by the assistant, asks more directed questions to clarify if needed, and performs the physical examination.

Stage 3 is for medical decision-making. The provider and patient formulate diagnoses and treatment plans together. The assistant records all diagnoses for the visit and enters any orders that require the provider's approval. This is an excellent opportunity to update the problem and medication lists, and also to complete Hierarchical Condition Category (HCC) coding for risk-adjustment purposes, with provider assistance [27]. The patient is invited to ask questions while the provider and assistant help to ensure the patient understands the results of the visit.

For *stage 4*, the provider leaves the room, spending a few minutes for careful review and editing of the visit note before signing off and completing the documentation for the visit. The assistant remains in the room with the patient, providing patient education, visit summary (if not accessible on the patient portal), referral and refill instructions. Follow-up visits are scheduled per established protocols. The provider moves on to a second exam room, where another clinical assistant has performed stage 1 of the visit, and the process repeats.

The Role of Medical Assistants and Nurses

Team-based care does not involve charting by traditional medical scribes. Instead, the process is more accurately viewed as a team "co-visit" with nurses and medical assistants managing preventive care and updating chronic illness management tasks. Clinical assistants begin to explore patient concerns and document in the electronic health record using pre-approved templates. Provider oversight of this process ensures careful documentation of clinical decision-making and accurate order entry. Notations made by assistants and physicians provide attestation so it is clear which parts of the documentation were provided by whom. Redesigned workflows encourage staff to contribute to direct patient care, expanding their experience compared to traditional practice models.

The Role of Good Data

Predictive analytics and risk stratification uncover current and future potential high-risk and rising-risk populations through examination of cost and utilization data. Aggregates from disparate sources like electronic health records, reference labs, regional health information exchanges (HIEs), registries, and claims data can be used to prioritize interventions based on chronic conditions, health status, and gaps in care. This has been done successfully in research organizations like those associated with Partners Healthcare [28].

Data must be presented to care teams clearly and succinctly for targeted, timely population health management efforts. Actionable information and decision support can be inserted directly into clinical workflows, informing care teams in real-time when new, community-based information is available. Technology can be used to support teams in providing the right care for the right patient at the right time; indeed, CMS is emphasizing the importance of strong data exchanges with other providers through application programming interfaces (APIs) and regional health information exchanges (HIEs) that make possible a transition from volume to value [29].

Advanced Team-Based Care Implementation

Team-based care is all about empowering teams to achieve a set of shared goals around managing total cost of care and improving clinical outcomes for patients. Once they have mastered the core principles of the model, teams may want to consider ways to leverage the model further by applying it to their own unique circumstances and existing protocols.

Assess Current Protocols

Team based care has the potential to work alongside existing protocols that were developed for specific clinics. Examples of such administrative protocols include patient notification of results, approaches to in-basket work, and the role of the front desk in direct patient care. Clinical protocols include those related to strep testing, urinalysis, glucose monitoring, blood pressure checks, and ear lavage. Practice managers and clinical teams can take a careful inventory of current protocols to ensure they are relevant; some protocols may need to be re-written to reflect the changes to policy that have been established under the team-based model of care.

With the extra time generated from team-based care, primary care teams are able to identify and reach out on a regular basis to rising risk populations. This creates the opportunity to build in behavioral interventions that prevent costly complications from chronic diseases. Care management that is embedded and integrated into the primary care practice team allows for closer communication with those patients and families that require additional support.

Findings about the Team-Based Model of Care

The author consulted on the implementation of several team-based care models in health care organizations across the United States. The following findings about the impact of this process were observed as feedback over the course of a six-month follow-up period after each implementation project. During this time, they spoke with providers over videoconference during monthly check-in meetings.

Provider Capacity

Broadly, implementations of team-based models of care were associated with increased provider capacity. Fig. 11.1 shows an example of the change in visit capacity with team-based care. We saw an increase in appointments from 16 to 24, representing a 50% increase in capacity. In addition, we heard that there was time for longer, more detailed visits with patients who need them. This figure shows that provider/patient time was optimized with more opportunity for discussion and personal connection.

An internal medicine practice in the Northeast experienced increased preventive care services, increased visit capacity, and enhanced care management activities within the first 6 months. They implemented universal PHQ-9 screening for depression at patient check-in, increasing documentation of screening from a baseline of 2–40% over the course of 3 months.

The practice experienced increased same-day visit access and a reduction in their appointment waiting list. This was associated with a 58% increase in their visit capacity in the first 6 months. The practice RN care manager is now embedded in their care team, attending pre-visit planning sessions and meeting in person with higher-risk patients at the end of their office visits, strengthening patient relationships and rapport. Her increased autonomy allowed her to develop a plan to divert patients experiencing exacerbations of chronic conditions from frequenting the emergency department to calling their care manager first. This gave their care team a chance to problem-solve with the patient directly.

A primary care practice in the Midwest developed a protocol for tracking and recording diabetic eye exam results by front desk personnel, with documented screening for retinopathy rising from 21% to 42% in the first 30 days of implementation. Similarly, a family medicine practice in the Southeast effectively doubled their rates of tetanus vaccination for the entire year within 30 days of making a few simple changes to their workflow. Several teams based in the same multi-specialty health system noted an immediate reduction in call volume and in-basket work with a more hands-on approach that resulted from implementation of the team-based model.

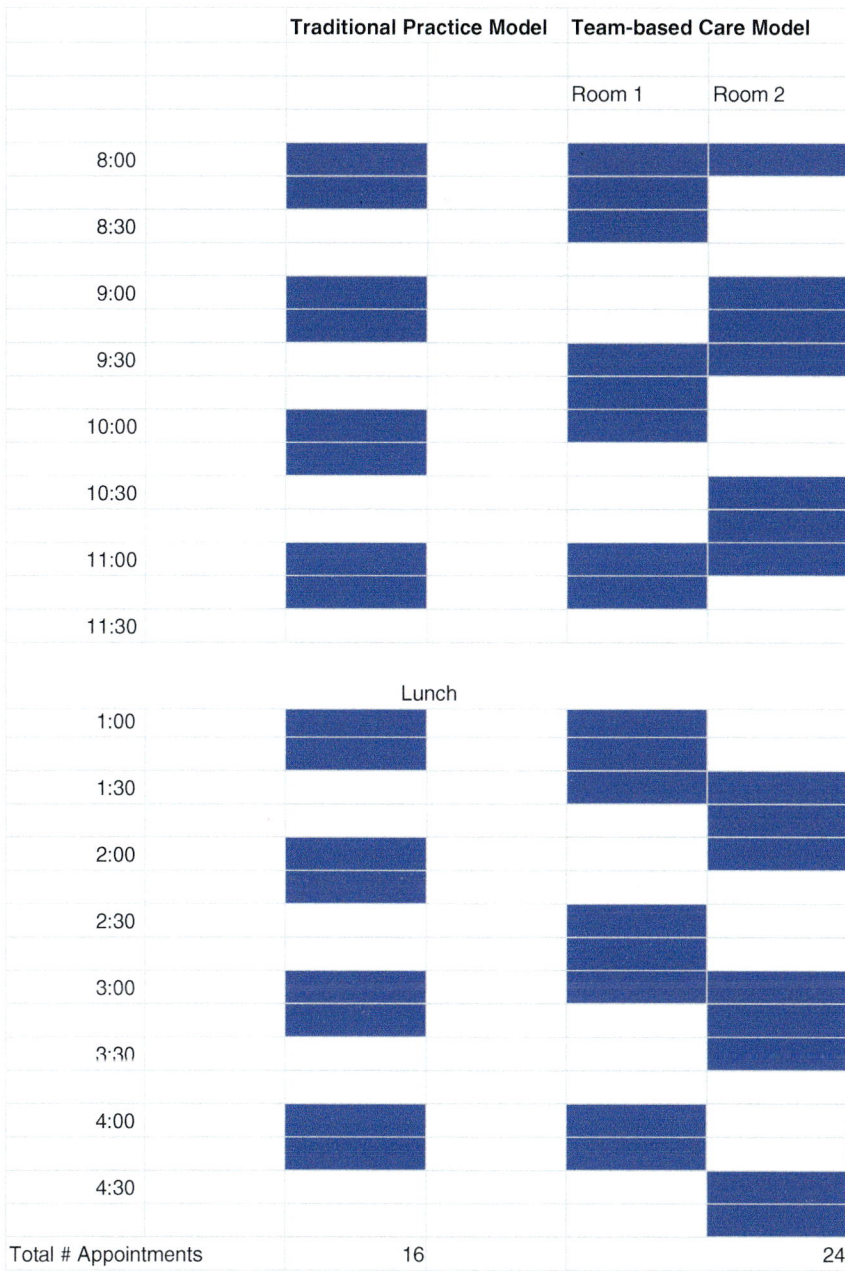

Fig. 11.1 Traditional practice model v. Team-based Care model

Patient Experience

Patients reported experiencing additional one-on-one time with their physicians. More patients requested patient portal access after team-based visits in one practice. Others noted that the care team was seen as an extension of the physician; one patient said to the medical assistant, "If I don't hear everything the doctor says, I can call back and ask you about it". Another patient said she "really liked having all the attention focused on *me*". Another reported feeling "more taken care of". A last patient wrote that "It's like a family environment".

Another practice started receiving phone calls from patients in advance of their appointments, having heard about the new model and eager to be included. More patients agreed to have lab work drawn in advance of their visits, so results could be reviewed, and any necessary adjustments explained in the room with the physician.

Provider and Staff Experience

Staff reported being happy with the increased interaction with patients and families. Nurses reported feeling valued and heard for the first time in years. "I feel more directly involved in patient care; I am actually using my nursing skills," said one nurse. Another said, "You are listening to us now. That's a big deal."

Front desk staff reported feeling empowered to complete process measures and accomplish non-clinical and administrative tasks. They reported being able to leverage critical thinking skills and reflecting on their objectives more often. Others noted that "(they) love the huddle; it works!" and felt as though the office felt more like a team.

Physicians were also very happy with team-based care. One physician had been using "pajama time" to work on clinical documentation after putting her children to bed. She commented that the team-based care model had reduced this work and "changed her life". Another physician used to take vacation days to catch up on paperwork and yet never quite completed everything. "We are seeing high rates of depression and burn-out. There's a reason for that, but there are also fixes. This (team based care) is one of those fixes."

Conclusion

Team-based care increases efficiency in value-based payment models. Putting relationships back at the center of health care is important as we acknowledge the shift in paradigm away from fee-for-service medicine. There are many other applications for this model outside of the primary care setting. Team-based care concepts may be leveraged for success in ambulatory surgical models as well as in specialty clinics, especially those that focus on complex care and chronic illness management. Research into the health outcomes and cost of care that is associated with a shift to team based care is needed to convince the payer world that team-based care and value-based care are more efficient and worth fostering.

References

1. Papanicolas I, Woskie LR, Jha AK. Health care spending in the United States and other high-income countries. JAMA. 2018;319(10):1024–39.
2. Trustees Report Summary. 2020 [cited 2020 Dec 18]. https://www.ssa.gov/oact/trsum/
3. 2019 Annual Report of the Boards of Trustees of the Federal Hospital Insurance and Federal Supplementary Medical Insurance Trust Funds, Washington, D.C., April 22, 2019.
4. Tikkanen R, Abrams M. U.S. Health Care from a Global Perspective, 2019: Higher Spending, Worse Outcomes? The Commonwealth Fund. January 2020.
5. Realizing the Full Potential of Primary Health Care. OECD 2019.
6. Petterson SM, Liaw WR, Phillips RL, Rabin DL, Meyers DS, Bazemore AW. Projecting UD primary care physician workforce needs: 2010-2025. Ann Fam Med. 2012;10(6):503–9.
7. Hauer KE, Durning SJ, Kernan WN. Factors associated with medical students' career choices regarding internal medicine. JAMA. 2008;300:1154–64.
8. Focus on Spending on Primary Care. First Estimates. OECD; 2018.
9. Phillips RL, Bazemore AW. Primary care and why it matters for U.S. health system reform. Health Aff. 2010;29(5):806–10.
10. CMS Press Release. HHS News: HHS to deliver value-based transformation in primary care: the CMS primary cares initiative to empower patients to drive better value and results. April 22, 2019. (was 16).
11. Phillips RL, Pugno PA, Saultz JW, et al. Health is primary: family medicine for America's health. Ann Fam Med. 2014;12(Suppl 1):S1–S12.
12. Gelmon S, Wallace N, Sandberg B, Petchel S, Bouranis N. Implementation of Oregon's PCPCH program: exemplary practice and program findings. https://www.oregon.gov/oha/pcpch/Documents/PCPCH-Program-Implementation-Report-Final-Sept-2016.pdf.
13. Goroll AH, Berenson RA, Schoenbaum SC, .Gardner LB. Fundamental reform of payment for adult primary care: comprehensive payment for comprehensive care. J Gen Intern Med 2007;22(3):410-415.
14. Organization for Economic Cooperation and Development. Fiscal sustainability of health systems: bridging health and finance perspectives. OECD Health; 2015.
15. Anderson G, Hussey P, Petrosyan V. It's still the prices, stupid: why the U.S. spends so much on health care, and a tribute to Uwe Reinhart. Health Aff. 2019;39(1):87–95.
16. Advanced Primary Care: A Foundational Alternative Payment Model (APC-APM) for Delivering Patient-Centered, Longitudinal, and Coordinated Care. American Academy of Family Physicians. April 2017.
17. Koller C, Brennan T, Bailit M. Rhode Island's novel experiment to rebuild primary care from the insurance side. Health Aff. 2010;29:5.
18. New England Direct Primary Care Alliance 2020. https://www.nedpca.org/
19. Larson HM, MD Family Medicine, LLC https://heidilarsonmd.com/
20. Sinsky C, Willard-Grace R, Schutzbank A, Sinsky T, Margolius D, Bodenheimer T. In search of joy in practice: a report of 23 high-functioning primary care practices. Ann Fam Med. 2013;11(3):272–8.
21. Primary Care Insights 2019. https://primarycareinsights.com/the-four-core-principles-of-team-based-care/
22. Gardner RL, Cooper E, Haskell J, Harris DA, Poplau S, Kroth PJ, Linzer M. Physician stress and burnout: the impact of health information technology. J Am Med Inform Assoc. 2019;26(2):106–14.
23. Hopkins K, Sinsky C. Team-based care: saving time and improving efficiency. Fam Pract Manag. 2014;21(6):23–9.
24. STEPS forward: implementing team-based care. AMA Toolkit, Practice Improvement Strategies, 2017.
25. McGough PM, Jaffy MB, Norris TE, Sheffield P, Shumway M. Redesigning your work space to support team-based care. Fam Pract Manag. 2013;20(2):20–4.

26. Shaw RJ. Nurse-led protocols provide quality care for hypertension, chronic disease. Ann Intern Med. 2014;161:113–21.
27. Pope G, Ellis R, Ash A, Ayanian J, et al. Diagnostic cost group hierarchical condition category models for Medicare risk adjustment: final report. Prepared for Health Care Financing Administration. Dec 21, 2000.
28. About Procedure Order Entry (PrOE) - Partners care decisions [internet]. My CMS. [cited 2020 Dec 18]. http://caredecisions.partners.org/partners-care-decisions/procedure-order-entry-proe/
29. CMS Fact Sheet: Primary Care First: Foster Independence, Reward Outcomes. April 22, 2019.

12. Impacting Risk Communication: Educating Providers to Improve Informed Consent Conversations in Procedural Sedation

Raquel M. Schears and Fernanda Bellolio

Key Learning Points
- Procedural sedation (PS) is routinely performed in the emergency department.
- Not all providers are familiar with the most common and serious risks related to procedural sedation.
- All providers should strive to deliver evidence-based care to patients including for PS in obtaining informed consent and communicating risk.
- Realize the basis of informed consent and shared decision-making begins with providers knowing the data and communicating it in conversations with their patients.
- Recognize the importance of patient-centered research which relies on evidence-based medicine and values and preferences of the patient.

Executive Summary

Procedural sedation (PS) is routinely performed in the emergency department (ED) to facilitate potentially painful procedures by administering agents to alleviate pain, reduce anxiety, and ameliorate suffering. Given the frequent use of PS by EPs, as well as the continued development of research and clinical evidence for this practice, we conducted two systematic reviews and meta-analyses to determine the incidence of adverse events during PS in the ED, including the frequency of events associated with individual medications and different medication combinations.

We identified a gap on the quality of care when assessing the baseline knowledge of clinicians conducting PS. Not all providers were familiar with the most common and

R. M. Schears (✉)
Department of Emergency Medicine, University of Central Florida, Orlando, FL, USA

F. Bellolio
Department of Emergency Medicine, Mayo Clinic, Rochester, MN, USA

serious risks related to procedural sedation at the time of obtaining informed consent from patients. Hence we provided an educational intervention that stressed the evidence-based risks of PS we had uncovered in the literature, and gave providers reminder cards and access to resources on how to incorporate adverse events' information when communicating risk effectively with patients' undergoing procedures. Providers showed improvements in their knowledge base on posttest 6 months later. However, this was not enough, as we had not reached the patients, and a decision aid was created to supplement the clinician/patient conversation when obtaining informed consent. The DA is a visual tool to allow patients to picture risks of PS that may be relevant to consider when making a decision. ED providers indicate that they still use the DA with patients to keep their risk communication on track when obtaining informed consent for PS.

Employing a collaborative process, we backfilled a quality of care gap using current high quality evidence-based research, designed audiovisual tools in support of the learning process, and implemented a decision aid as the hallmark to a unified approach for patients undergoing PS.

Introduction

Procedural sedation (PS) is routinely performed in the emergency department (ED) to facilitate potentially painful procedures by administering agents to alleviate pain, reduce anxiety, and ameliorate suffering [1]. PS involves the use of short-acting analgesic and sedative medications to relieve distress, remove awareness, and prompt amnesia albeit temporarily to give clinicians a brief window to perform procedures effectively while monitoring the patient closely for potential adverse effects.

As emergency physicians (EPs), we are uniquely trained and qualified to provide all levels of sedation (moderate and deep). ED-based PS has been shown to be safe when performed by trained EPs [2–5]. Moreover, we have the skill sets for managing the airway, conducting resuscitation and initiating mechanical ventilation that are necessary to provide safe patient care should an adverse event occur. Expertise in PS is included as a core competency in emergency medicine (EM) residency training and pediatric EM fellowships [1].

The use of various analgesic, sedative, and anesthetic agents has been outlined in several guidelines [1, 6, 7]. Numerous classes and combinations of medications are commonly used for PS in the ED [2, 8–21]. The use of short-acting sedative agents such as propofol [22, 23], etomidate [21, 21–27], and ketamine [28–30] has gained widespread acceptance. The American College of Emergency Physicians (ACEP) has developed a clinical policy regarding PS [1]. However, adverse event reporting for PS has been heterogeneous.

For over a decade, most clinicians have assumed that the definitive procedure, itself, and not the sedation to accomplish it, impacted the ED length of stay and complication rates. Example: sedation to facilitate the fracture reduction and cast placement of a patient with a fracture, or sedation to perform electrical cardioversion in a patient with an arrhythmia. The focus on the definitive procedure overlooked the underlying confounder of varied consent regimens typically directed by the individual EP as opposed to having one standardized informed consent process for PS that could eventually even be facilitated by other providers. Thus, the penultimate component of care, the means of obtaining informed consent for sedation required to accomplish procedures was not homogeneously performed, and was missing as a variable of care in most published studies. Adequate sedation and procedural understanding has come to light as the possible driver of ED length of stay and patient experience, resulting in extended ED care costs and potentially patient morbidity.

Most likely, the sedation costs were bundled with the care provisions for the definitive diagnoses that are fairly common reasons to seek care in the ED. However, the clear sequence of events: 'first sleep and then manipulate' quality mantra is undeniable. In the past, general consent for the definitive procedure may also have obviated explicit consent for sedation, or led to the mistaken belief that seeking pain relief was covered by a presumption that patients' presenting to the ED were giving consent for treatment, just by being there, in a more paternalistic approach. Although most patients would agree they want separate assurance that their procedure will be as pain-free as possible, they are accustomed to naturally turning to their assigned care team to get reassurance, analgesics and procedural details. Therefore, we purposefully involved a multidisciplinary team of health care providers, and crafted our provider baseline knowledge survey, educational intervention, and posttest survey. Having nursing buy-in for the study, and their participation with both providers and patients, although not formally measured, solidified the relational coordination [31] and the iterative process expertise necessary to design and implement this project. RNs were energized to start small with a doable project, to increase awareness of PS risks specifically, and to champion the overhaul of our informed consent process incrementally. Moreover, when queried regarding risk disclosure, patients have indicated in consent studies and courtroom proceedings they want more information, not less [32–34]. After all, the priority is given to the definitive procedure for which patients' are motivated (by pain) and not free-will to seek care in the ED in the first place.

Although The Joint Commission's (JC) hospital accreditation program recommendations is subject to Centers for Medicare and Medicaid Services (CMS) approval and pricing perspectives, Serious Adverse Effects (SAEs) of procedural sedation in the ED are not captured as a review criteria. In fact, litigation incurred by missed fractures is far more common and costly to hospitals than defending providers against perceived communication shortcomings in discussing sedation risks for the reduction of known fractures. As such, litigation often defines the institutional liabilities that in turn refine the JC's criterion list for review. Also licensed physicians are permitted to bill for either the definitive procedure or sedation, not both under federal reimbursement rules. Perhaps this constraint relates to the rarity ($<1\%$) of serious airway adverse events and need in those circumstances to initiate costly life-saving interventions, which can be more easily audited for occurrence and potential for associated downstream costs. Nonetheless, a gap in quality of care exists in the way the risk and benefits are explained to patients, and we found that not all providers are familiar with the most common and serious risks related to procedural sedation. This is likely related to a lack of standardized, formal training in obtaining informed consent and a lack of published data specific to the risks of procedural sedation in the ED setting.

There are many ways to gain consent for procedures, sedation included, that can range from presumed consent with incapacitated patients or emergency exceptions for patients presenting in extremis to the ED, to verbal affirmation for minors with their parents, or written consent forms that can be customized to serve an educational role for use before and after definitive procedure is completed. Positioning the care team, to be able to engage the questions of patients and families, as they arise when undergoing procedures, is important.

PS performed in the ED is distinctive from other settings in that the procedures performed are likely to be more painful and urgent in nature. Over the past decade, PS in the ED has been in a relative steady state regarding the guidelines set forth and the monitoring performed [1]. In addition, there has been a move to standardize reporting of adverse sedation events [35]. Despite the advance in monitoring and medication selection, there is no single 'safe' and 'risk-free' medication for PS [18, 20–22, 36].

Given the frequent use of PS by EPs, as well as the continued development of research and clinical evidence for this practice, we conducted two systematic reviews [31, 36] to determine the incidence of adverse events during PS in the ED, including the frequency of events associated with individual drugs and different drug combinations. The results of the review provided useful information for providers when performing PS in a given patient, when engaging in risk communication and shared decision-making. Results should also support the validity of the informed consent process and patients-centered focus to advance quality of care.

Methods

First, two large systematic reviews and meta-analysis of current data on procedural sedation in adults and children were conducted. The reviews adhered to recommendations made in the Preferred Reporting Items for the Systematic Reviews and Meta-Analyses (PRISMA) statement. Eight databases were searched including: MEDLINE, EMBASE, EBSCO, CINAHL, CENTRAL, the Cochrane Database of Systematic Reviews, Web of Science, and Scopus. We included published literature on randomized controlled trials and observational studies of procedural sedations in the ED.

Subsequently, the incidence data on procedural sedation was summarized for incorporation into the risk conversation for informed consent to be considered both current and highly evidence-based. Next, a brief survey (pretest) was designed and administered through email, including staff physicians, resident physicians and advanced practice providers (NP/PA) working in our Academic ED. These surveys were analyzed with simple statistics, comparing percentages of the responses. The survey tool was used to assess the baseline knowledge of providers regarding known serious adverse events (SAEs) for PS reflected in the medical literature. Then we provided a tutorial on the actual incidence data (from the systematic reviews) on SAEs in PS. A reminder card of the sedation risks and incidence data was developed and distributed for clinical reference to participants and is available as a supplementary file in a prior publication [31]. Additionally, we created a video [31] that demonstrates how to obtain informed consent for PS with a simulated patient.

To capture learning and new awareness, we obtained a posttest assessment 6 months later, sent to 70 participants. The posttest survey was standardized to the pretest items. We also evaluated access to the online information, and we inquired about whether the reminder card, and AV aids helped providers navigate informed consent conversations. Posttest responders could also write in an open text box feedback and ideas for which they'd like to see educational activities developed in the future.

We analyzed both surveys with descriptive statistics. Participation on the surveys was voluntary with responses kept anonymous and data confidentiality maintained. The motivation to participate was accomplished in fulfilment of quality of care project requirements convened for resident graduation from the EM academic program. As well, staff physicians and NP/PAs were encouraged to support resident projects and be faculty mentors helping to advance the quality of care for ED patients.

The second phase of implementing a new informed consent pathway for PS included development of a pictorial (iconic array format) decision aid (DA) which grew out of anecdotal concerns that the general written informed consent for PS in the ED, was insufficient to document the patients' active involvement in the consenting process. Moreover, there was previously no take-home information the patient could refer back to in review of their actual consent agreement or sedation experience post discharge. Hence, the DA for PS in the ED was developed through 3 rounds of Delphi exercise, in effect to 'picture' the data previously captured in worded risk versions, was to broaden understanding in interactions with patients undergoing informed consent for PS. Communication and design experts collaborated to create a pictorial document with accurate data presentation for point of care consideration. This document went through an iterative and collaborative vetting process including patients and clinical stakeholders to arrive at the final version.

Results

The systematic review and meta-analysis of procedural sedation in adults included 55 studies and nearly 10,000 sedations. The incidence of severe adverse events requiring emergent interventions were rare with one case of laryngospasm in 883 sedations (4.2 per 1000), 1.6 per 1000 intubations, and 1.2 per 1000 aspirations respectively. The most common adverse event was hypoxia in 40.2 per 1000 sedations, vomiting in 16.4 per 1000 sedations and hypotension in 15.2 per 1000 sedations [31]. We did not find any reported deaths in this cohort of sedations in the ED. Although there was no 'risk-free' medication or method identified, portrayal as 'over 99% safe 'is the same as 'less than 1% airway risk' may not be considered suitable nor equal disclosure for all. Since there are well documented medical literacy challenges of the general public, ED clinicians must put effort into managing individual patient concerns thoughtfully to arrive at their understanding meaningfully.

Our review regarding pediatric procedural sedations found similar results than the adult review. We found 41 studies including 13,883 procedural sedations. The most common adverse events were: vomiting 55.5 per 1000 sedations, agitation 17.9 per 1000, hypoxia 14.8 per 1000 sedations and apnea 7.1 per 1000. The incidences of severe respiratory events were: laryngospasm in 2.9 per 1000, 4 intubations among 9136 sedations and 0 cases of aspiration among 3326 sedations [36]. We concluded that SAE were infrequent in children, however it is important to be prepared when conducting PS in the ED. Both systematic reviews provide quantitative risk estimates to facilitate risk communication, informed consent and resource allocation. Understanding better the type and incidence of adverse events allow us to have the right resources at the bedside when performing PS, for example have an airway cart, respiratory therapist, pharmacist, the right number of nurses, etc.

Pretest data demonstrated that of ED providers (staff, residents and NPs/PAs, $N = 49$, response rate 65%, 75 surveys sent) who responded to our survey, 88% either agree or agree with reservation that they are fully aware of the common and serious adverse events associated with adult procedural sedation and 90% either fully agree or agree with reservation that they are confident in their knowledge and ability to relay these risks to patients during the informed consent process. However, when asked specifically to choose from a list which three events occur mostly commonly, the top three most common adverse events were selected by 65%, 37% and 6% of respondents respectively. Similarly, when asked to identify from a multiple-choice list how often serious events (laryngospasm, intubation and aspiration) occur, only 39% responded correctly. We believe this data shows that while providers may be aware of associated risks, their knowledge of the frequency with which they occur could be improved upon.

The PS posttest data showed confounding of the reminder cards and are subject to possible Hawthorne effect and/or participation bias from repetition purposely loaded in educational interventions (presentation and AV aids) with nearly all participants (staff, residents and NP/PAs, $N = 50$, response rate 71%, 75 surveys sent) able to identify the top three most common adverse events and correctly pick from a multiple-choice list how often the most serious SAEs occur. Most participants (88–90%) continued to indicate that they were fully aware of the most common events but their answers for the most common adverse events and frequency of the most serious SAEs associated with adult procedural sedation showed well over the 50% improvement rate in the average posttest scores we had targeted for significance. Interestingly, although the participants remained equally confident in their knowledge and ability to relay these risks to patients during the informed consent process, the majority (80%) affirmed the educational tools had helped them communicate risk to patients (Y/N) and 100% of participants could also accurately identify (multiple choice) where to find the informed consent materials for PS in the physical ED and on the intranet. Several participants also indicated an interest in shared decision making and how to use DAs effectively in the ED for other clinical entities as a future topic for educational advancement.

Specific graphical representations of PS SAE risks, risk probability, and the spectrum of sedation events (percentile basis) for aiding provider communication when educating patients regarding risks of PS were also created in the study frame. An iterative process (modified Delphi) and 3 rounds of deliberation were employed by the study group and stakeholders to use information in arriving at the final DA version. We overall found similar rates for SAEs in adults and children in both systematic reviews and through feedback from the stakeholders, having 2 separated visual tools for these 2 age groups was confusing and not liked by providers. Because the overall magnitude of risks were similar, we created one single visual aid with both pediatric and adult risks combined using the worst case scenario as the represented numbers. Figure 12.1 shows the incidence of adverse events in procedural sedation in the ED [37].

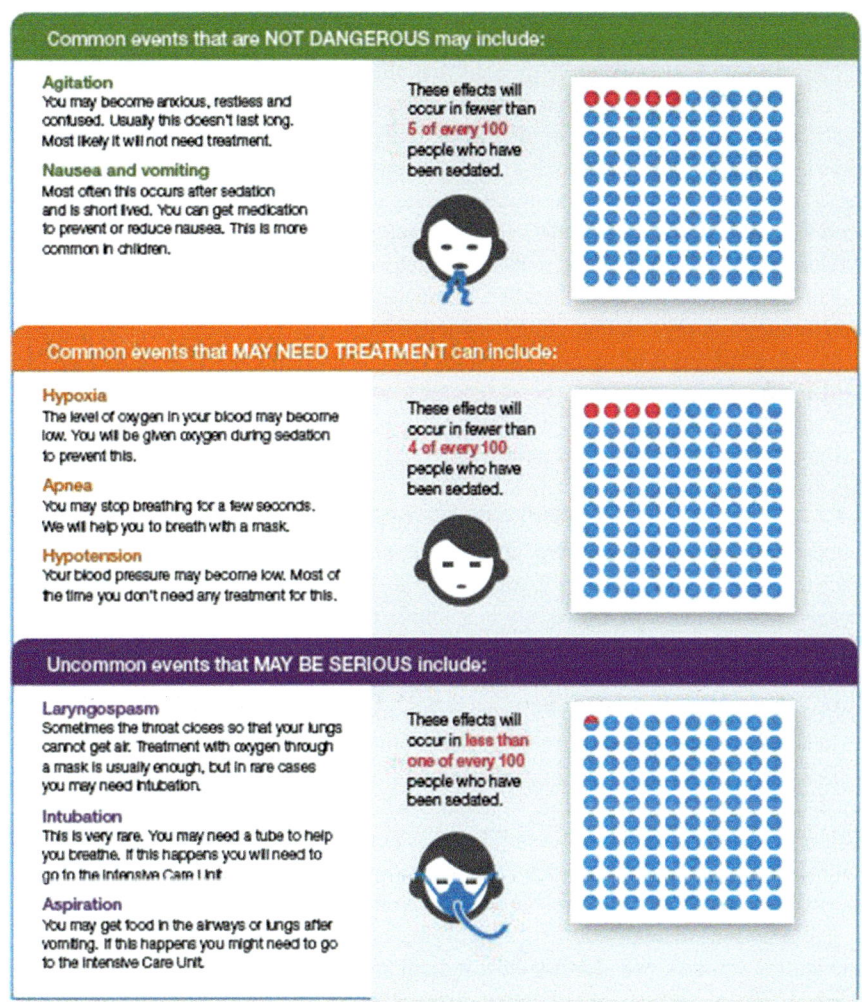

Fig. 12.1 Incidence of adverse events in procedural sedation in the ED [37]. Reprinted with permission from Mayo Clinic and from Bellolio MF, OJ e Silva L, Alencastro Puls H, Hargraves I, Cabrera, D. The research to practice continuum: Development of an evidence-based visual aid to improve informed consent for procedural sedation. Journal of Clinical and Translational Science 2017, 1(5), 316-319. DOI:10.1017/cts.2017.303. Used with permission of Mayo Foundation for Medical Education and Research, all rights reserved

Discussion

Everyday there are several adults and children who underwent procedural sedation in multiple Emergency Departments. In our ED there are more than 550 per year, and clinicians treating these patients were trained on how to perform informed consent through didactics, visual aids and pocket cards that summarize the adverse events of PS to prepare them for informed consent discussions. The communication of the need and benefits of PS seemed more obvious than the risks and the alternatives including not providing adequate sedation or pain relief. Restoring normal heart rate through electrical cardioversion, reducing fractures, realigning joints, and draining abscesses had a common denominator goal: to accomplish the maneuvers necessary in as pain-free a way as possible. Risk communication regarding sedation was more straightforward for clinicians exposed to the card, but remained challenging for providers armed with only words to transmit the risks of PS that would reliably deliver on the patients' expectation of evidence-based guidance to make an informed decision.

Evaluation of provider baseline knowledge of the risks of PS (pretest) was found to be subpar in terms of identifying either the uncommon but serious SAEs probabilities or picking out the three most common non-serious SAEs from a list. Despite this, most providers' indicated they were fully aware of the most common SAEs and serious SAEs associated with adult procedural sedation. Providers also indicated they had confidence in their knowledge of the adverse events related to adult procedural sedation and ability to relay these risks to patients during the informed consent process. Six months later, after an educational intervention, ED introduction of electronic accessible reminder cards, and an instructional video on how to incorporate risk communication effectively in a simulated consent conversation with an ED patient, providers demonstrated that although they had learned the correct answers (posttest) on SAE incidence questions, as a group they continued to maintain a high degree of confidence in their PS knowledge and ability to communicate risk with patients when obtaining informed consent. This overconfidence may have derived from a practical reliance on the cards and AV tools since nearly all of providers on posttest, indicated they found these resources helpful in PS risk conversations with patients. We think the posttest reliability was potentially confounded by Hawthorne effects. Providers had been repeatedly encouraged to study up and there was wide accessibility of our teaching resources both in the ED and online.

Through multidisciplinary work involving bedside providers, patients and communication experts, we developed a patient decision aid (DA) tool, specifically geared to PS to supplement rather than replace clinician counselling about treatment options. DAs are known to promote patient engagement in medical decision making, collaboration between patients and their care team, increase knowledge and align patient choices with their preferences. Therefore, the information included in DAs can significantly impact patients' decisions. For this reason, patients and clinicians expect the information in DAs to be highly evidence-based and rigorously selected and summarized.

As a testament of institutional endorsement of the improvements to informed consent process and evidence-based medicine, the project won awards and departmental recognition for advancing patient-centered care. The card and DA for PS used by the respective ED providers and patients in navigating consent conversations to articulate risk, achieve understanding and document informed consent for PS are still in use today. Trained providers are interacting with patients predicted to be undergoing procedural sedation using the evidence-based visual aids as these tools helped in improving knowledge for both patients and providers while obtaining informed consent. It is possible that the goal of improving risk communication in a unified evidence-based manner, may impact patient experience. Moreover, if the use of a visual aid increases patient understanding meaningfully, the effect needs to be measured. Patient-centered research is the next step to validate the impact patients' have on the visual aid tool for informed consent in the ED.

Lessons Learned

Lessons for medicine and management reveal the generalizability of first gaining incidence data on a phenomenon, in our case SAEs associated with PS, and then employing that data in user-friendly ways to educate providers and patients. Our AV tools and final iconic array DA version reformatted incidence data in a way both provider and patient could digest in the short window ahead of a definitive procedure, and were determined to be helpful by providers when communicating risks of sedation when obtaining informed consent specifically for PS. This relatively small change initiative can decrease the variance in care, resulting in positive physician improvements including education and a protocolized way to communicate risk to patients, to truly achieve informed consent for PS. The use of *relational coordination* [38] came with the leveled approach to the project, initially focused on defining the knowledge gaps related to sedation risks among clinicians (RNs, MDs, and NP/PAs) and secondarily examining the previously unpinned risk conversation and overhauling it with medical staff for improvement. The data and educational information focused on both the providers and patient feedback. Although we did not gather patient satisfaction scores with our educational interventions, the future is bright for obtaining patient-centered data to help develop collaborative care processes that incorporate an assessment of patient experience from ED patrons who have undergone PS and the new informed consent process that relies on shared AV aids.

The stakeholders in this process improvement were tied in from the beginning by the need to meet requirements. For residents, this was the stipulation that they needed to complete a quality assurance project to graduate from the residency program. For staffers, they were motivated by the requirement that all providers must attain a silver level certification for a quality project as judged by the institution-wide Quality Care Academy. Thus, fulfilling goals as part of requirements for graduation or academic promotion and retention became the professional motivation for participation. Because of these overlapping expectations, the involved participants did not need to be involved at all points of the care in progress. Faculty mentors and resident mentees came up with the original idea to study the informed consent process, specified to PS, and then worked together. Once the study was developed, contributions from nursing and other clinical providers with varying levels of experience, could be sorted out in weekly open study discussions to incrementally implement versions of the AV aids and their incorporation into the planned care process for PS ongoing during the study window in the ED.

By being involved and considered valued as an equal member of the team brought in on a rolling basis there was encouragement, but also an awareness to not be wasting people's time. This actually created focused participation and a time horizon for implementation that held a level of accountability for participants, doing their part. This team building process also allowed exposure to AIDET (Acknowledge, Introduce, Duration, Expectation, and Thank you) conferences and role play to improve managing patient and family's expectations or dissatisfiers. *Managing expectations of families* is key to the positive impact of *AIDET training* [39]. This built strong group dynamics and since the frontline was in it to win it, for 'their area of expertise' it empowered them to speak up.

Certainly, the first few hours after the definitive procedure may have complications relating to the sedation which might be missed if the patient is no longer in the ED. This follow up window could be captured by RN callbacks to check on the status of discharged patients after their procedure. However, hospitals have been reluctant to inquire after discharged patients fearing the follow up may extend institutional liabilities.

Conclusion

Serious adverse events during procedural sedation that need airway support are exceedingly rare. Quantitative risk estimates obtained from evidence based incidence data, provided the base information presented in graphic formulations which progressed from text and color coded tables to synthesized pictorial representations in a visual aid simplified for use by providers to facilitate risk communication in order to obtain informed consent. Notably, the decision aid tool born of high quality clinical research has achieved integration into routine clinical care in the ED for the last several years. Patient centered projects and those open to multidisciplinary collaboration, are the ones that best translate into clinical practice.

References

1. Godwin SA, Burton JH, Gerardo CJ, et al. Clinical policy: procedural sedation and analgesia in the emergency department. Ann Emerg Med. 2014;63(2):247–58. https://com-jax-emergency-pami.sites.medinfo.ufl.edu/files/2015/03/Godwin-et-al-Clinical-policy-Procedural-sedation-and-analgesia-in-the-emergency-department.-2014.pdf
2. Burton JH, Miner JR, Shipley ER, Strout TD, Becker C, Thode HC Jr. Propofol for emergency department procedural sedation and analgesia: a tale of three centers. Acad Emerg Med. 2006;13(1):24–30. https://doi.org/10.1197/j.aem.2005.08.011.

3. Harvey M, Cave G, Betham C. Contemporary sedation practice in a large New Zealand emergency department. N Z Med J. 2011;124:36–45. https://www.researchgate.net/profile/Martyn_Harvey2/publication/51732868_Contemporary_sedation_practice_in_a_large_New_Zealand_emergency_department/links/565f959508aefe619b28b14d/Contemporary-sedation-practice-in-a-large-New-Zealand-emergency-department.pdf
4. Sacchetti A, Senula G, Strickland J, Dubin R. Procedural sedation in the community emergency department: initial results of the ProSCED registry. Acad Emerg Med. 2007;14:41–6. https://doi.org/10.1197/j.aem.2006.05.023.
5. Taylor DM, Bell A, Holdgate A, MacBean C, Huynh T, Thom O, Augello M, Millar R, Day R, Williams A, Ritchie P, Pasco J. Risk factors for sedation-related events during procedural sedation in the emergency department. Emerg Med Australas. 2011;23(4):466–73. https://doi.org/10.1111/j.1742-6723.2011.01419.x.
6. Gross JB, Epstein BS, Bailey PL, Gilbertson L, Connis RT, Nickinovich DG, Cote CJ, Zerwas JM, Davis FG, Zuccaro G. Practice guidelines for sedation and analgesia by non-anesthesiologists. Anesthesiology. 2002;96:1004–17. Available from: http://bvanesthesia.com/images/Sedation.pdf
7. Baker SN, Weant KA. Procedural sedation and analgesia in the emergency department. J Pharm Pract. 2011;24:189–95.
8. Sawas A, Davis V, Youngquist S, Ahern M, Johnson D, Wilson C, et al. Combined ketamine and propofol sedation vs propofol sedation for emergency department procedures: a prospective randomized trial [abstract]. Acad Emerg Med. 2011;18:S233.
9. Andolfatto G, Willman E. A prospective case series of single-syringe ketamine-propofol (Ketofol) for emergency department procedural sedation and analgesia in adults. Acad Emerg Med. 2011;18(3):237–45. https://doi.org/10.1111/j.1553-2712.2011.01010.x.
10. Chudnofsky CR, Weber JE, Stoyanoff PJ, Cologne PD, Wilkerson MD, Hallinen DL, Jaggi FM, Boczar ME, Perry MA. A combination of midazolam and ketamine for procedural sedation and analgesia in adult emergency department patients. Acad Emerg Med. 2000;7:228–35. https://doi.org/10.1111/j.1553-2712.2000.tb01064.x.
11. Dewar A, Gray A, Open M, Leal A, Main A. Procedural sedation and analgesia in a large UK emergency department: a 5-year review [abstract]. Acad Emerg Med. 2012;19:738.
12. Miner JR, Biros M, Krieg S, Johnson C, Heegaard W, Plummer D. Randomized clinical trial of propofol versus methohexital for procedural sedation during fracture and dislocation reduction in the emergency department. Acad Emerg Med. 2003;10(9):931–7. https://doi.org/10.1197/S1069-6563(03)00310-5.
13. Miner JR, Moore J, Clarkson E, Plummer D, Hess J, Nelson R, et al. Randomized, blinded, three-arm clinical trial of propofol, 1:1 Ketofol, and 4:1 Ketofol for procedural sedation in the emergency department [abstract]. Acad Emerg Med. 2011;18:S233–4.
14. Hohl CM, Sadatsafavi M, Nosyk B, Anis AH. Safety and clinical effectiveness of midazolam versus propofol for procedural sedation in the emergency department: a systematic review. Acad Emerg Med. 2008;15(1):1–8. https://doi.org/10.1111/j.1553-2712.2007.00022.x.
15. Messenger DW, Murray HE, Dungey PE, van Vlymen J, Sivilotti ML. Subdissociative-dose ketamine versus fentanyl for analgesia during propofol procedural sedation: a randomized clinical trial. Acad Emerg Med. 2008;15(10):877–86. https://doi.org/10.1111/j.1553-2712.2008.00219.x.
16. Ruth WJ, Burton JH, Bock AJ. Intravenous etomidate for procedural sedation in emergency department patients. Acad Emerg Med. 2008;8(1):13–8. https://doi.org/10.1111/j.1553-2712.2001.tb00539.x.
17. Cicero M, Graneto J. Etomidate for procedural sedation in the elderly: a retrospective comparison between age groups. Am J Emerg Med. 2011;29(9):1111–6. https://doi.org/10.1016/j.ajem.2010.08.004.
18. Hoffman RJ, Barnett G. Does sedation with combined ketamine/propofol (Ketofol) result in fewer adverse events than ketamine or propofol alone? [abstract]. Ann Emerg Med. 2011;58(4):S227. https://doi.org/10.1016/j.annemergmed.2011.06.175.

19. Miner JR, Gray R, Delavari P, Patel S, Patel R, Plummer D. Alfentanil for procedural sedation in the emergency department. Ann Emerg Med. 2011;57(2):117–21. https://doi.org/10.1016/j.annemergmed.2010.08.010.
20. Jacques KG, Dewar A, Gray A, Kerslake D, Leal A, Lees F. Procedural sedation and analgesia in a large UK emergency department: factors associated with complications. Emerg Med J. 2011;28(12):1036–40.
21. Chan KK, Ho HF. Etomidate and midazolam for procedural sedation in the emergency department of Queen Elizabeth Hospital: a randomized controlled trial. Hong Kong. J Emerg Med. 2017;15(2):75–87. https://doi.org/10.1177/102490790801500203.
22. Black E, Campbell SG, Magee K, Zed PJ. Propofol for procedural sedation in the emergency department: a qualitative systematic review. Ann Pharmacother. 2013;47:856–68. https://doi.org/10.1345/aph.1R743.
23. Swanson ER, Seaberg DC, Mathias S. The use of propofol for sedation in the emergency department. Acad Emerg Med. 1996;3:234–8. https://doi.org/10.1111/j.1553-2712.1996.tb03426.x.
24. Burton JH, Bock AJ, Strout TD, Marcolini EG. Etomidate and midazolam for reduction of anterior shoulder dislocation: a randomized, controlled trial. Ann Emerg Med. 2002;40(5):496–504. https://doi.org/10.1067/mem.2002.126607.
25. Falk J, Zed PJ. Etomidate for procedural sedation in the emergency department. Ann Pharmacother. 2004;38(7-8):1272–7. https://doi.org/10.1345/aph.1E008.
26. Keim SM, Erstad BL, Sakles JC, Davis V. Etomidate for procedural sedation in the emergency department. Pharmacotherapy. 2012;22(5):586–92. https://doi.org/10.1592/phco.22.8.586.33204.
27. Patanwala AE, McKinney CB, Erstad BL, Sakles JC. Retrospective analysis of etomidate versus ketamine for first-pass intubation success in an academic emergency department. Acad Emerg Med. 2014;21(1):87–91. https://doi.org/10.1111/acem.12292.
28. Green SM, Roback MG, Krauss B. Laryngospasm during emergency department ketamine sedation: a case-control study. Pediatr Emerg Care. 2010;26:798–802. https://doi.org/10.1097/PEC.0b013e3181fa8737.
29. Jamal SM, Fathil SM, Nidzwani MM, Ismail AK, Yatim FM. Intravenous ketamine is as effective as midazolam/fentanyl for procedural sedation and analgesia in the emergency department. Med J Malaysia. 2011;66(3):231–3. http://e-mjm.org/2011/v66n3/Intravenous_Ketamine.pdf
30. Sener S, Eken C, Schultz CH, Serinken M, Ozsarac M. Ketamine with and without midazolam for emergency department sedation in adults: a randomized controlled trial. Ann Emerg Med. 2011;57(2):109–14. https://doi.org/10.1016/j.annemergmed.2010.09.010.
31. Bellolio MF, Gilani WI, Barrionuevo P, Murad MH, Erwin PJ, Anderson JR, Miner JR, Hess EP. Incidence of adverse events in adults undergoing procedural sedation in the emergency department: a systematic review and meta-analysis. Acad Emerg Med. 2016;23(2):119–34. https://doi.org/10.1111/acem.12875. Epub 2016 Jan 22
32. Spatz ES. The new era of informed consent: getting to a reasonable patient standard through shared decision making. JAMA. 2016;315(19):2063–4.
33. Gabay G, Bokek-Cohen Y. Infringement of the right to surgical informed consent: negligent disclosure and its impact on patient trust in surgeons at public general hospitals—the voice of the patient. BMC Med Ethics. 2019;20(1):77. Published 2019 Oct 28. https://doi.org/10.1186/s12910-019-0407-5.
34. Yek JL, Lee AK, Tan JA, Lin GY, Thamotharampillai T, Abdullah HR. Defining reasonable patient standard and preference for shared decision making among patients undergoing anaesthesia in Singapore. BMC Med Ethics. 2017;18(1):6. Published 2017 Feb 2. https://doi.org/10.1186/s12910-017-0172-2.
35. Mason KP, Green SM, Piacevoli Q, International Sedation Task Force. Adverse event reporting tool to standardize the reporting and tracking of adverse events during procedural sedation: a consensus document from the world SIVA international sedation task force. Br J Anaesth. 2012;108:13–20.

36. Bellolio MF, Puls HA, Anderson JL, Gilani WI, Murad MH, Barrionuevo P, Erwin PJ, Wang Z, Hess EP. Incidence of adverse events in paediatric procedural sedation in the emergency department: a systematic review and meta-analysis. BMJ Open. 2016;6(6):e011384. https://doi.org/10.1136/bmjopen-2016-011384. PMID: 27311910 PMCID: PMC4916627
37. Bellolio MF, Silva LOJE, Puls HA, Hargraves IG, Cabrera D. The research to practice continuum: development of an evidence-based visual aid to improve informed consent for procedural sedation. J Clin Transl Sci. 2017;1(5):316–9. https://doi.org/10.1017/cts.2017.303publication.
38. Gittell JH. "New Directions for Relational Coordination Theory" in the Oxford Handbook of Positive Organizational Scholarship, 2011.
39. Braverman AM, Kunkel EJ, Katz L, Katona A, Heavens T, Miller A, Arfaa JJ. Do I buy it? How AIDET™ training changes residents' values about patient care. J Patient Exp. 2015;2(1):13–20. https://doi.org/10.1177/237437431500200104.

Factors Influential in Seeking Care for Neonates with Congenital Heart Disease

13

Glenn J. Pelletier

Key Learning Points
- Congenital heart disease is the most common birth defect.
- Prenatal diagnosis of critical congenital heart disease contributes to improved outcomes.
- Prenatal counseling, perinatal planning, and timely expert care for neonates with congenital heart disease are essential for optimal outcomes.
- Alignment of all stakeholders in the referral process for expectant mothers who carry a fetus with congenital heart disease is essential for efficient, state-of-the-art care.
- Personal choice for expectant mothers carrying a fetus with congenital heart disease is a strong influence in the decision about where to seek care for their unborn child or neonate.
- Insurance contracts had a remarkably low influence on where mothers sought prenatal and postnatal care for their children with congenital heart disease.
- During the prenatal evaluation for CHD in a fetus, a mother's confidence in the program's reputation, staff professionalism, and care and concern exhibited by the medical team strongly influenced the decision about where to seek care.
- Strong, working, professional relationships between mothers and members of the care team and among care team members are very important to mothers when deciding about who will care for their children with congenital heart disease.

G. J. Pelletier (✉)
Nemours A. I. duPont Hospital for Children, Nemours Cardiac Center, Wilmington, DE, USA
e-mail: glenn.pelletier@nemours.org

Executive Summary

Congenital heart disease (CHD) is the most common birth defect occurring in approximately 1% of live births [1]. Prior to 1980 the imaging technology and the understanding of congenital heart malformations versus normal development were not refined [2]. Therefore, prenatal diagnosis of CHD was not clinically available. However, with technological advances in echocardiographic imaging and experience interpreting the images detection of fetal heart abnormalities in utero is now widely available. Current estimates rate diagnostic accuracy for detecting complex congenital heart disease prenatally at 95% when the studies are performed and interpreted by skilled personnel [2]. Despite these improvements in technology and diagnostic skill, the rate for prenatal detection of CHD ranges from approximately 70% to 85% [3, 4]. One obstacle to prenatal detection of CHD is access to this care limited by lower socioeconomic strata and a rural home address [3, 4]. The value of prenatal diagnosis of CHD is not simply the timing of the diagnosis. Rather, there are clear benefits including parental decision-making, learning and counseling, potential in utero treatment options, preparing for a smooth transition from fetal to neonatal life, and evidence for improved outcomes for babies with complex CHD who receive a prenatal diagnosis [5–7].

Important to this delivery of perinatal care for unborn and newborn children with CHD is organization of a referral system in which all stakeholders align to achieve the best possible outcomes for the patients. This group of stakeholders includes the mother, the fetus, obstetricians, perinatologists, maternal fetal medicine specialists, cardiologists, congenital heart surgeons, care coordinators, pediatricians, family members, health insurers, and hospital systems. Central to coordinating such complex care that involves an array of people from many disciplines is first to understand the preferences and values of the pregnant mother. While the specific choices made by mothers may vary, we hypothesized that common themes exist and drive their healthcare decisions for their fetuses and future newborns. To investigate our theory we conducted a survey of 563 mothers who had fetal echocardiograms with a cardiology consultation from 2011 to 2016. Physician referral to a specific congenital heart center (73%) and patient choice (89%) were the two most influential factors in the decision made by these mothers who sought care for their fetuses with CHD and ultimately their newborn children. This information may inform strategies for growth and development of CHD services by focusing on building stronger relationships with referring physicians and their patients.

Introduction

Early detection of CHD using fetal echocardiography is a medical advance that has been in broad use for over three decades and continues to evolve. When combined with prenatal counseling, appropriate perinatal planning, and timely care delivered in a congenital cardiac center with appropriate expertise, improved survival of infants with critical CHD (CCHD) has been achieved [8–13]. For noncritical structural heart lesions, fetal echocardiography allows for early diagnosis and creation of a plan for delivery and postnatal follow up before the baby is born. Similarly, detection of arrhythmias in a fetus enables a pediatric cardiologist to treat the problem in utero potentially preventing cardiovascular impairment in the newborn period.

With the burgeoning attention to healthcare outcomes and their geographic and health system variation across the country [14] stakeholders including patients, providers, and payers seek the best results available. Consequently, health systems and physicians alike keenly focus on improving patient survival and quality of life with the fewest medical errors possible. The drive to reach these goals necessarily leads to competition within the healthcare marketplace.

This study focuses on a cardiac center located in the Delaware Valley (DV), where this competition for pediatric cardiology and cardiac surgery services is intense. The DV is a geographic parcel including Philadelphia and its surrounding Pennsylvania counties, four New Jersey counties that surround Camden, New Castle County in which Wilmington is located and Cecil County Maryland. Nemours Cardiac Center (NCC) is located in Wilmington, Delaware and is part of the Nemours Children's Health System (NCHS). It operates in a competitive marketplace in which there are eight congenital heart centers in a region demarcated within a 150-mile radius of Wilmington. Within the Delaware Valley NCC is one of three programs to provide services for CHD. The population in DV is approximately six million people with a relatively stable birth rate [15]. Based on the estimated incidence of CHD per live births (~1%), there are approximately 800 children born with CHD in DV each year. The objective for NCC is to provide congenital heart care services to a larger share of this population.

NCC celebrated its 20th anniversary in 2018. During this era, the program evolved to provide a full complement of services for congenital and pediatric heart disease. These services include complex neonatal surgery, surgery for adults with congenital heart disease, heart failure care including ventricular assist device therapy and transplantation, both diagnostic and interventional catheterization, electrophysiological testing and intervention, fetal heart care and outpatient cardiology services across the DV. Both inpatient and outpatient care is delivered by a fully integrated team of nurses, physicians, technicians, practitioners, and administrative staff. Amidst this competition, our group sought to determine the factors, which influence the choice of physician and hospital by mothers who are carrying fetuses diagnosed with congenital heart disease.

Methods

This study uses data from the NCC, given its unique position in the Delaware Valley and being one of three centers to provide services for CHD. All fetal echocardiograms (1324) performed at the NCC from 2011–2016 were queried in the institutional database. Duplicate studies (314), incomplete studies (2) and studies in which no CHD was detected in the fetus (445) were eliminated. The remaining 563 patient studies formed the basis for this investigation. We contacted each mother who had a fetus diagnosed with CHD and asked them to participate in a telephone survey (Box 13.1) designed to ascertain the factors important to them in deciding which physician and health system to choose for their child's care. All mothers had health insurance.

Eighty-nine respondents (16%) completed the survey.

> **Box 13.1 Survey Questions**
> I am (name) from the NCC at AI duPont Hospital for Children in Wilmington and am calling to ask you to participate in a short survey to help inform us about the factors that influence mothers' or families' decisions to seek care at the cardiac center. Our goal is to obtain information that will help us better serve you and other families in the future. To learn this information we have a few questions to ask you. It will only take a few minutes of your time.
>
> 1. For your prenatal fetal echocardiogram to assess your child's heart problem were you free to decide where to receive care and from which doctor?
>
> 2. Did your health insurance plan determine which hospital or doctor you could go to for the echocardiogram to assess your child's heart problem?
>
> 3. Did another doctor, nurse or healthcare provider refer you to a specific cardiologist (heart doctor) or hospital to have the echocardiogram done to assess your child's heart problem? If yes, which type of healthcare provider?
>
> 4. If you visited with a pediatric cardiologist (heart doctor) during your pregnancy to get the echocardiogram, did that visit(s) influence your decision about where (at which hospital) your child would receive care for the heart problem?
>
> 5. If you visited with a pediatric cardiologist (heart doctor) during your pregnancy to get the echocardiogram, did that visit(s) influence your decision about which pediatric cardiologist (heart doctor) would care for your child's heart problem?
>
> 6. Did family members influence your decision about which hospital to go to for the fetal echocardiogram and later care of your child's heart problem?
>
> 7. Did family members influence your decision about which pediatric cardiologist (heart doctor) to choose for the fetal echocardiogram and later care for your child's heart problem?
>
> 8. Did the distance from your home to the children's hospital where you got the fetal echocardiogram or later care for your child's heart problem help you to choose that hospital?
>
> 9. Did the availability of family members close to the children's hospital you chose for care of your child's heart problem help you to make that choice?
>
> 10. During your pregnancy if you visited the hospital(s) where your child could receive care for the heart problem, did the facility influence your choice of where your child would receive that care?
>
> 11. During your pregnancy if you visited the hospital(s) where your child could receive care for the heart problem, did the people you met influence your choice of where your child would receive that care?
>
> 12. Did the location of the hospital where you planned to deliver your baby help to determine where your child would receive care for the heart problem?
>
> 13. Are there any other factors that helped you determine where your child would receive care for the heart problem?

Results

Ten survey respondents (11%) chose the largest regional competitor over NCC for their child's care. Three of these ten mothers (3.4% overall) cited the presence of a labor and delivery unit within the children's hospital as the primary reason for their choice. These mothers further explained that being within the same facility as their newborn child offered comfort to them. In contrast, two respondents (2%) opted for their child to receive care for congenital heart disease at NCC despite having visited and considered the largest regional competitor during the prenatal period.

The algorithm for this database query including the empirically derived three most likely responses is shown in Fig. 13.1. Among the 89 survey respondents, patient choice (89%) and physician referral (73%) were the most common influences in a mother's decision about where to seek prenatal care for a fetus with CHD. Payer contracts had a small impact on this decision (15%). Frequencies of affirmative responses to the specific survey questions are shown in Table 13.1. Prenatal pediatric cardiology visit to determine either site or physician for follow up care (65%), prenatal visit with care providers from the FHP (66%), and prenatal tour of the facility (50%) all had a moderate influence on the mothers' decision for where to seek care. The distance from home to the CHD center (40%), the distance

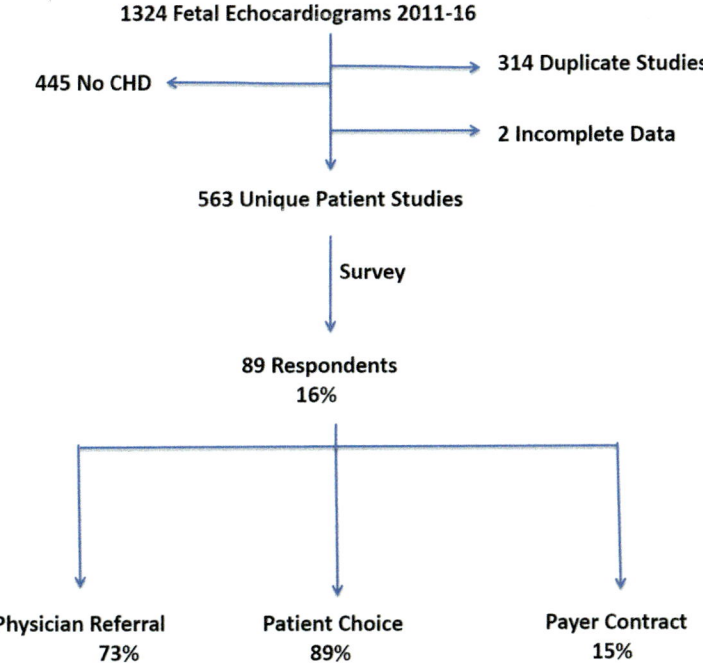

Fig. 13.1 Algorithm flowchart to query the fetal echocardiogram database and frequency of three empirically derived factors that influence maternal choice for congenital heart disease care of their children

Table 13.1 Survey results showing frequencies for factors that influence maternal choices for prenatal and postnatal care of a child with CHD

Influential factor	Frequency (%)
Patient choice for site or physician for initial fetal evaluation for CHD	89
Referral[a]	73
Prenatal pediatric cardiology visit for site or physician	65
Prenatal visit with care providers[b]	66
Prenatal tour of facility	56
Distance from home to site for CHD care	40
Distance between hospital for delivery and the children's hospital for CHD care	38
Desire for extended family help in postnatal period	30
Payer contract	15
Extended family's impact on choice of site for CHD care	15
Extended family's impact on choice of pediatric cardiologist	4

CHD congenital heart disease
[a] Referrals from maternal fetal medicine physicians, obstetricians, pediatricians, midwife, nurse, other physician
[b] Care providers include pediatric cardiologist, pediatric cardiothoracic surgeon, echocardiography technician, fetal care coordinator, fetal nurse practitioner

Table 13.2 Survey results showing additional factors that influenced maternal choice for CHD care in response to question 13 in the survey

Additional factors that influenced maternal choice for CHD care
• Hospital or cardiac program reputation
• Family accommodations to room-in with baby or availability of a Ronald McDonald House close to hospital
• Prior personal experience with physician, cardiac program or the children's hospital
• Staff professionalism
• Quality of care
• Outcomes
• Expertise specific to child's CHD type
• Level of care and concern demonstrated by staff
• Confidence instilled from meeting staff, visiting the facility, or researching the program
• Strong relationship between MFM and cardiac center physicians

from the hospital for delivery and the CHD center (38%), and a desire for extended family available to help in the postnatal period (30%) each had low levels of influence in the decision-making process for mothers. In addition to payer contracts (15%), extended family's impact on choice of CHD center site (15%) and pediatric cardiologist (4%) exerted minimal influence on the mother's decision for care. Table 13.2 shows the responses to the final survey question, "Are there any other factors that influenced your decision about which physician or hospital you chose to care for your child?" These varied responses can be summed into factors such as program's reputation, prior personal experience with the program or hospital, quality of care, outcomes, available expertise, and level of care and concern exhibited by staff that instilled confidence in the mother that her child would receive the best care. In addition, evidence for strong relationships between MFM and cardiac center physicians and staff professionalism had positive influences in selecting the site and physicians to provide care for the child with CHD.

Lessons Learned

Prenatal services to manage CHD in fetuses and postnatal care delivered to newborns and infants with heart disease have improved greatly over the last several decades. While there is survival benefit to prenatal diagnosis plus an organized care plan for the child born with CCHD and planning advantages for postnatal care once a child is born with noncritical CHD, fetal echocardiograms and prenatal consultation with pediatric cardiologists and cardiac surgeons are not accessible to all mothers. That statistically only 7–8.5 out of 10 mothers carrying a fetus with CHD get a prenatal diagnosis in part because of socioeconomic position or a rural home location highlights the inequity in access to care. However, for those mothers who have access to prenatal cardiology services and the option to plan for the postnatal care for their children this study shows individual choice is the primary factor that determines where mothers and their children receive their care. Similarly, referral from a physician who is involved in the mothers' health care has an important influence as well.

Contrary to general opinion, for mothers in the DV who sought prenatal cardiology services and subsequent care for their children at NCC, health insurer restrictions on who provides the care and where was a small factor in the decision. From the open-ended question, "Are there any other factors that helped you determine where to receive care for your child's heart problem?" two themes emerged. The first is confidence the mothers felt from a visit to NCC for a prenatal evaluation. From the program's reputation for outcomes, quality, and expertise to the initial impressions of staff professionalism and levels of care and concern for the mother and her fetus, those mothers who chose NCC did so because it felt like the right place for them. Second, relationships matter. The mothers' relationships with physicians in NCC or NCHS, and knowledge of a strong collaboration between MFM and NCC physicians were important factors in choosing where to receive care.

Based on the survey results, NCC could improve its regional market share to care for mothers and their fetuses with CHD by placing strong emphasis on developing durable relationships with referring physicians, particularly maternal fetal medicine providers and by striving to make every patient encounter an opportunity to build confidence in the care delivered to children with heart disease. Undoubtedly, achieving these goals will require steady and persistent effort with the return on investment realized over years. However, not to address the needs and preferences of pregnant women who carry fetuses with CHD and have a choice about where they seek care in the DV will likely jeopardize the potential for NCC to grow its fetal cardiology program.

Reflecting on this project from a management perspective there are three domains I will evaluate below in the context of principles and practices fundamental in business administration. First, my leadership style of the group that completed the project had a higher relational component versus a task component. As such, I performed with listening, informing, and asking behaviors more than telling group members what to do. I am most familiar with this leadership style, but I also prospectively anticipated with this management approach I could cultivate a sense of fair process in which participation and contributions by all team members would be valuable to the success of the project and we would enhance our work from the collective intelligence of the group. The team was intentionally small. I chose the pediatric cardiologist who directed the FHP at NCC and a clinical systems coordinator who had extensive knowledge of referral patterns for all echocardiograms within the NCC and ready access to the database. Using relational coordination [16], I introduced the inter-connectedness of the many stakeholders within the referral process for fetal echocardiograms. The goal here was to get team members to see the relationships among the stakeholders and prompt ideas to strengthen weaker links and capitalize on strong associations. The initial enthusiasm for the project was encouraging. Team members volunteered for tasks and committed to a timeline.

Unfortunately, team performance, the second domain to review, waned over time. Some technical delays in consolidating the data caused slow forward progress initially and perhaps created declining interest. Although the team members participated in constructing a RC (relational coordination) map, there was no buy-in to carry the concept further. Accountability without authority was a difficult challenge to overcome. Despite my explanation of the project, its rationale, and the potential value to NCC and the whole organization, dedication to the work seemed to dissipate. My intuition tells me the lack of accountability was rooted in an opinion that this project was simply, "Glenn's school project." Alternatively, my leadership style may have contributed to the struggle to hold the team accountable. Perhaps if I better understood the individual team members' personalities, strengths and weaknesses, I could have recognized who best to lead with relational techniques and for whom I needed to adopt a telling/directing style. Another possible contributor to declining interest is team selection. I selected team members with credentials I judged to be pertinent for this project. A pediatric cardiologist with expertise in fetal echocardiography and a coordinator well versed in referral patterns and the database for echocardiograms would be strong assets to the group, I thought. However, recruiting people with a desire to contribute to the project proved to be more valuable than those with particular expertise. Support for this practice is compelling. By the time we extracted the data and honed down the number of patients we would survey, the existing team members were disengaged. I recruited a physician's assistant (PA) and a medical student, both eager to help, to conduct the survey and collate the responses. This portion of the project ran smoothly and efficiently.

The third domain is lessons I learned from organizing and leading this project. Team building begins with member selection and member selection must include some gauge of motivation and work ethic assessment. Generally, those that want to do the work and are enthusiastic about the project will likely perform well. The contrast between the PA and medical student versus the coordinator and the cardiologist is striking. Despite no prior knowledge of the project and a time crunch to finish the work, the PA and medical student far out performed the initial team members who had experience and expertise in the subject matter. Once the team is assembled, a leader should get familiar with how members work best. Do they need encouragement? Will they respond well when someone delegates a task to them?

Are they inclined to problem solve independently? Do they need to be persuaded or sold on an idea? Do they work best when told what to do? As a surgeon, I use this adaptable leadership style in the operating theater and it works quite effectively. Perhaps one difference between the operating room and an organizational project is a heightened attentiveness to the work at hand because the situation is frequently life or death in cardiac surgery. Such an urgency that calls for focus and attention to detail is difficult to replicate for a project that spans months or years. However, the challenge for a leader is to maintain the focus and enthusiasm for the work and to see the project to completion. In this case, knowing the team members well is important to achieving the goal.

Conclusion

Prenatal diagnosis of congenital heart disease is a medical advance that yields substantive benefits to the mother, the fetus, and the newborn. It is, however, the first step in a complex care process that demands fluid communication and extensive coordination among numerous stakeholders. Initiation of the process is highly dependent upon a mother's choice for who will provide the care and where. As part of that decision, mothers emphasize a need for confidence in the care they could receive from providers at a specific hospital, and look to those providers to work together collaboratively and with them specifically to achieve the best possible outcome.

As became evident in organizing and completing this study to examine factors influential in seeking care for neonates with CHD, relational coordination and skilled leadership are essential. Similarly, providing complex healthcare such as perinatal services for a mother and fetus with CHD would benefit from a focus on establishing strong relationships between providers and patients and a coordinated approach to deliver that care specific to the patient.

References

1. Hoffman JIE, Kaplan S. The incidence of congenital heart disease. J Am Coll Cardiol. 2002;39(12):1890–900.
2. Strainic J, Stiver C, Plummer S. Prenatal diagnosis of congenital heart disease. In: Martin RJ, Fanaroff AA, Walsh MC, editors. Neonatal-perinatal medicine. Philadelphia: Elsevier, Inc; 2020. p. 1320–33.
3. Hill GD, Block JR, Tanem JB, Frommelt MA. Disparities in the prenatal detection of critical congenital heart disease. Prenat Diagn. 2015;35:859–63.
4. Bucholz EM, Sleeper LA, Newburger JW. Neighborhood socioeconomic status and outcomes following the Norwood procedure: an analysis of the pediatric heart network single ventricle reconstruction trial public data set. J Am Heart Assoc. 2018;7:e007065. https://doi.org/10.1161/JAHA.117.007065.
5. Berkeley EMF, Gowns MB, Karr S, Rappaport V. Utility of fetal echocardiography in postnatal management of infants with prenatally diagnosed congenital heart disease. Prenat Diagn. 2009;29:654–8.

6. Mahle WT, Clancey RR, McGaurn SP, Goin JE, Clark BJ. Impact of prenatal diagnosis on survival and early neurologic morbidity in neonates with hypoplastic left heart syndrome. Pediatrics. 2001;107(6):1277–82.
7. Rychik J, Ayres N, Cuneo B, Gotteiner N, Hornberger L, Spevak PJ, Van der Veld M. American Society of Echocardiography guidelines and standards for performance of the fetal echocardiogram. J Am Soc Echocardiogr. 2004;17(7):803–10.
8. Tworetsky W, McElhinney DB, Reddy VM, Brook MM, Hanley FL, Silverman NH. Improved surgical outcome after fetal diagnosis of hypoplastic left heart syndrome. Circulation. 2001;103:1269–73.
9. Bonnet D, Coltri A, Butera G, Fermont L, Le Bidois J, Kachaner J, et al. Detection of transposition of the great arteries in fetuses reduces neonatal morbidity and mortality. Circulation. 1999;99:916–8.
10. Donofrio MT, Skurow-Todd K, Berger JT, McCarter R, Fulgium A, Krishnan A, Sable CA. Risk-stratified postnatal care of newborns with congenital heart disease determined by fetal echocardiography. J Am Soc Echocardiogr. 2015;28:1339–49.
11. Holland BJ, Myers JA, Woods CR Jr. Prenatal diagnosis of critical congenital heart disease reduces risk of death from cardiovascular compromise prior to planned neonatal cardiac surgery: a meta-analysis. Ultrasound Obstet Gynecol. 2015;45:631–8. https://doi.org/10.1002/uog.14882.
12. Peyvandi S, De Santiago V, Chakkarapani E, Chau V, Campbell A, Poskitt K, et al. Association of prenatal diagnosis of critical congenital heart disease with postnatal brain development and the risk of brain injury. JAMA Pediatr. 2016;170(4):e154450. https://doi.org/10.1001/jamapediatrics.2015.4450.
13. Morris SA, Ethen MK, Penny DJ, Canfield MA, Minard CG, Fixler DE, Nembhard WH. Prenatal diagnosis, birth location, surgical center, and neonatal mortality in infants with hypoplastic left heart syndrome. Circulation. 2014;129:285–92. https://doi.org/10.1161/CIRCULATIONAHA.113.003711.
14. Wennberg JE, Bubolz TA, Fisher ES, Gittlesohn AM, Goodman DC, Mohr JE, et al. The Dartmouth Atlas of Health Care in the United States. In: McAndrew Cooper M, editor. Dartmouth atlas of health care. Chicago: American Hospital Publishing, Inc; 1996. p. 2–34.
15. Center for Disease Control and Prevention. Birth Data [Internet] 2020. http://www.cdc.gov/nchs/nvss/births.htm.
16. Gittel JH, Fairfield KM, Bierbaum B, Head W, Jackson R, Kelly M, et al. Impact of relational coordination on quality of care, postoperative pain and functioning, and length of stay. Med Care. 2000;38:807–19.

Creation of the LSU Health Shreveport Complex Cranial Surgical Center of Excellence: Needs Served, Process to Obtain, and Lessons Learned

14

Sandeep Kandregula, Audrey Demand, Patrick Ingraffia, Krystle Trosclair, and Bharat Guthikonda

Key Learning Points
- Establishing a Center of Excellence requires immense interest, profound knowledge of managing a healthcare institution and a collaborative effort of all parties involved.
- Identifying the lacunae and needs for a Center of Excellence is the first step to addressing the problem.
- Strategic location, monetary support, academic excellence and clinical interdependency are key factors for any academic center to flourish.
- Goal setting requires engaging the team players with diverse aspirations and incorporating these perspectives to achieve common aims.
- A Center of Excellence requires leadership that is engaged with the team.

Executive Summary

In this chapter, we present the fundamental elements of writing an application to establish a Center of Excellence (COE) in Complex Cranial Surgery for the LSU Health Shreveport Department of Neurosurgery. We share our experiences of problems addressed, strengths cultivated, and lessons learned along the way. We also provide a brief explanation of the reasons to form a COE, the essential criteria and elements needed to initiate and support COE development, and the necessary environment to cultivate in order to ensure COE success. We believe this information will be helpful to managers considering establishing a COE in the clinical setting. This intervention has been associated with opportunities for healthcare advancement and improved patient outcomes while increasing clinical team morale, effectiveness, and productivity around the globe.

Introduction: Background and Problem Description

LSU Health Shreveport is one of three medical schools in the state of Louisiana (along with LSU Health Sciences Center—New Orleans and Tulane University). Neurosurgery has historically been a main clinical and academic strength at LSU Health Shreveport. A Center of Excellence is a specialized program housed within a medical organization that houses high concentrations of specialists and subspecialists to work together in an interdisciplinary fashion [1]. Our Center of Excellence, although rooted in the Department of Neurosurgery, will focus primarily on skull base surgery. Skull base surgery is a subspecialty within neurosurgery that involves the surgical management of complex vascular and tumor pathology, along the base of the skull. These surgical cases are considered challenging primarily due to the location of the pathology as well as the proximity of these lesions to the deep brain structures and the main vasculature supplying the brain and cranial nerves. The risks in these surgical procedures are quite high, and the consequences of morbidity are often significant decrease in or complete loss of quality of life. Pathologies that are treated by a skull base team include but are not limited to: skull base meningiomas, acoustic neuromas, pituitary adenomas, craniofacial neoplasms, CSF leaks (spontaneous, traumatic, or post-operative), aneurysms, arteriovenous malformations (AVM), cavernous malformations, trigeminal neuralgias, and Chiari malformations. In many centers (including ours), the skull base team will also manage other complex intracranial surgical problems such as awake craniotomy for glioma or metastatic tumor removal, extracranial to intracranial (EC-IC) bypass, microvascular decompression for trigeminal neuralgia, and removal of deep-seated brain masses.

Our primary purpose for forming a Center of Excellence (COE) was that our team wanted to formalize and strengthen an already existing collaborative effort to help solidify our center's standing as the premier intracranial surgery center in Louisiana. Given the absence of other competitive centers in the vicinity, our team saw this opportunity as somewhat of a "blue ocean" in Louisiana.

A second and related piece of background is that the management of our university hospital is currently being taken over by Ochsner Health, a healthcare organization based in south Louisiana. Their flagship institution is in New Orleans, and they have branched out to several other communities in Louisiana with hospitals and outpatient clinics. In October of 2018, they overtook operations of the LSU Health Shreveport's University hospital with the intention of making operations more efficient and profitable. This transition also provides a timely framework for improving neurosurgery further within our institution.

Why Should We Develop a Neurosurgical Center of Excellence?

Collaborative efforts and interdisciplinary medicine result in better outcomes. Khan et al. studied the outcomes of malignant glioma in two different settings [2]. They reported an improved outcome in the patients treated by subspecialized neurosurgical oncologists. Albright et al. reported in their study that neurosurgical subspecialization in pediatric neurosurgery improved patient survival [3]. Similarly, McLaughlin et al. reported improved outcomes in pituitary adenoma patients who received surgery in a multidisciplinary environment and suggested that this is achieved at a Center of Excellence [4]. Establishing these centers requires dedicated neurosurgeons, otorhinolaryngologist-head and neck surgeons, maxillofacial surgeons, nurses trained in neurocritical care, and interventional neuroradiologists [5]. Organizational change is most effective at changing the core identity of the organization when the change incorporates members from several distinct subsets of the organization [6].

LSU Health Shreveport would like to increase the patient volume and surgical case volume of complex intracranial pathology to gain access to world class clinical methods and machinery. Studies suggest that patient outcomes are associated with treatment delivered in high volume centers with commensurate resources compared with low volume centers [7]. Evidence-based care around interprofessional collaboration is likewise associated with improved outcomes [8]. This is especially relevant in cranial base surgery and surgery involving the head more broadly [5, 9]. The goal of this project is to formalize a collaborative, multi-disciplinary, symbiotic relationships that drive high-volume care delivery. Through collaborative multidisciplinary teamwork, and strategic marketing, we hope to become the premier complex cranial surgery center for all of Louisiana.

Methodology: Developing a Center of Excellence for Complex Cranial Surgery

In this section, we will briefly discuss the strengths, and thus tools/methods, used to assemble our application to become an official Center of Excellence, as well as the additional factors that the leader of this movement found to be particularly helpful. We use principles of system engineering to guide our framing [10]. These principles hold that the system can be defined at various scales/levels; in this chapter, the central part of the system is defined as a lone department (LSU Health Shreveport Department of Neurosurgery) which is interdependent on many other systems to function efficiently. We began by assessing the current system in place in the surgical department and developed an organized approach of presenting them in order to gain the support of the accrediting institution. We also developed a proposed management structure for the Center of Excellence.

For the LSU Health Shreveport Department of Neurosurgery, we used a framework built around the five dimensions of (1) strategic location, (2) a strong referral system, (3) clinical interdependency, (4) academic excellence, and (5) monetary support, as displayed in Fig. 14.1.

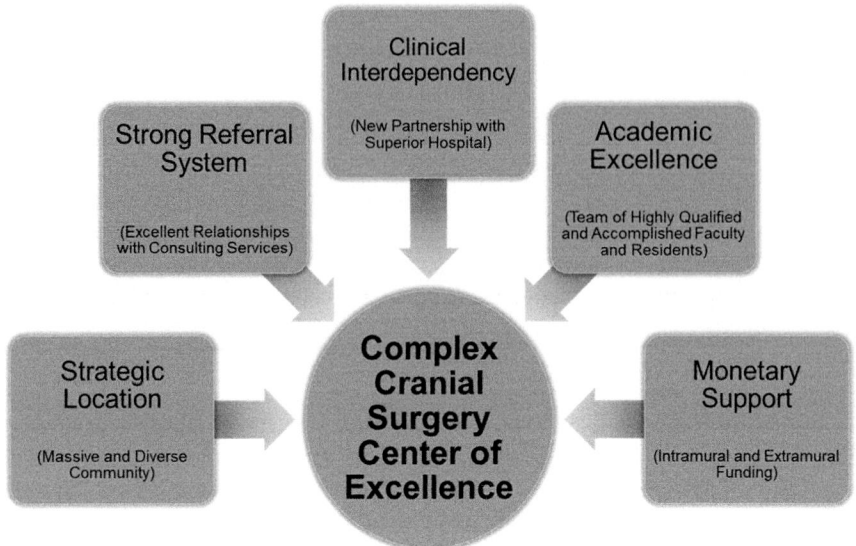

Fig. 14.1 Essential systems for creating a complex cranial surgery center of excellence

Strategic Location

Our department is the sole tertiary care neurosurgical center for north Louisiana, southern Arkansas, and east Texas. Shreveport is located 3 hours east of Dallas, TX, 3.5 hours north of Baton Rouge, LA, 3 hours southwest of Little Rock, AR, and 3 hours west of Jackson, MS (Fig. 14.2). This prime location is essential and strategic in our department's and overall institution's ability to draw patients from such a wide catchment area.

Neurosurgery at our institution has historically been steadfast in its commitment to managing all neurosurgical patients from anywhere that referrals/transfers are sent to our institution regardless of payor mix. Skull base and complex intracranial surgery have also been a strength of our department. Over the past decade, we have worked together in a multi-disciplinary manner amongst departments within our medical school to provide high-level care for these patients with complex intracranial problems. However, creating the formal collaborative relationships between other hospital departments is a more recent endeavor at our institution.

Strong Referral System

Our community and regional neurosurgeons are colleagues with whom we already have well-developed relationships. As with most private practice and hospital-employed neurosurgeons, they have practices that are almost exclusively focused in spine surgery. They do not have the desire or interest to do much complex

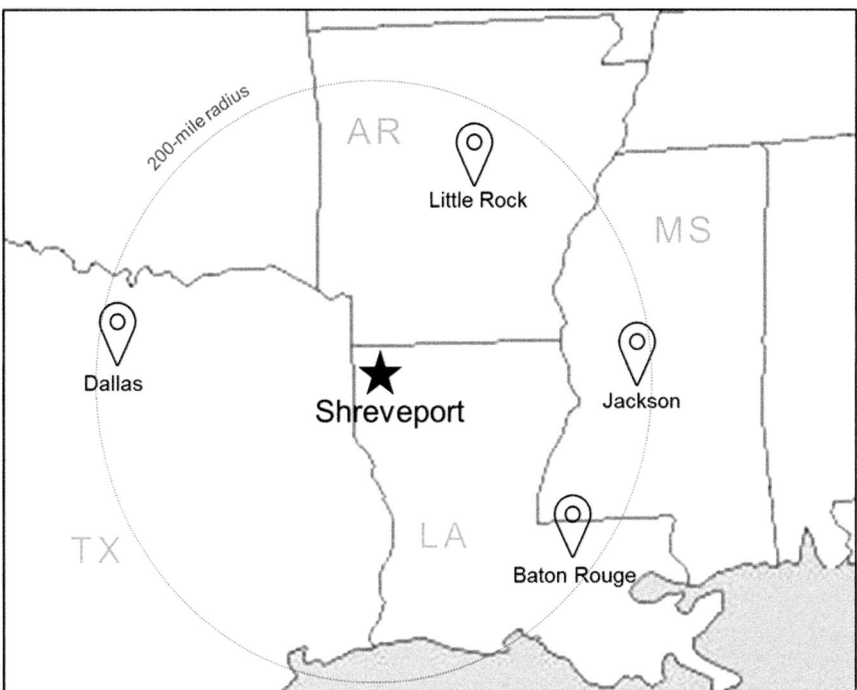

Fig. 14.2 Map depicting strategic location of LSU Health Shreveport's Complex Cranial Surgery Center of Excellence

intracranial surgery. This is primarily because those cases tend to take longer, patients are hospitalized for longer, and the cranial surgery reimbursement (especially per time spent) is less than spinal surgery. This combination of our extreme interest and our community colleagues' relative (and in some cases, extreme) disinterest is an ideal combination for us to formalize this niche as our own. This allows our relationship with them to be very symbiotic rather than competitive. We provide an option for them to triage these patients, and it is good for us in that it allows us to maximize our volume of these complex cases. As part of the plan for the Center of Excellence, we plan to formalize our existing collaborative relationships with many other key departments both in our institution and in the regional area, a strategy that we hope will help to pull patients in from Houston, Dallas, or other regional tertiary care academic medical centers.

Clinical Interdependency

Establishing clinical interdependency with local health care organizations also helps to allow centers of excellence the freedom to specialize. Connecting to a larger health system that can manage the day to day administrations allows an organization to focus on a narrow range of skills and capitalize on economies of scale that are associated with doing the same thing for a larger consumer base. In the case of LSU, our hospital, this was made possible with the merger with Ochsner Health, an experienced healthcare organization that has historically done well at running hospitals in a profitable and efficient way.

Fortunately the relationships between core team members were already fairly strong in the department. The existing team included surgical sub-specialists such as ENT (with endoscopic sinus/skull base surgeons, neuro-otologists, and head and neck surgeons), interventional neuroradiology (for definitive management of certain vascular pathologies and adjunctive management/embolization of others), and oral and maxillofacial surgery (OMFS) for management/reconstruction of facial/mandibular related problems with the complex pathologies that we treat.

We envision the Center of Excellence as working closely with other departments, specialists and subspecialists that are essential to the team that produces skull base surgeries [4]. Endocrinology, for example, is particularly relevant to managing our patients with pituitary tumors. Regulating hormonal function both in the perioperative and long-term period is imperative to this patient population [3]. Though many of the pathologies that we manage in skull base/complex intracranial surgery are benign, some are malignant and some benign problems may require adjuvant or stand-alone radiation. As such, both radiation oncology and medical oncology are also essential members of an ideal team.

Neuro-ophthalmology is also a key field in skull base surgery. They are crucial to visual assessment of our skull base patients, especially those with pituitary pathology. Neurology and neuropsychology teams will also be very helpful to assist with management of the non-surgical neurologic symptoms that this patient population may have either before or after surgery. For our vascular patients, the neurology team is also crucial to the non-surgical management of these conditions. Psychological assessment and counseling will also be a key component of care that will help with overall quality of life in these patients with significant intracranial pathology. Neuropathology is also a department that we envision working closely with as many of these patients will have tumors that require a clear histopathological diagnosis. Their input will often dictate the adjuvant treatment, if any, that patients will undergo after surgical intervention.

Lastly, the evaluation of this patient population involves constant radiographic assessments (mainly through CT scans, MRI scans, and angiograms). For this reason, close relationships with the neuroradiology department benefits the core team (Fig. 14.3). Often, the imaging we perform will be not only anatomy-based but also function-based (with functional MRIs being a common imaging modality for lesions in eloquent areas of the brain).

Having everyone together under the umbrella of our Center of Excellence will also allow a one-stop-shop for our patients. As mentioned above, our patients sometimes travel from hours away to see the needed physicians. Our goal is to have a multi-disciplinary center (in both name as well as space) that will allow our patients to be seen by all physicians involved in their care, have all needed imaging and

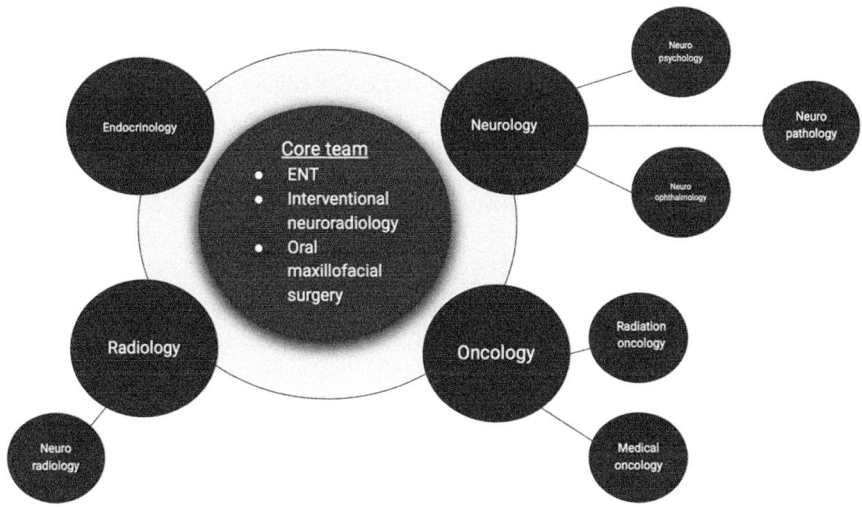

Fig. 14.3 The various specialties and subspecialties relevant to the core team of the Complex Cranial Surgery Center of Excellence

laboratory studies done, and, when needed, have their pre-operative assessment all done in one trip to Shreveport. Many times, patients with complex intracranial pathologies will not be financially well off, and having everything done in one trip to Shreveport will be particularly valuable for such patients.

Having all departments in one center will facilitate referral protocol between departments that will allow us to evaluate patients in a timely fashion and determine their treatment plan in a collaborative manner. Often, these surgical procedures are also performed as a team with two or more of the listed departments. The consolidated referral process will help to centralize patient care and reduce patient transport and remote collaboration. We anticipate that this will improve the quality of the team that together provides comprehensive care to the patients.

Academic Excellence

Education is central to the mission of our institution. A pillar of our department is resident and fellow education. Our COE would allow us to take this education to even another level. This would provide an organized foundation upon which our residents/fellows could improve their clinical skills and execute high quality research projects.

We plan to have a monthly educational complex cranial conference which would be led by our skull base fellows. These forums will be used to discuss upcoming cases of interest. We will use these spaces to collaborate on developing clear surgical or non-surgical plans and review recent cases/complications.

Our team's educational outreach would not be limited to our residents/fellows. We would also provide community outreach education targeted towards patients and referring physicians in the so-called Ark-La-Tex region (Southwest Arkansas, Northwest Louisiana, and East Texas).

Monetary Support

In addition to the many generous donors who have contributed to the LSUHS Department of Neurosurgery over the years, the department has also been fortunate to consistently maintain ample clinical revenue, even despite COVID-19 related setbacks. In addition, our department has invested considerable time and effort into applying for extramural funding to help support various research endeavors. Thus, lack of monetary support will not be a limiting factor for the establishment of the Complex Cranial Surgery Center of Excellence.

Managing the Change

The leadership framework of the COE would include a central Director and two Co-Directors (one likely from another clinical department and one from a research background). We would plan for the leadership to turn over every 2–3 years with election of new officers by the team members. There will be no formal term limits. Despite neurosurgery being the primary home of the concept of the COE, it would be our goal to distribute key leadership roles amongst all of the specialties involved in the center. We want everyone to have a stake in the COE and want the leadership to reflect this as well. The stakeholders will be the team members from each of the different departments. We are fortunate to have the buy-in of the necessary key personnel from each department. To reiterate, we are all people who have worked together and departments which have worked together for some time. The formalization of a COE will allow our intermittent collaboration to become more organized and streamlined, leading to better patient care, improved research productivity, and enhanced education.

The Business Proposition

By setting up the COE in our center at LSU we hope to attract additional patient numbers for other aspects of the health center. This will help to offset the cost of this investment with additional patient service revenue, increased ancillary service revenue (such as imaging, physical therapy, and speech therapy), and increased institutional visibility throughout our region.

Patient care will be the central focus of our Center of Excellence, but fantastic opportunities for research can stem from this central aim. Treating more complex intracranial pathology patients would create a lot of opportunity for a research program. Skull base surgery is a very technically challenging subspecialty within neurosurgery, and the field has advanced in terms of collaborative patient management over the past 20 years. Much of the research in our field used to involve advancing the technical components of our subspecialty. However, with a robust comprehensive database/registry, our COE will have the opportunity to evaluate patient outcomes, cost-effectiveness, and complication management in a much better, more ordered fashion. This endeavor will also allow us to study the intervention of incorporating our department as a Center of Excellence, which will contribute to the field of medical management research.

For data management, we plan to use RedCap, which is a medical registry software that would allow us to actively maintain data related to demographics, severity of pathology, surgical management, surgical outcome, long and short-term complications, and cost of care in a prospectively maintained data registry. We would also maintain imaging studies, pathology slides, and surgical videos as a part of our registry. This thorough data collection plan will make the processes of research more straightforward, which will in turn facilitate publications out of the health center. Recording this data will also allow us to identify longitudinal trends in patient outcomes. We plan to have one full time employee to maintain and continuously update this database. This cost will be offset by the reputation gained by becoming a leading research institution for complex intracranial surgery.

Lessons Learned by Our Leadership

Preparing an application for a COE was a great overall experience for our team. I have been a member of the faculty at LSU Health Shreveport since completion of my neurosurgical training in 2007. It is the only job that I have had since completing my training. Over the years, I have felt that I have become a part of the family of LSU Health Shreveport and specifically of our department. This Center of Excellence is something that we have wanted to do for several years. Formal business education has allowed us the opportunity to build the COE in a way that is structured and time tested.

Establishing a core team of changemakers was (and remains) vital for the success of the center of excellence. At the outset of this project it was especially important to get all of the key stakeholders in the center and in administration to be a part of the planning process. I found particular success in developing shared goals with all of the stakeholders and team members. This helped various departments to put all of their aspirations for the project on the table and negotiate a single set of goals based on shared values.

Relationships remained the most important part of the process of developing the center. In 2019, I became chairman of our Department of Neurosurgery at LSU Health Shreveport. The fact that I had been in the department during difficult times significantly helped my leadership ability in both the department and in the development of this Center of Excellence. My experience in our institution has allowed me to create relationships through the clinical departments, research arenas, and institutes of education. The advantage of being in a relatively small academic medical center is that I was able to formulate relationships with key people and collaborators in many departments very early in my career. I have continued to build upon these relationships over many years. These relationships, more than anything else, allowed this center to come together smoothly.

The leadership structure for our center was very well received by the team members. My institutional knowledge and commitment to the development of the Center of Excellence made me the first candidate for leadership. That said, it is important to note that we took measures to divorce leadership from the long term success of the project to make the project durable over time. The structure of having a co-director and having rotating leadership every 2 years showed everyone on the team that this was not a one-team mission and that other departments would have their turn being the "face of the Center of Excellence".

To this end, this center is yet another example of how influential the culture of a team is for success. Our team's culture is excellent because it is a collection of positive people who all want the same things: to provide exceptional surgical and medical care for critically ill patients, to elevate the research platform of our skull base team and the institution as a whole, and to provide the best possible teaching for our residents and fellows in our programs. Fortunately we could not identify one dissenter or difficult-to-convince team member. I was so lucky to have this team structure and I also realize how unique this culture is for any team.

As time goes by, it will be my role as the center director and center founder to maintain this culture. As long as we all are interested in pushing forward our mission and achieving the common goal of higher quality patient care, I believe that this outstanding culture can be maintained.

I have also tried to make culture change and improvement towards positive culture a primary change initiative in my role as neurosurgery department chair. It is amazing how much more can be achieved by a group when the culture is positive. Our resident ACGME surveys have never been better, and our faculty growth is progressing well, and I believe that the EMBA teachings that I have benefitted from have also let me be able to relay these teachings to both our center and my department.

I feel so fortunate to have had the opportunity to have made so much progress towards the goal of obtaining a Center of Excellence designation during my EMBA program. This was an incredibly beneficial experience for our department, and we believe it will be a great accomplishment for our institution and health system.

We are also creating opportunities for the junior members to flourish in their academic and clinical practice which in turn helps to achieve the common goal of establishing a Center of Excellence (Fig. 14.4). We think that fostering relationships, allowing junior members to lead and flourish, and being fair are all parts of team success. We have tried to incorporate all of these qualities in developing our center. We are also genuinely fortunate to have the support of our administration, which is key to moving forward any initiative. This again highlights the importance of people and the importance of relationships. We think that knowing the people,

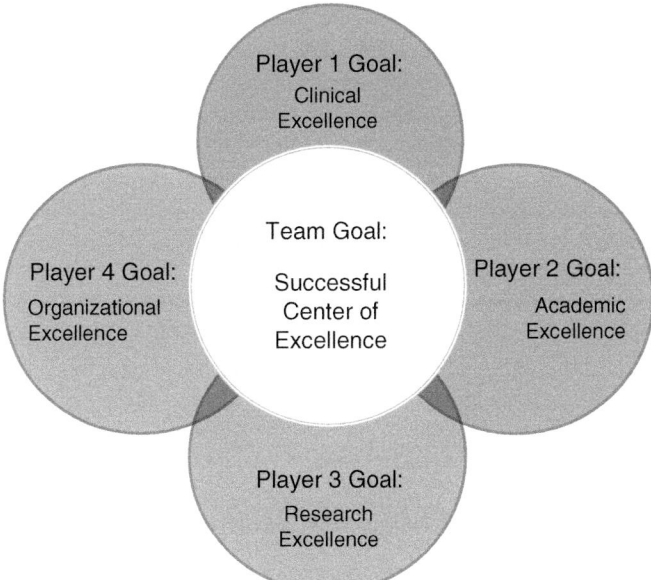

Fig. 14.4 Shows goal alignment between players in our medical team

being familiar with key relationships, and being kind/fair/inclusive are the keys to facilitating a collaborative effort such as obtaining a multi-disciplinary center.

We were fortunate to stick to our timeline that we proposed during the initial planning phase. We had regular meetings over the last year towards the goal of formulating a final proposal for the center. When we were satisfied that we had all aspects of the center addressed, we submitted this to the LSU system for initial approval. Fortunately, we were able to obtain approval through the first local institutional phase. The proposal is currently under review by the Louisiana Board of Regents. Approval from the Louisiana Board of Regents will be the final step in the process of obtaining formal center designation. Their review was tentatively planned for the late spring/early summer, but was delayed by COVID-19. Our team now anxiously awaits the submission/review process from the Louisiana Board of Regents.

Conclusion: Summary and Future Directions

In this chapter, we aimed to provide the fundamental elements and potential challenges to be considered when establishing a Center of Excellence (COE) in Complex Cranial Surgery. We provided a brief explanation of the reasons to form a COE, the essential strengths needed to initiate and support a COE, and the necessary environment to cultivate in order to ensure common goals and objectives of the team as a whole and individuals. More specifically, a center for excellence thrives when it is established in a strategic location, with plenty of monetary support, in conjunction with an experienced healthcare system, with strong interdisciplinary relationships and with a strong intent of the team to excel.

Although we are still awaiting the formal approval of our COE, we anticipate its official title being granted in the near future. In the meantime, we are continuing to provide excellent patient care, strengthen our collaborative relationships, and grow as a team. Once our COE is formally established, we look forward to expanding our efforts toward the betterment of our community, healthcare team, and trainees by orchestrating and participating in various philanthropic and educational endeavors. Our plans include, but are not limited to: community health fairs, research symposiums, educational workshops, fundraisers, and eventually, offering funding opportunities for education and medical support for our staff and patients.

References

1. Elrod JK, Fortenberry JL. Centers of excellence in healthcare institutions: what they are and how to assemble them. BMC Health Serv Res. 2017;17(Suppl 1) https://doi.org/10.1186/s12913-017-2340-y.
2. Khan UA, Bhavsar A, Asif H, Karabatsou K, Leggate JRS, Sofat A, et al. Treatment by specialist surgical neuro-oncologists improves survival times for patients with malignant glioma. J Neurosurg. 2015;122:297–302.
3. Albright AL, Sposto R, Holmes E, Zeltzer PM, Finlay JL, Wisoff JH, et al. Correlation of neurosurgical subspecialization with outcomes in children with malignant brain tumors. Neurosurgery. 2000;47:879–87.
4. McLaughlin N, Laws ER, Oyesiku NM, Katznelson L, Kelly DF. Pituitary centers of excellence. Neurosurgery. 2012;71:916–26.
5. McLaughlin N, Carrau R, Kelly D, Prevedello D, Kassam A. Teamwork in skull base surgery: an avenue for improvement in patient care. Surg Neurol Int. 2013;4:36.
6. Hendy J, Barlow J. The role of the organizational champion in achieving health system change. Soc Sci Med. 2012;74:348–55.
7. Mesman R, Westert GP, Berden BJMM, Faber MJ. Why do high-volume hospitals achieve better outcomes? A systematic review about intermediate factors in volume–outcome relationships. Health Policy. 2015;119:1055–67.
8. Martin JS, Ummenhofer W, Manser T, Spirig R. Interprofessional collaboration among nurses and physicians: making a difference in patient outcome. Swiss Med Wkly. 2010;40(3536) https://doi.org/10.4414/smw.2010.13062.
9. Tonn J, Schlake H, Goldbrunner R, Mileski C, Helms J, Roosen K. Acoustic neuroma surgery as an interdisciplinary approach: a neurosurgical series of 508 patients. J Neurol Neurosurg Psychiatry. 2000;69:161–6.
10. Kolker A. Management science for healthcare applications. In: Wang J, editor. Encycl Bus Anal Optim. Hershey, PA: Business Science Reference; 2014. p. 1446–56.

Obtaining Center of Excellence Accreditation of a Robotic Program in a Safety Net Academic Hospital

Shaneeta M. Johnson and Omar K. Danner

Key Learning Points
- Clear articulation of the vision and ability to persuade others to work towards a shared goal.
- Strategies to deal with obstacles and barriers which are an expected part of any project and should be dealt with strategically.
- Communication with those who may be resistors to change is paramount and crucial.
- Delegation is necessary to increase team involvement, empower the team, and complete tasks more efficiently.
- Relationships, built properly, persist, and are the catalyst for the change envisioned.

Executive Summary

Introduction of Topic/Background Information

Patient safety and quality care are the true benchmarks of accreditation as a Center of Excellence. This designation represents the focus and attention to detail demonstrated by a healthcare system in delivering high-quality care. Accreditation of the program as a Center of Excellence ensures that the program is working towards maintaining the highest standards of care for Minimally Invasive Surgery [1]. The

S. M. Johnson (✉)
Department of Surgery, Satcher Health Leadership Institute, Morehouse School of Medicine, Atlanta, GA, USA
e-mail: shajohnson@msm.edu

O. K. Danner
Department of Surgery, Morehouse School of Medicine/Grady Memorial Hospital, Atlanta, GA, USA

purpose of highlighting the successful accreditation of a Robotic Surgery (RS) program is to show the large impact the establishment of a successful Robotics program can have on the patients, faculty, and community experience, and healthcare system's botto-line. Minimally invasive surgery has numerous patient and healthcare organizational benefits. However, it may be limited to those with the economic means to afford such procedures, unless safety-net hospitals can provide access to these cutting-edge minimal access procedures. Accreditation of the Robotic Surgery program will validate the importance of delivering superior quality care, providing significant financial gains, reducing healthcare disparities, improving patient comfort and recovery time, and aligning with the strategic direction of academic medical institutions, hospitals, and healthcare systems.

Benefits of Robotic Surgery

Low-income and underrepresented minority populations are at increased risk of developing many common chronic diseases that warrant surgical intervention including prostate cancer, colon cancer, obesity, ovarian cancer, cardiovascular disease, lung cancer, and others. Minimally invasive surgery to treat these diseases has shown numerous benefits, such as lower complication rates, decreased pain, less opiate use, shorter recovery time, and decreased hospital length of stay. However, studies demonstrate that low-income and underrepresented minorities have decreased access to these advanced minimally invasive procedures and technology such as robotic surgery on a consistent basis [2]. This particular community is already at significantly increased risk for increased complications, poorer clinical outcomes, readmission to the hospital, and the need for reoperation. Open surgery is associated with longer lengths of hospital stay, increased wound complications, wounds that may require weeks to heal, higher levels of pain, amplified need for opiate use, and greater risk for reoperation. These factors all translate into higher financial costs that are being borne by local, state, and federal governments.

Environment

Grady Hospital (GH), the largest safety-net hospital in the state of Georgia, serves a significant population of underserved persons in metro Atlanta. GH sees more than 130,000 patients per year through its Emergency Department. Of these visits, the vast majority meet the criteria for classification as low-income, underrepresented patients. In 2012 analysis, the estimate was that more than 22% of Georgians were uninsured, this amounts to 1.8 million people and accounts for the seventh highest uninsured rate in the country [3]. GH has a significant group of patients who are also homeless. This poses unique and substantial challenges for providing medical and social care. Often, the patients we serve have no housing available after their surgical intervention and hospital stay, which makes simple issues such as care of surgical wounds and obtaining optimal nutrition for healing exceedingly difficult. This places a heavy burden upon the treating hospital facility.

In 2016, through a national grant process, we obtained and were able to provide GH with cutting-edge Robotic Surgery technology. GH acquired a Da Vinci surgical robot platform that year, making it one of only a handful of safety-net teaching centers with access to advanced robotic surgical technology for use in its patient population.

Current Status of Program and Benefits

Since the inception of the robotic surgery program at GH in February 2017, staff surgeons have completed nearly 700 cases robotically. Our data analysis has shown dramatic improvements in clinical outcomes and length of stay (LOS) reduction. We have seen decreased rates of wound infections, substantially reduced pain scores and need for opiate use, and increased patient satisfaction. These patients are discharged from the hospital sooner, return to their jobs earlier, and require decreased amounts of medication, particularly pain medicine. Considering the current opioid epidemic, this is a major advantage, and the majority of RS patients go home with minimal to no prescription for narcotic agents. Improvements in hospital LOS have been very significant with 2 to 10-day shorter stays consistent with data nationally. This has translated into improved patient satisfaction as well as a significant hospital cost reduction due to a decrease in inpatient bed days. Additionally, hospitals are able to treat more patients due to the increased availability of surgical beds related to shorter LOS and decreased need for admission. This means even greater access to healthcare for vulnerable patient populations.

With the introduction of RS in an organized, multispecialty fashion, we have been able to show improved value with streamlined costs. In fact, our LOS is on average greater than 5 days less than the overall hospital postoperative LOS. This has given healthy cost savings to our healthcare system. Our mortality, readmission, infection rates, complication rates are all lower than the overall hospital average for similar open procedures. Additionally, we have seen a rapid proliferation of surgeons in the program with expansion from 3 to 17 surgeons since its short inception. The number and breadth of cases have also rapidly expanded. In the first year of implementation, the program was projected to perform 50 cases and instead was able to complete 178 cases. The program has now completed more than 700 cases and there are 10 surgical subspecialties represented. This has increased market share, patient demand in these subspecialties, and resident training opportunities, and expanded the footprint of both medical institutions and the healthcare system.

These advances are in direct alignment with the strategic vision and plans of Morehouse School of Medicine. The plans of the system are to capitalize on and further the advancements made within this program and replicate the successful program components in other service lines. This supports GH's vision of being the leading public academic hospital in the country.

Reason for Accreditation

Accreditation of the RS program at GH by the Surgical Review Corporation will validate the success of this program, improve quality outcomes, and provide certification of the excellent level of service administered at the facility. From a hospital administrative viewpoint, we expect that it will give a more comprehensive view of the program and invite the involvement of non-surgical departments and specialties in the service delivery model. This designation will represent the dedication demonstrated by the hospital to deliver high-quality care. Accreditation of the program as a Center of Excellence authenticates the early successes of the program. It will also serve as a blueprint for other safety-net hospitals to establish similar programs and provide the same high level of care to their patients.

While minimally invasive surgery has been shown to be associated with many benefits, many of the patients served by these safety-net hospitals are unable to take advantage of these benefits due to a lack of access to RS technology and trained providers. Strengthening and accrediting such a program allows us to continue to address and help reduce healthcare disparities. This affords patients of lower socioeconomic status and\or lack of adequate insurance afford the highest level of service and receive standard of care treatment. This is in direct agreement with moves within the healthcare system to eliminate any barriers of access to care.

Robotic Surgery Center of Excellence designation will also affect patient safety and their experience. Protocols will be developed and solidified to ensure the highest standards of patient safety. Additionally, the patient experience must be a central focus and kept at a superior level.

Accreditation requires the establishment of documented protocols of training for residents, operating staff, and surgeons. These protocols will ensure the maintenance of the highest levels of training and safety. We expect to see improved operational efficiency, improved finances, and decreased long-term costs resulting from the rigorous standards implemented during accreditation. An added benefit is the continued financial benefits seen in decreased length of hospital stay, decreased narcotic use, and other cost reduction due to decreased wound-related complications.

Additional policies and research protocols regarding advanced robotics use and the implementation of an RS program in a safety-net academic hospital will require further development. The overall goal is to be able to benefit the unique patient population served by GHS. Lastly, along with accreditation, we plan to develop and solidify educational curriculums for resident, surgeon, and operating room staff training.

Methodology

Stakeholders and Resources

In order to accomplish this goal, we identified key stakeholders and then implemented a timeline. We identified the required resources and made plans to acquire and/or implement these resources.

We held monthly robotic steering committee meetings are held to evaluate the program, establish guidelines, and improve processes and workflow. Additionally, we proactively gathered and evaluated clinical and quality outcomes data.

Stakeholders

The key stakeholders selected were the leaders of the hospital and both medical institutions. In order to engage these key leaders, regular updates on the program, its growth, and successes, as well as the timeline for accreditation, were presented. The value brought by assimilation of these leaders for a project such as this one is the congealing of a program to improve patient care outcomes among vulnerable patients, resident education, and hospital operational metrics such as length of stay. The key stakeholders were made aware of the project and supportive of this drive towards accreditation.

Executive Change Team

Table 15.1 shows the key members and their roles and responsibilities.

Resources

Table 15.2 lists the resources required.

Table 15.1 Executive team members and responsibilities

Key team members	Role and responsibilities
Shaneeta Johnson MD Chair Robotic Committee	Chair, Robotic Committee, Director of Minimally Invasive and Bariatric Surgery, MSM Responsible for overall program leadership, credentialing of surgeons and residents, and leading the program through accreditation
Executive Perioperative Director	Executive Perioperative Director Responsible for Operating room operations. Critical in ensuring policies needed for accreditation are created and implemented
Robotic Team Lead/Coordinator	Robotic Team Lead/Coordinator Responsible for the daily administration of the robotic team and training of staff. Develop staff training manuals and policies
Quality Data Analyst	Quality Data Analyst Responsible for collecting and analyzing data for outcomes, quality, and demographics. Will obtain data from the robotic program and collate this data.
General Surgery Resident	General Surgery Resident Acts as a liaison with the surgical and gynecologic residencies
Ad-hoc: COO GH, Chairman of Obstetrics and Gynecology	Crucial relationships within the organizations

Table 15.2 Resources needed

Resource	Method of securing
Time	Dedicated meetings with the team (every 3 weeks) to assess completion of deliverables and milestones
	Monthly robotic committee meetings
Funding	Site Visit and Application fees required—Will be obtained from Operating Room budget
Additional Personnel—Robotic First Assistant	Job has been posted in Human Resources to secure this additional personnel who will also play a role in obtaining accreditation

Project Plan

Meetings were begun almost a year prior in March 2019 and held every 3 weeks with the launch team to evaluate progress and completion of milestones. Initially, the estimated accreditation completion date and submission of the application were in October 2019. However, it took until February 2020 to complete. Following this, the initial application was begun.

Unexpected Obstacles

As expected there were obstacles encountered during the project. These included the loss of the executive champion, resistance to change, and barriers to forward progression.

Loss of Executive Champion

In April 2019, we lost our executive champion which lead to the need to regroup and refocus the team. This led to the development of new connections and influence within the C suite which had to be redeveloped and aligned to allow for the re-establishment of an advocate in the executive suite.

Resistance to Change

As expected, the program was met with resistance from those who do not fully recognize the benefits of robotic surgery such as shorter hospital stays and improved outcomes as these benefits are typically realized by the corporation and payors.

Barriers to Forward Progression

In order to ensure the success of the program there was a temporary pause to ensure that faculty were properly credentialed and all quality processes and procedures were in place. After review, the program was continued fully and has thrived and flourished.

Evaluation of the Program

Competitive Advantage and Key Success Factors

The program was evaluated for organizational strategy, competitive advantage, and key success factors. The organization is committed to offering the same standard of care to its underserved patient population. It is a multi-institutional program that provides RS training while remaining in alignment with the organizational goals of the GHS (Fig. 15.1).

Relational Coordination Analysis

We used relational coordination as a robotic steering team, to evaluate the program's strengths and weaknesses from our point of view [4]. We determined that we need to improve our relationships with Anesthesia, Robotic Staff, OR Leadership and the C-Suite. The relational coordination analysis showed the following (Fig. 15.2):

- **Weak relational coordination based on relational map analysis**:
- Anesthesia had the weakest relational coordination.
- Corporate (Robotic) staff also had weak relational coordination.
- OR leadership and C-Suite had moderate relational coordination.
- **Strong relational coordination based on relational map analysis**:
- Strongest relational coordination is seen with patients, OR staff, and surgeons.

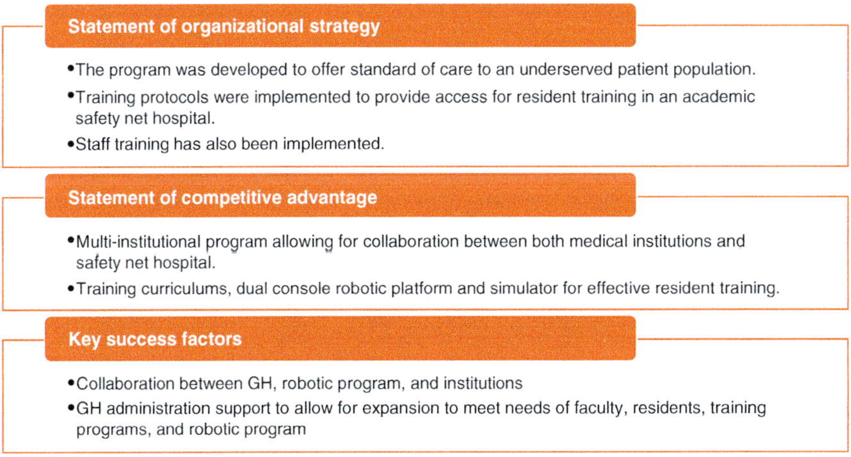

Statement of organizational strategy
- The program was developed to offer standard of care to an underserved patient population.
- Training protocols were implemented to provide access for resident training in an academic safety net hospital.
- Staff training has also been implemented.

Statement of competitive advantage
- Multi-institutional program allowing for collaboration between both medical institutions and safety net hospital.
- Training curriculums, dual console robotic platform and simulator for effective resident training.

Key success factors
- Collaboration between GH, robotic program, and institutions
- GH administration support to allow for expansion to meet needs of faculty, residents, training programs, and robotic program

Fig. 15.1 Evaluation of organizational strategy, competitive advantage and key success factors

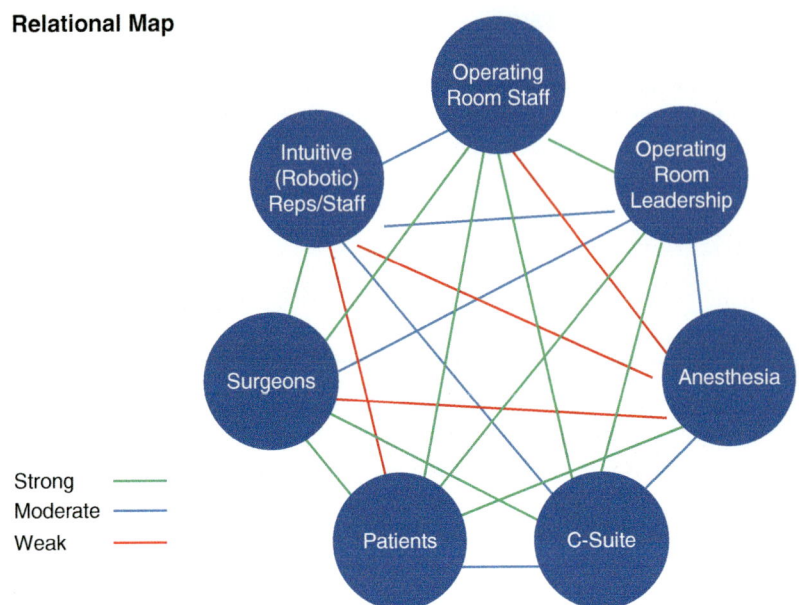

Fig. 15.2 Relational coordination map

Organizational Alignment

We analyzed the organizational alignment using several different frameworks including Seven S Factor analysis, Sweet Spot Analysis, and Evaluation of the Environment [5].

Seven S Factor Analysis
Seven S factor analysis demonstrated that there was a significant structure to the program with a participatory and engaged team. This has led to the growth of the program and the team. However, it was constrained by a lack of alignment with the administration of the hospital. Another constraint was that the technology now needed to be upgraded to current technology which is projected to incur financial costs of approximately $2 million [6] (Table 15.3).

Sweet Spot Analysis
Sweet spot analysis also demonstrates of this program is in alignment with the organization. It allows for the delivery of a high standard of care to a patient population who would not otherwise have access to this level of care. However, these patients require the best care possible in order to have improved outcomes and decrease cost to the health system. Therefore, with GH being able to offer this level of care to patients' requirements, this represents a definite sweet spot (Fig. 15.3).

Table 15.3 Seven S factor analysis

Seven S factor	Support capabilities	Constrain capabilities
Strategy	Advanced technology available to provide the standard of care for patient care and resident training	Need alignment with goals of GH Administration
Structure	Robotic steering committee—surgeons, OR leadership, ancillary services	Constrained by fully blocked schedule affecting utilization
Skills	Multiple surgical specialties available to provide care utilizing the robotic platform	Difficulty with the recruitment of faculty and residents due to outdated technology
Systems	Third gen technology with dual console and simulator	Prior generation technology with equipment becoming unavailable
Style	Participatory robotic committee	Need alignment with goals of GH Administration
Staffing	Capable robotic team leader Physician Champion OR leadership	Need a dedicated robotic coordinator—recommended best practice Need First assistant—best practice
Shared values	Commitment to providing the standard of care in an academic safety-net hospital	Need alignment with goals of GH Administration

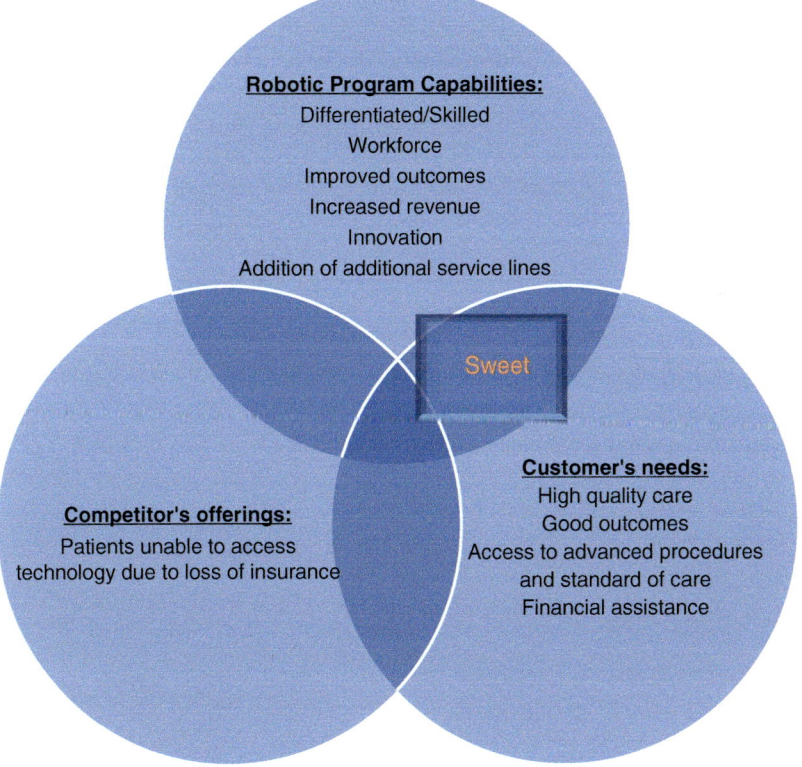

Fig. 15.3 Sweet spot analysis

Sizing Up the External Environment

Remote Environment

An economic evaluation of the external environment revealed some startling facts, namely 22% of Georgians had no insurance in 2014 [7]. In fact, GH sees a significant number of uninsured or government-insured patients. This vulnerable patient population has a higher Medicare case mix index (CMI) indicating an increased level of acuity. Furthermore, the surgical CMI for GH (5.3303) is higher than local competitor facilities, such as Emory University Hospital (3.7419), WellStar Kennestone Hospital (3.6162), and Northside Hospital (2.9942). It is comparable to the CMI of Atlanta Medical Center (6.0247) [8].

Social evaluation of the remote environment shows a high percentage of African-Americans. In fact, it is estimated that "African-Americans make up just over half of the city's residents. But a recent study found that 80% of black children here live in neighborhoods with high concentrations of poverty, which often have poor access to quality medical care, while 6% of white children do. Several of the neighborhoods with predominate minority communities have poverty rates higher than 40%" [9].

Politically, the external environment is overshadowed by the fact that the state of Georgia has not expanded Medicaid. This significantly affects the patient population served at GH as well as throughout the metro Atlanta metro region.

The remote environment shows significant changes in the technological arena, especially in the field of surgery where robotic surgery has had exponential growth in its adoption nationally. There continue to be significant advances in technology that promise to improve the care that we deliver for patients. The metropolitan area of Atlanta serves as a headquarters and training site for medical devices and equipment companies as well as a place for innovation and technology such as the surgical robotic platform to grow exponentially.

Operating Environment

Evaluating the operating environment for customers, competitors, and creditors revealed that the customers who were patients and referring doctors were now requesting and expecting a higher level of patient care. This includes increased access to less invasive technology and advanced procedures. GH is poised to deliver this advanced level of care.

Results

Project Deliverables and Milestones

1. Letter of support from GH Administration—Requested.
2. Robotic Privileges Credentialing Documentation—The credentialing process underwent marginally necessary revision in 2019 and again in 2020.
3. Documentation of robotic cases number—The program has completed more than 700 cases which are all recorded within a dashboard evaluating metrics of quality, length of stay, volume, mix, and robotic-specific metrics.
4. Surgeon Documentation—125 cases lifetime and 30/year—Completed and updated ongoing.
5. Documentation of Chair of Robotic Committee—The robotic committee was established in September 2016 and meets monthly with minutes.
6. Surgeon accreditation documentation—All surgeons completed a robotic privileging process.
7. Documentation of Consultative Support from:
    A. Intensive Care.
    B. Interventional Radiology.
    C. Cardiology.
    D. Endocrinology.
    E. Infection Disease.
    F. Nephrology.
    G. Pathology.
    H. Pulmonology.
    I. Surgical ICU
    J. Anesthesia.

   All services within the hospital support the program.

8. Obtained JCAHO policy regarding ACLS 24/7 coverage—JCAHO policies were requested to demonstrate compliance.
9. Documentation of Regular Staff training—We have implemented monthly staff training for RS for staff and residents.
10. Service Contract with Intuitive Surgical—A service contract with Intuitive surgical was instituted.

11. Evidence of 12 hours of CME/3 years—The Chair of the Committee spearheaded along with the robotic committee the proposed strategy and developed robotic symposiums and other educational activities in robotic surgery.
12. Documentation of GH General Surgery & GYN Call Schedule—Present.
13. Demonstration of RS pathways for:
    A. Anesthesia—Monitoring and airway.
    B. Post-operative care—pain management and airway.
    C. Antibiotic management.
    D. Urinary Catheter early removal.
    E. Discharge instructions—early identification of complications.
    F. Preoperative patient preparation and education.

These pathways are in existence and will be placed within the documentation.

14. Program Coordinator—A program coordinator was interviewed and hired. Her duties include training, coordination, scheduling, and education.
15. Staff Training—Instituted monthly including pathways and checklists to demonstrate competence.
    A. Complications.
    B. Equipment and Surgical Instruments.
    C. Clinical Pathways.
16. Preoperative Education—Formalized process and Consent.
17. Maintain Outcomes Database—Evaluate SRC database and determine if we will participate—pending.

Results and Impact

Metrics

We have been collecting data on every robotic surgical case performed at GH. In addition to surgical metrics such as operative time, the number of cases, anesthesia time, hospital length of stay, and robotic console time we also evaluate quality metrics such as outcomes, complications, infection rates, and mortality. Additionally, we track payor mix, cost of instrument use, county of residence, and operating room turnover time.

Growth

The robotic surgery program has seen tremendous growth and improved results in our underserved patient populations. The program involves hospital administrative support, medical institutional support, surgeons, nurses, operating room leadership, information technology, quality data and outcomes, financial personnel, anesthesiologists, and other partnerships. The program has seen a 29% volume growth in surgeries performed from 2017 to 2018 and a 13% growth from 2018 to 2019. We have had significant increases in the number of surgeons and staff trained and successfully implemented this program to address the disparity of care for this underserved community (Figs. 15.4 and 15.5).

Outcomes

The program has seen tremendous length of stay improvements. This results in significant cost savings for the organization. Additionally, instrument costs were tallied and determined to be better than national data.

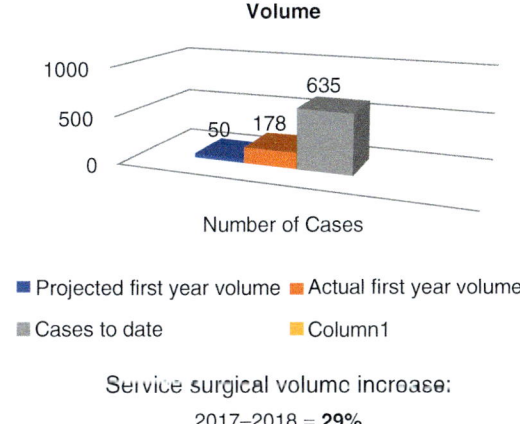

Fig. 15.4 Surgical case volume increase

Surgical subspecialties:

Initial:
1) General Surgery
2) Gynecology Oncology
3) Urology

Current:
1) General Surgery
2) Gynecology Oncology
3) Urology
4) Hepatobiliary Surgery
5) Surgical Oncology
6) Thoracic Surgery
7) Colon and Rectal Surgery
8) *Cardiac Surgery*
9) Pelvic and Reconstructive Surgery
10) Benign Gynecology

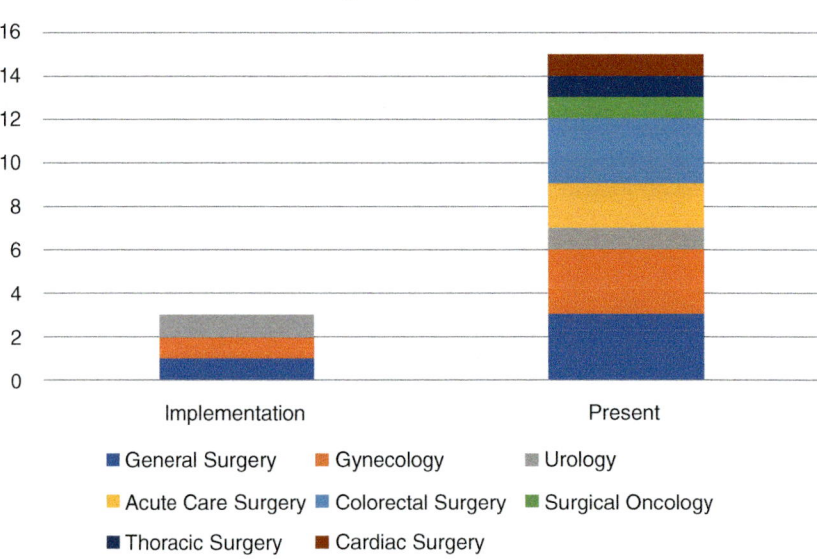

Fig. 15.5 Surgical specialty increase

Discussion/Lessons Learned/Reflections

Leadership Reflections

This was a daunting, yet very rewarding task. It required assembling a multidisciplinary team that met frequently to complete a very task-oriented project with great significance for the hospital system, its associated academic institutions, and metro Atlanta.

Assessment of Leadership

Change, especially in the face of naysayers is incredibly challenging. This is especially difficult when there is a loss of administrative support. The project experienced this with the loss of a strong supporter in the person of the Executive Champion. It is important to demonstrate motivation and passion for the program and mission during times of change. We were able to identify institutional leadership who were incredibly supportive of the robotic program and its impact on training the learners.

Dealing with opposition can also be especially difficult. The unique program has undergone continuous evaluation and shown tremendous success. Reaching out to those with opposing views, including them in the successes of the program, and also utilizing "going to the Gemba" techniques has assisted in establishing common ground. Finally, bringing other leaders on board who are able to increase collaboration seems to be the most successful method to date.

Requiring accountability from the team is crucial. In fact, team members are expecting this accountability and it also gives them the opportunity to demonstrate their prowess and accomplishments.

Assessment of Team Performance

The strengths of the team are many. The team shares a common vision for the program and its success. The team was also very motivated, organized, and responsible. There are different strengths possessed by the members of the team that complement each other.

The team was expected to complete individual and team assignments within this change project. This was embraced by this motivated team. They were participatory in analyzing the strengths and weaknesses of the program and making strides to the goal of accreditation. Each of the team members was independent in completing requirements.

This project elucidated several key learning objectives.

1. The ability to clearly articulate a vision and persuade others to work towards this goal is imperative in leadership.
2. Obstacles and barriers are an expected part of any project and should be dealt with strategically.
3. Communication with those who may be resistors to change is paramount and crucial.
4. Delegation is necessary to increase team involvement, empower the team, and complete tasks more efficiently.
5. Relationships, built properly, persist. I have learnt many leadership lessons from the prior executive champion and others in leadership.

Conclusion/Summary

While daunting, strategic vision and plans once properly approached can lead to significant wins. Leadership and organizational management strategies are paramount in developing team-based approaches for the effective completion of goals and objectives. Many leadership lessons were required during this process and continue to be obtained. The healthcare system has benefited greatly from the introduction of this team-based consulting project focus. Even more importantly, the patients that we care for have benefited the most.

Since the inception of the robotic surgery program at GH in February 2017, over 700 cases robotic cases have been performed. Our health system has seen dramatic improvements in patient outcomes with decreased LOS, reduced pain score and narcotic requirement, and increased overall patient satisfaction. We have experienced decreased rates of wound infections, and other quality metrics since the introduction of the RS program. More expeditious hospital discharges along with a quick return to work offer a significant benefit to patients, employers, and the health care system in the form of additional available inpatient beds. As it relates to the raging opioid epidemic, RS offers a major advantage, and the majority of RS patients go home with a minimum to no prescription for narcotic agents. Coupled with the significant potential cost savings at our hospital, the benefits and merits of RS portend a bright future and greater penetration for this exciting, revolutionary technology in the field of medicine and healthcare quality improvement.

References

1. https://www.surgicalreview.org/facilities/. Why achieve accreditation? Last accessed 3/2/2021.
2. Kim J, ElRayes W, Wilson F, et al. Disparities in the receipt of robot-assisted radical prostatectomy: between-hospital and within-hospital analysis using 2009-2011 California inpatient data. BMJ Open. 2015;5(4):e007409. https://doi.org/10.1136/bmjopen-2014-007409.
3. https://www.kff.org/health-reform/fact-sheet/the-georgia-health-care-landscape/. The Georgia Health Care Landscape. Last accessed 3/2/2021.

4. https://www.mckinsey.com/business-functions/strategy-and-corporate-finance/our-insights/enduring-ideas-the-7-s-framework#. Enduring Ideas: The 7-S Framework. Last accessed 3/2/2021.
5. Hoffer GJ. Transforming relationships for high performance: the power of relational coordination. Palo Alto, CA: Stanford University Press; 2016.
6. Ho C, Tsakonas E, Tran K, et al. Robot-assisted surgery compared with open surgery and laparoscopic surgery: clinical effectiveness and economic analyses [Internet].CADTH Technology Report, No. 137. Ottawa (ON): Canadian agency for drugs and technologies in health; 2011.
7. https://opendatanetwork.herokuapp.com/entity/0400000US13/Georgia/health.health_insurance.pctui?year=2013&age=18%20to%2064&race=All%20races&sex=Both%20sexes&income=All%20income%20levels Last accessed 3/2/2021.
8. https://www.ahd.com/georgia American Hospital Directory. Last accessed 3/2/2021.
9. https://www.npr.org/sections/health-shots/2018/04/04/599253766/atlanta-struggles-to-fulfill-mlks-legacy-in-health-care "Atlanta Struggles to fulfill MLK's legacy in Health Care". Last accessed 3/2/2021.

Part IV

Value Creation in Health Care II: Improving Clinical Efficiency and Lowering Costs

Vascular Diagnostic Laboratory Improvements Through Effective Data Management

16

Evan C. Lipsitz

Key Learning Points
- Perform a quick screen using the Payback method to assess project viability.
- Perform an analysis of incremental costs and revenues associated with a project including an analysis of sunk costs and opportunity costs.
- Analyze and articulate fixed and variable cash outflows as well as revenue over the project term.
- Perform a discounted cash flow analysis including net present value calculations to assess a project's value under different conditions including cost of capital and with sensitivity analysis under best, middle, and worst conditions.
- Perform a stakeholder analysis to identify all interested and impacted parties. Assemble a project team and use the principles of relational coordination to map, leverage, and build relationships.
- Use leadership principles to have the project team articulate, pitch, and formally present the project to all interested parties.

Executive Summary

This chapter describes a project whose purpose was to justify, acquire, and implement an advanced imaging and data management system at a large academic medical center within the non-invasive vascular diagnostic laboratory. Major steps in the project included understanding and providing appropriate financial justification for the project using accounting principles, identifying stakeholders and their interests,

E. C. Lipsitz (✉)
Division of Vascular and Endovascular Surgery, Department of Cardiothoracic and Vascular Surgery, Montefiore Medical Center and the Albert Einstein College of Medicine, Bronx, NY, USA
e-mail: elipsitz@brandeis.edu

bringing stakeholders together to work towards a common goal and establishing a timeline and metrics. The majority of the work centered around providing financial justification for the project, using principles of relational coordination to ensure engagement of stakeholders and leadership learnings to guide the process as a whole. These learnings and principles can be applied to related projects of any scale and may serve as a template for those wishing to consider such projects.

Introduction of Topic/Background Information

This project was designed to demonstrate the need for, acquire, and implement an advanced imaging and data management system for the non-invasive vascular diagnostic laboratory at a large academic medical center. The vascular lab performs non-invasive, ultrasound based anatomic testing as well as non-invasive physiologic tests that assess vascular pathologies. Physiologic studies include lower extremity pulse volume recordings (a measure of overall flow at various levels in the extremities) and Photoplethysmogaphy (to measure flow in the digits). Anatomic studies include duplex (an ultrasound-based measure of blood flow) that can be applied throughout the body including the aorta, as well as carotid, extremity, visceral and renal arteries. These studies are also performed in the venous system and for the surveillance of all interventions, both open surgical and endovascular. The lab is extensively utilized by the emergency department, all inpatient services, outpatient medical practices in addition to our own vascular and endovascular service. At the time of the project we were performing approximately 31,000 studies per year across our three major campuses and several outpatient sites (Table 16.1). The process and workflow were inefficient, costly, cumbersome, error prone, and archaic with low satisfaction by all stake holders. In short, the existing system no longer met the needs of our medical center.

The lab has grown significantly over the past several years based on increasing volume at existing sites and the addition of an additional busy outpatient office and surgical facility, which functions effectively as a fourth major lab. Growth at existing sites is estimated at approximately 5% per year over the past 5 years. This growth occurred during a time when the organization acquired several local hospitals and group practices, making future growth rates more difficult to predict.

Table 16.1 Vascular Lab studies by site (2015)

Site	Number of studies
Hospital 1	17,641
Hospital 2	7520
Hospital 3	3530
Ambulatory Center	2178
Other Satellite Labs	151
Total	31,020

The large volume and need to provide inpatient services mandate that individual labs are maintained at each of the three main hospital campuses. The introduction of the fourth major site (ambulatory center) ensures that diagnostic evaluations are completed in a single visit, improving patient flow and convenience by reducing the need for additional visits.

The Vascular Lab and its' large volume of studies is a major revenue source for the institution. There are also significant costs associated with its operation. Efficient functioning of the lab has a significant impact on the institution's financial status. For example, delays in testing and/or reporting can lead to increased length of stay, delays in operative procedures, and Emergency Department overload.

Our organization is a large, urban, academic medical center that supports an evolving major regional health system with several recent hospital acquisitions and affiliations. The institution also recently assumed operational control of its affiliated medical school. This rapid expansion has led to resource constraints since labor and capital are largely deployed towards expansion projects. We are also constrained by our payer mix consisting of approximately 83% government insurance, forcing us to operate at greater efficiency than most other academic medical centers. We serve a population with significant medical and social needs and for a time were the first and only pioneer Accountable Care Organization in our State.

The project is long overdue. There are no disagreements on the merits. The queue of much needed projects in the hospital is long. The current system (OldLab) involves manual data entry by lab technicians, produces pictures on paper that are not digitally stored or available, requires computer sign-off of reports that are generated on paper, does not allow for viewing of preliminary reports by referring physicians. The system is outdated, inefficient, error prone, and is currently unsupported by the vendor.

We chose NewLab as our system of choice after extensively vetting against a variety of other systems by multiple stakeholders. The benefits of this system are numerous and are expected to have a far-reaching impact across the Medical Center including significant cost savings, efficiency, and study quality. These current status and anticipated impacts are highlighted to follow.

Vascular Laboratory: Current System

A comprehensive Vascular Laboratory solution includes image acquisition, management and storage. It also requires a mechanism for physician interpretation of the images, generating a report to referring providers and making the images and reports available to all interested providers. This includes access via the electronic medical record (EMR). Finally, long term data storage is essential. Ideally, the system would also have a mechanism for generating reports on performance and outcomes. OldLab was a new build by its company and is a beta version. This system lacks image management and storage functions. It is designed only for generating written reports. Images must be generated, reviewed and maintained through a separate mechanism. Reports are uploaded into our EMR via a complex mechanism that required a build and maintenance by our information technology (IT) department. There is no dedicated long-term image storage solution and one-off solutions are required to perform this function. A description of the current workflow follows. Processes that can be improved upon with the new system are shown in italics.

An order is generated in the EMR (inpatient or outpatient) and sent to the lab. The patient is then scheduled for the procedure and presents to the lab at the assigned time. Patients arrive on their own for outpatient studies and are brought by transport for inpatient studies. When the patients arrive in the lab they are registered by the clerical staff. The technologist who will perform the study then begins the *pre-study evaluation,* which consists of greeting the patient and transferring patient information manually into the ultrasound machine. The *study* itself is then performed, with times that may range from 20–90 min depending on the type and complexity of the study. Various measurements are taken and *recorded manually* during the study. The images are then *printed in black and white* on rolls of 3-inch-wide photographic paper as they are acquired. An overall average *study* time is approximately 40 min. The technologist then completes the *post-study evaluation*, which consists of manually entering the data (blood flow velocities and vessel measurements). The printed images are then *cut into strips* creating anywhere from 4–16 strips of 3×3 inch photos which *are stapled to the reports* that are *printed* on standard letter size paper. These strips should not exceed 11 inches in length, allowing a series of three images per strip maximum. This facilitates storage of the paper files. The original color images, and any video clips that are obtained must be *loaded onto disks* and are *filed in a separate individually managed database*. Color is used to represent speed, direction and character of blood flow. Rendering these images in black and white leads to diminution of this important information. Neither the printed images, nor the clips are *available for review* except by making a physical trip to the lab. Once sent for storage, retrieving these hard copy images requires a *complex process*. Again, depending on the type and complexity of the study there may be multiple measurements that need to be entered which is time-consuming and prone to errors. The final part of the *post study evaluation* is for the technologist to enter the preliminary findings and submit for *review by the interpreting physician*.

Since the images are available on paper only the interpreting physician must physically *go to the lab* for a detailed review of the images. The reports have a *cumbersome structure* with *lengthy (up to 4–5 pages) reports* that are difficult to read through. The system does not allow for posting of preliminary reports and therefore these reports are frequently *faxed* leading to further wasted paper. In order to sign off and finalize the report the physician must sign onto the current system on the computer while reviewing the paper images, make any edits, and sign it.

Vascular Laboratory: Proposed System (NewLab)

The major improvements that are anticipated follow. The *pre-study evaluation* will no longer require that any manual entry of patient information be performed. The data will be electronically transferred from the hospital EMR to the ultrasound machine via an electronic interface. During the *study* various measurements are directly transferred to the NewLab software and recorded electronically. Manual entry by the technologist is not required. We expect that the majority of the benefit will be realized in the *post study evaluation* for several reasons. The measurements recorded during the study will automatically populate the report, saving time and potential errors resulting from manual entry of a large number of measurements. The reports are structured based on the measurements with minimal requirements for searching through drop down menus and free texting. The reports are streamlined, easy to read, intuitive, and in most cases, only one page in length.

The reports and original images are then sent to an inbox where they are available for review by the interpreting physician, on any computer with internet access. Preliminary reports are posted on the electronic medical record and marked as such for referring physicians to see. The interpreting physician is able to review the report, side by side with the images and generate a final report in an efficient manner. All of the information including the report and the original images are stored in the EMR for immediate review by any treating physician resulting in improved patient flow in both the inpatient and outpatient settings.

Methodology

Providing justification for such a large-scale project that will require investment of both upfront costs and labor is essential. This justification must include financial, relational, and global stakeholder considerations. The presentation of the project requires appropriate leadership and presentation of the information noted above to all stakeholders that makes a cohesive case for moving forward.

The first task was to generate evidence that the project should be considered. The proposed system is essentially a software acquisition that requires significant investment in updated hardware to support the database. Two methods of hardware acquisition will be considered. In the first, we will purchase outright and host within our own system. In the second, we will utilize remote servers and pay a fee for usage and storage.

The first step was to perform a quick screen using the Payback method which suggested that the project may pay for itself after 1–2 years and should at least be considered. The analysis is described by the following equation:

Investment required / Annual net cash inflows = \$1,140,000 / \$836,720 = 1.36 years

The next step was to perform an incremental analysis, which is the best way to assess the revenues/costs of the new system versus the old system. With incremental analysis, we only have to consider changes in costs and revenues and thus do not have to consider variables that remain unchanged. The incremental revenues and costs associated with the project follow here.

Incremental Costs

1. Upfront cost of the NewLab software system. This includes materials and labor for installation and training. Training can be accomplished within a few days, is performed on site, and without major disruption of workflow.
2. Cost of new hardware. This will involve the purchase of computers only, as all current ultrasound machines are compatible with the new system. This hardware can be bought by the institution, or hosted remotely on an amazon server. In the past, our institution, like many others, has not been enthusiastic about remote hosting due to privacy and security concerns. As this procedure becomes more of an industry standard, the option remains viable.
3. Maintenance, service costs for NewLab.
4. Electronic data storage costs, which may be handled as in 2 above, either in house or remotely hosted.

Incremental Revenues/Cost Savings

1. Decrease in time per study (direct labor (DL), technicians). The time-savings will occur in all three phases of these lab studies. At the front end, demographic data entry to the ultrasound machine and hence the study is automated, and technicians do not have to enter it directly, which is tedious and prone to errors. During the study measurements (of blood flow velocity and vessel diameter for example) are directly imported into the report, eliminating time and transcription errors. On the back end the reports are structured within templates that are based on the type of study and data acquired. Again, there is no need for transcription and the interface is far more intuitive and user friendly. Savings on direct labor would allow the lab the lab to perform the same number of studies as they presently do with a fewer number of technicians, and less cost (see below).
2. More studies can be performed (increased capacity) thus increasing revenue. Projections of study volume can be found later in the report.
3. Deceased costs for direct materials (DM). These include paper costs, both for photographic paper and plain paper and ink as noted above.

Other Intangible Cost Savings

1. Decreased administrative assistant direct labor time. Staff will not have to spend time faxing preliminary reports, which currently do not appear in the electronic medical record in our system. Since the faxing does not account for a large amount of the clerical staff's effort, time saved by eliminating this process will neither allow for reduced staffing nor elimination of any overtime pay. Therefore, this will not result in an incremental cost saving based on wage expense.
2. Maintenance, service, and electronic storage costs for the existing system. Paper storage costs and the cost of individually maintaining a database will be eliminated. Storage will be combined with other hospital storage functions and can take advantage of the inherent synergies.
3. Eliminate time spent by senior staff and technical director creating storages discs. This too is unlikely to result in cost savings since wage expense is unchanged as noted above. It will however free up time for more important tasks.
4. Eliminate need for storage space for voluminous reports and transport to storage space.

Sunk Costs

The cost of existing system can be viewed as a sunk cost. It cannot be recouped and has no salvage value.

The ultrasound machines are already purchased and will be used throughout the duration of their useful life. These will not change with the new system and do not distinguish between the current and future state.

Opportunity Costs

There are no significant opportunity costs other than the cost of capital discussed later. The opportunity costs of recouped storage space are small, off site, and are not directly traceable to the Lab.

While these methods strongly suggest that the project should be considered they are inadequate as a complete analysis as they include no consideration for the time value of money, nor do they help delineate financing options that are impacted by the liquidity of the organization. For these and other reasons a detailed Net Present Value (NPV) Analysis using discounted cash flows was felt to be the most useful tool for evaluating the project.

Articulation of Variable and Fixed Cash Outflows over the Project Term

Since the project involves the comparison of an existing (OldLab) to a proposed new system (NewLab) we will articulate the cash flows for each scenario. Cash outflows that will not change with the introduction of a new system and are listed as "non-incremental".

Existing System (OldLab)

Variable Costs Include
Direct Materials including photographic and plain paper (used to print reports), and ink.

Fixed Costs Include
Technician time per study (direct labor, fixed cost within a relevant range).
   Storage for archiving of paper reports.

Proposed System (NewLab)

Variable Costs Include
Direct Materials, the new system will eliminate photographic paper, plain paper and ink traceable to printing images and reports.

Fixed Costs Include
Technician time per study (direct labor, fixed cost within a relevant range).
   Electronic storage costs, the cost structure will depend on whether the solution is hosted on our own servers, or outsourced to third party servers.

Non-incremental Cash Outflows
Disposable supplies (direct materials) including ultrasound gel, towels, etc. These costs are negligible and even with a moderate increase or decrease in the number of studies performed are essentially non-differential in this relevant range.
   Ultrasound machines and maintenance.
   Fixed allocated Manufacturing and Overhead (MOH) costs (utilities, space, etc.)
   Finance and Administrative; Sales, General and Administrative costs (SG&A).

Articulation of Revenues (Cash Inflows) over the Project Term

There are three cash inflows that may be associated with this project. Two of these are cost savings and one is direct revenue. Cost savings result from first, reduced study times and greater efficiency, and second savings of direct materials. The third is direct revenue from additional patient volume per year.

Cash Inflow 1: Cost Savings from Greater Efficiency

This will be manifested as cost savings in technologist time (direct labor). Since the number of studies performed is quite large, and the time-savings reflect a significant reduction in time spent, the overall savings stand to be enormous. These can be quantitatively assessed using a time driven activity-based costing (TDABC) analysis (see below) [1]. The benefit of direct labor reduction can be realized in one of three ways. One is reduction in total staffing requirement. A second is in reduced overtime pay. A third is reduced dependence on per diem technicians. In reviewing the lab costs, the need for overtime work and per diem technician usage is infrequent and is deemed unlikely to significantly distinguish between the current state and the proposed state. This leaves reduction in staffing needs as the primary cost (savings) driver. Since the technicians are salaried employees, costs are essentially fixed within a certain relevant range. A technician can only do a certain number of studies per year, any additional demand for studies would have to be met with additional technician hiring. Thus, greater efficiency can lead to a significant reduction in total technician costs.

In addition, since technicians are salaried employees and occupy a designated number of allocated positions, any cost benefit would not be realized until one or more positions are left unfilled or eliminated. Therefore, the cost savings analysis must be considered within these relevant ranges that are based on staffing needs. A TDABC analysis is shown here.

Lab performs 31,000 studies/year (Table 16.2).

Technician utilization = 31,000 studies × 60 min/study = 1,860,000 min of studies/2,657,349 total lab minutes available = 70% utilization.

This utilization makes sense since it allows for variability in the system including random daily variation, the need for portable exams (technician must travel to the patient), bursts of activity (e.g. from the emergency room), and covering technicians' lunch hours (Table 16.3).

Table 16.2 TDABC analysis-utilization

Hours of operation		Total hours of operation	Total minutes of operation
Lab is open 10 h/day/weekday=		2537	
Lab is open 8 h/day/weekend day and holidays=		890	
Total		3427	205,646
Staffing	# of technicians	× total hours Total technician hours	Total technician minutes
# Technicians in lab/weekday=	15	2537 38,057	
# Technicians in lab/weekend=	7	890 6232	
Total		44,289	2,657,349

Table 16.3 TDABC analysis-cost pool

	# of technicians	Average technician salary + fringe	Cost per given # of technicians
Unit cost per technician = salary +fringe (30.5% of salary)	1	$93,960	$93,960
	22	$93,960	$2,067,120

Table 16.4 TDABC analysis-study times

	OldLab			NewLab		
Per study costs	Min	DL rate ($/min)	Cost ($)	Min	DL rate ($/min)	Cost ($)
Pre-study	5	1.11	5.56	3	1.11	3.33
Performing study	40	1.11	44.45	35	1.11	38.89
Post study	15	1.11	16.67	5	1.11	5.56
Total	60		66.68	43		47.78

Cost pool (minute at 70% utilization) = costs/total min = $2,067,120/1,860,000 min = $1.11/min (Table 16.4).

Using this information alone we can calculate a TDABC cost savings of
Cost savings per study $18.89
Cost savings for 31,000 studies $585,638.66

Looking at this calculation another way, on average each technician can perform 1400 studies per year (31,000 studies/22 technicians = 1400), assuming maximum capacity utilization in the current system.

With the time savings of 17 min per study with the new system (and assuming the same 70% utilization) the total technician-minutes needed to accomplish the same number of studies is 31,000 studies × 43 min/study = 1,333,000 min × 0.70 = 933,100 min.

We can then solve for how many technicians would be needed to perform these 31,000 studies:

1,333,000/1,860,000 = new # technicians/22 technicians
0.717 × 22 = new # technicians = 15.7 technicians (16 total technicians)

Note also that these technicians would be performing more studies per technician per year as a result of the efficiencies (time-savings) of the new system: 31,000/16 = 1937 studies per technician per year.

Using unit costs, we can figure out the cost savings for the relevant range at various levels of staffing (Table 16.5).

We have made several assumptions in developing this model. They include the following.

Other parts of the process map, such as scheduling the procedure, transportation to and from the unit, billing, support staff, utilities, and depreciation will not change with the new system

The number of studies performed per year is unchanged.

Insurance reimbursement structure and amount will not change.

We used average technician salaries as there is not significant variability.

Table 16.5 TDABC analysis-cost savings

	# of technicians	Average technician salary+fringe	Cost per given # of technicians	Cost savings at given # of technicians
Unit cost per tech = salary +fringe (30.5% of salary)	1	$93,960	$93,960	NA
	16	$93,960	$1,503,360	$563,760
	17	$93,960	$1,597,320	$469,800
	18	$93,960	$1,691,280	$375,840
	19	$93,960	$1,785,240	$281,880
	20	$93,960	$1,879,200	$187,920
	21	$93,960	$1,973,160	$93,960
	22	$93,960	$2,067,120	$0

Table 16.6 Direct Materials-cost savings

Cost	per month ($)	per year ($)
Plain paper	200	2400
Thermal paper	1200	14,400
Ink	500	6000
Storage (paper, disc)	200	2400
Total	2100	25,200

There is no change in technician salary.

The distribution of studies by type will not change with the new system, i.e. there will not be greater number of more or less time-consuming studies with the new system.

Clerical work (faxing) will decrease, but not to a degree that would result in decreased staffing requirement.

We have rounded off numbers to simplify viewing the results, e.g. 31,020 studies per year rounded to 31,000 studies.

Cash Inflow 2: Cost Savings from Direct Materials

The second major cost savings will result from eliminating the need for certain direct materials most prominently including photographic paper, plain paper, and ink. These can be articulated as follows: (Table 16.6).

There are additional minor and somewhat more difficult to quantify costs associated with disposal of these materials as well as potential environmental benefits to eliminating them.

Cash Inflow 3: Direct Patient Service Revenue

The third cash inflow is patient service revenue for the various studies done in the lab. Analysis of this revenue is somewhat complex. There are two components to patient service revenue. The first is the technical component, which is billed by the hospital and reflects all operational costs including the cost of capital equipment, disposable supplies, technologist and staff salaries, overhead costs, etc. *Our analysis includes only the technical component of revenue, using an average charge of $2500.*

The second revenue is the professional component, which is billed by the reading physician and covers the professional service of study interpretation. The average professional charge is closer to $100. While important, since it sits in a different cost center (faculty practice) and does not directly cover the technical component, we have not included it as a part of this analysis. Any significant impact on professional charges would result from a change in the number of studies performed and the work effort of the interpreting physicians is unlikely to be significantly altered within the relevant range.

Within the technical component of patient service revenue there are also several complexities that relate to the reimbursement models within our current health care system. The most important of which is whether the patient is an inpatient (admitted to the hospital) or an outpatient (outpatient or in the Emergency Department). Outpatients are billed and reimbursed with a discrete and traceable technical charge, as noted above. For hospital inpatients, the cost of these studies is included in a Diagnosis Related Group (DRG) lump sum payment of the Inpatient Prospective Payment System (IPPS) made to the hospital, which covers all costs associated with the patient's hospital stay. As such, the discrete technical component revenue is not directly traceable to the Vascular Lab for inpatients. It must be assigned in manner similar to assigning overhead costs. This payment methodology highlights the importance of identifying cost savings measures in the evaluation of such a large-scale project that has significant implications for the cost and efficiency of inpatient care. The percentage of outpatients and Emergency Department patients for which revenue is traceable is approximately 40% + 10% = 50%. Inpatients comprise approximately 50% of the patients having studies.

The anticipated gains from a new system would be in the area of efficiency and timely reporting, which should also result in decreased length of stay (discussed later). Finally, a number of patients in our system are capitated, a trend that will likely continue throughout our health system. In these cases, the organization accepts a lump sum payment for the care of a patient, and similar to the inpatient technical fee scenario noted above, the revenue stream for a given study may be difficult to trace and the cost savings and efficiency aspects highlighted accordingly.

We can estimate the average unit revenue per case by taking the total collections of $19,000,000 and dividing by 31,000 studies giving us $613 per study. We can then use this number later in revenue projections if additional studies can be performed.

Discounted Cash Flow Analysis

The following NPV analysis assumes a cost of capital of 6%, over 5 years, for the condition where we buy the hardware and host the system ourselves (Once pay). We assume an additional 1000 outpatients in the first year and every year thereafter resulting from greater efficiencies and growth of the health system and that all revenues accrue at the end of each defined period (Table 16.7).

Table 16.7 Discounted cash flow analysis where we own the hardware and host the system

	Purchase	Year 1	Year 2	Year 3	Year 4	Year 5
Cash outflows						
Initial Investment (software)	$(400,000.00)					
Initial Investment (hardware)	$(500,000.00)					
Repairs, Maintenance, Training (15% software)		$(60,000.00)	$(60,000.00)	$(60,000.00)	$(60,000.00)	
Cash inflows						
Incremental Patient Service Revenue		$613,000.00	$613,000.00	$613,000.00	$613,000.00	$613,000.00
Cost Savings (TDABC)		$469,800.00	$469,800.00	$469,800.00	$469,800.00	$469,800.00
Cost Savings from Direct Materials		$21,360.00	$21,360.00	$21,360.00	$21,360.00	$21,360.00
Total Cash Flows	$(900,000.00)	$1,044,160.00	$1,044,160.00	$1,044,160.00	$1,044,160.00	$1,104,160.00
Discount Factor	1.00	0.943	0.890	0.840	0.792	0.747
Present Value of Cash Flows	$(900,000.00)	$985,056.60	$929,298.68	$876,696.87	$827,072.52	$825,092.58
Net Present Value	$(900,000.00)	$85,056.60	$1,014,355.29	$1,891,052.16	$2,718,124.68	$3,543,217.26

In this scenario where we host the system ourselves, i.e. own the hardware

With 1000 additional outpatients the break-even point occurs at approximately 11 months.

The NPV at 5 years is approximately $3,540,000.

It requires an initial cash outlay of $900,000.

The following NPV analysis assumes a cost of capital of 6%, over 5 years, for the condition where we buy the hardware and remotely host the system, paying a click fee for every study performed (Incremental pay). We assume an additional 1000 outpatients in the first year and every year thereafter resulting from greater efficiencies and growth of the health system and that all revenues accrue at the end of each defined period (Table 16.8).

In this scenario where we use remote hosting, i.e. lease the hardware

With 1000 additional patients the break-even point occurs at approximately 7 months

The NPV at 5 years is approximately $2,980,000

It requires an initial cash outlay of $450,000.

Final Analysis Using Net Present Value to Determine if the Proposal Is Viable Along with Sensitivity Analysis Showing Estimations of Best, Middle, and Worst-Case Scenarios

Sensitivity analyses were performed to test assumptions that bear on profitability and net present value of the endeavor. In the original analysis, we made an estimation that new patient volume would increase by 1000 outpatients per year. The revenue and cost-savings were then calculated for this change and a 5-year net present values of $3.5 million and $3.0 million were calculated for the once-pay option and the incremental-pay option, respectively. To support the flow of an additional 1000 patients, we had to hire one additional technician beyond the necessary 16 technicians, for a total of 17 technicians. We estimated that each technician should be able to perform about 1900 studies per year (31,000/16 = 1937.5). Thus 1900 patients per technician constitutes the relevant range of fixed costs for the purpose of adding another technician. In other words, to support up to an additional patient volume of up to 1900 patients, one additional technician would be necessary.

Analysis 1: Patient Volume

It is estimated that the lab will service 32,000 patients once the new system is implemented (1000 additional outpatients than previously)—given that there is more demand for outpatient studies that cannot currently be satisfied. For the sensitivity analysis, we may conjure two additional hypothetical situations: one, a gain of an additional 2000 patients for a total of 33,000 patients per year (best-case scenario) and two, no change in total patient volume (worst-case scenario). Middle case scenario will be the current estimated 1000 additional patients.

Table 16.8 Discounted cash flow analysis: where we lease the hardware and the system is remotely hosted

	Purchase	Year 1	Year 2	Year 3	Year 4	Year 5
Cash outflows						
Initial Investment (software)	$(400,000.00)					
Remote hosting Click fee ($7.5 × # studies)	$(50,000.00)	$(240,000.00)	$(240,000.00)	$(240,000.00)	$(240,000.00)	$(240,000.00)
Repairs, Maintenance, Training (15% software)		$(60,000.00)	$(60,000.00)	$(60,000.00)	$(60,000.00)	
Cash inflows						
Incremental Patient Service Revenue		$613,000.00	$613,000.00	$613,000.00	$613,000.00	$613,000.00
Cost Savings (TDABC)		$469,800.00	$469,800.00	$469,800.00	$469,800.00	$469,800.00
Cost Savings from Direct Materials		$21,360.00	$21,360.00	$21,360.00	$21,360.00	$21,360.00
Total Cash Flows	$(450,000.00)	$804,160.00	$804,160.00	$804,160.00	$804,160.00	$864,160.00
Discount Factor	1.00	0.943	0.890	0.840	0.792	0.747
Present Value of Cash Flows	$(450,000.00)	$758,641.51	$715,699.54	$675,188.24	$636,970.04	$645,750.62
Net Present Value	$(450,000.00)	$308,641.51	$1,024,341.05	$1,699,529.29	$2,336,499.33	$2,982,249.95

Table 16.9 Best, middle, and worst-case scenarios

	Scenario		
	Worst	Middle	Best
Patient Vol Change	0	1000	2000
Total Patient Vol (first year)	31,000	32,000	32,900
Total Patient Vol (subsequent years)	31,000	32,000	33,000
Technicians (first year)	17	17	17
Technicians (subsequent years)	16	17	18
Revenue (loss) for first year	$0	$613,000	$1,164,700
Revenue (loss) change (subsequent years), per year	$0	$613,000	$1,226,000
Technician cost savings for first year	$469,800	$469,800	$469,800
Technician cost savings (subsequent years), per year	$563,760	$469,800	$375,840
Net present value (once pay) at 5 years	$1,268,259	$3,543,289	$5,760,489
Net present value (incremental pay) at 5 years	$738,816	$2,982,250	$5,168,561

Because we have estimated an additional 1000 patients in the model, we will have to hire one additional technician (total 17 technicians) to prepare for the first year. After the first year, we can modify this technician number to reflect the appropriate number that will be needed: 16 in the worst-case; 17 in the middle scenario; and 18 in the best-case scenario. For the table below we have utilized the once pay model (Table 16.9).

Note that in all instances, the incremental-pay option provides a less net positive value.

Note also that in the first year of the best-case scenario above, we cannot accommodate all 2000 additional patients because we only have 17 technicians. Accordingly, only 1900 additional patients can be done, thus missing out on additional potential revenue. This will be remedied in subsequent years.

If patient volume remains unchanged (worst-case scenario), then the lab still enjoys a positive net present value for the investment in the new system (under both the once-pay or incremental-pay options) over 5 years. However, it should be noted that under this scenario, the net present value does not turn positive until the end of the third year of operations for either once-pay or incremental-pay options. In contrast, in the other two scenarios, a positive net present value is realized at the end of the first year.

One may suggest that the 'worst case' scenario is actually a loss of patient volume. This is certainly true; however, this might occur as a result of a change in market forces under the old system *or* the new system. In that case, while revenue is lost in total, comparative revenue between the two systems will be unchanged and should not be factored into the calculation. There will still be fewer technicians and associated cost savings with the new system. Thus, in all situations of patient volume the new system will provide a positive net present value.

Analysis 2: Technician Costs

Technicians salaries have been stable with standard increases over several years. Whether the technicians receive an incremental raise related to the new system or for other reasons remains to be seen. We may assume that if OldLab stays the technicians will not receive a raise, and that they will only receive one if the lab switches to NewLab. In that case we may use a worst-case scenario of a 10% raise, the middle case of a 5% raise, and the best-case scenario of no raise in terms of cost.

In the best-case scenario of obtaining the new system with no raise for the technicians (estimated above), the cost savings for technicians will be $469,800 per year. This translates to a net present value of $3.5 million for the pay-once scenario and $3.0 million for the pay-incrementally scenario (all outlined above, base case). The remainder of the cases is outlined below: (Table 16.10).

Thus, even a 10% raise in the technician salary still provides a substantially positive net present value for switching to the NewLab. The NPV is positive starting in the first year of operations for all scenarios.

Analysis 3: Cost of Capital

We have estimated a cost of capital of 6% for this project. This value could be incorrect, and thus, a sensitivity analysis of varying this value is worthwhile, and the results are shown in the table below using the remote hosting model (Table 16.11).

Note that under all of the scenarios with cost of capital ranging from 2% to 20%, the NPV of both pay-once and pay-incrementally options is still substantially positive. It should be noted that in all of these scenarios, NPV is also positive even in the first year of operations.

Table 16.10 Incremental technician salary scenarios

	Technician salary		
	No raise	5% raise	10% raise
Technician Cost Savings/year	$469,800	$389,934	$310,068
NPV Once-Pay (5 years)	$3,543,289	$3,206,864	$2,870,440
NPV Incremental-Pay (5 years)	$2,982,250	$2,645,825	$2,309,401

Table 16.11 Cost of capital impact on the own and lease scenarios

	Cost of capital					
	2%	4%	6%	10%	15%	20%
NPV Pay-Once (5 years)	$4,076,030	$3,797,806	$3,543,289	$3,095,508	$2,630,074	$2,246,841
NPV Pay-Incrementally (5 years)	$3,394,719	$3,179,293	$2,982,250	$2,635,654	$2,275,500	$1,979,043

Sensitivity Analysis Conclusions

Under each of the worst-case scenarios outlined above, NPV remains positive over the 5-year term. The most influential factor studied above is patient volume as it has a substantial influence on the revenues and thus, net present value over the long term.

Articulation of Qualitative Factors that Require Consideration Along with the Financial Analysis

There are multiple qualitative issues that will be addressed by improving operational efficiency, workflow, through put and documentation of vascular lab studies. These are best appreciated from the viewpoint of the many stakeholders that are impacted by the functioning of the vascular lab. Probably the most important stakeholders are the outpatients who comprise the largest portion of customers. By increasing capacity, their studies are completed in a timelier manner. This is not trivial and can translate into improved outcomes. Outpatient providers are another group of customers who will appreciate reduced time to next appointment the patients they refer. Providers will also benefit from instant preliminary readings as well as more timely access to final results.

Emergency Departments in the health system have significant overcrowding issues. By increasing capacity many patients will be delivered a disposition more quickly. The system has an average door to doctor time of 1 h and 20 min and 2% left without being seen rate. A study by CEP America estimates that if 5 patients leave without being seen each day the hospital loses approximately $5 million per year [2]. This is from a loss of revenue from the ED visit as well as the 15% that would be admitted.

The next group of stakeholders comprise inpatients and the inpatient physicians and staff. By increasing capacity patients that are in the hospital will not need to wait for studies. This can have a profound impact on length of stay as treatment decisions as not delayed while awaiting test results. Often patients wait in hospital beds for a vascular study before discharge. In the DRG payment system this has a direct effect upon incurred costs with a fixed revenue. Although it is possible to attempt to quantitate this effect, it would be very difficult as there are a multitude of factors impacting length of stay. Increasing throughput will not only improve the patient and physician satisfaction but also have a financial impact on both medical and surgical inpatient wards.

Another no less important group of stakeholders are Vascular Laboratory Technicians and Interpreting physicians. Both groups have experienced significant frustration with OldLab in terms of its tedium and inefficiency. This results in significant workplace dissatisfaction and can contribute to the phenomenon of burnout that is an emerging and significant concern among all health care workers today. NewLab will improve workflow and as a more "intuitive" system should improve job satisfaction and performance and reduce fatigue. All of this will improve the ability to recruit and retain physicians and technologists, efforts that are currently hampered in part by the outdated technology. The improvements to the system should also have a positive impact on the job satisfaction of other groups as well, such as the Emergency Department staff referring physicians and referring physician office staff as noted above.

Compliance with regulatory issues is an important concern. The cost of the lab losing its accreditation would be difficult to measure accurately but there would be cash outflows based on penalties and decreased reimbursement in the future would be a very real possibility. Implementation of the new system will resolve issues and concerns around compliance with currently accepted image management and digital storage requirements, including HIPAA and safe data storage and transmission. Researchers and educators will have access to structured data that can be used in research projects. We will be able to implement Quality Improvement measures more efficiently and with greater impact. Another important factor to consider is the potential for a catastrophic system crash with loss of data in the existing system. As OldLab is a beta version it does not have the same level of support as other established systems, making such a scenario a real concern. The results of that situation would also be accompanied by significant costs including the costs of extensive repair vs. the costs of replacement, which would then require expedited replacement and implementation of a temporizing and bridging solution. The increased likelihood of errors with the current system also increases the likelihood of legal action and an unfavorable result based on poor documentation.

Another important aspect of NewLab is that it will allow for the posting of preliminary reports. These are not available with OldLab. These reports represent the technicians' preliminary findings documented as such and are generated prior to the reports being finalized by the reporting physicians. If however, there is a positive finding at the time of the study, the referring physician or primary team caring for the patient are also notified by direct communication with a phone call. It is very helpful, especially in the inpatient setting for referring and treating physicians to have an idea when exactly a study has been performed and that there were no immediately identified positive findings that warrant attention. This aspect also can help improve discharge planning and length of stay issues.

A final benefit of NewLab pertains to resident/fellow education and preparation for certification. It is now a requirement that all residents and fellows completing programs in Vascular Surgery be certified in Vascular Laboratory interpretation (RPVI) prior to sitting for the written, and subsequently oral boards. Their pathway and requirements to sit for this exam includes interpreting 500 studies in the lab under the supervision of a credentialed interpreting physician. At present, residents and fellows keep track of this and submit a manual record. NewLab has a separate functionality, not included in the clinical report that allows residents and fellows to track their readings and supervision and then to generate a structured report, which is stored in the system.

There are several challenges facing the implementation of this project. These include the up-front cost of system, the need to implement a new workflow, and any unforeseen changes in reimbursement or payment models that may impact the project. We believe that on balance, the financial and non-financial benefits of the project warrant supporting it fully.

Project Team, Process, and Evolution

The project team included interpreting physicians, the vascular lab medical director, vascular lab technical staff, the lab technical and administrative directors, hospital administration, the hospital IT staff, and NewLab. Physicians and lab staff provided the necessary medical and technical expertise to evaluate and facilitate the project. Hospital IT was responsible for integrating the system with our current information technology infrastructure including the electronic health record and radiology systems. NewLab was an important partner in terms of their need to provide value and product support. The Administration had to evaluate and ultimately fund the project. The scope of the project and large number of involved stakeholders necessitated and benefitted from an analysis of the relational coordination between these groups (Fig. 16.1) [3]. The creation of a relational coordination map provides an opportunity to assess the current state including the degree of coordination within and between groups as well as a chance to target relational interventions in a way that facilitates the overall project and its intended objectives. The improvements in organizational coordination are expected to produce benefits that are synergistic with the project and which will outlast the duration of the project benefitting the institution, employees and customers.

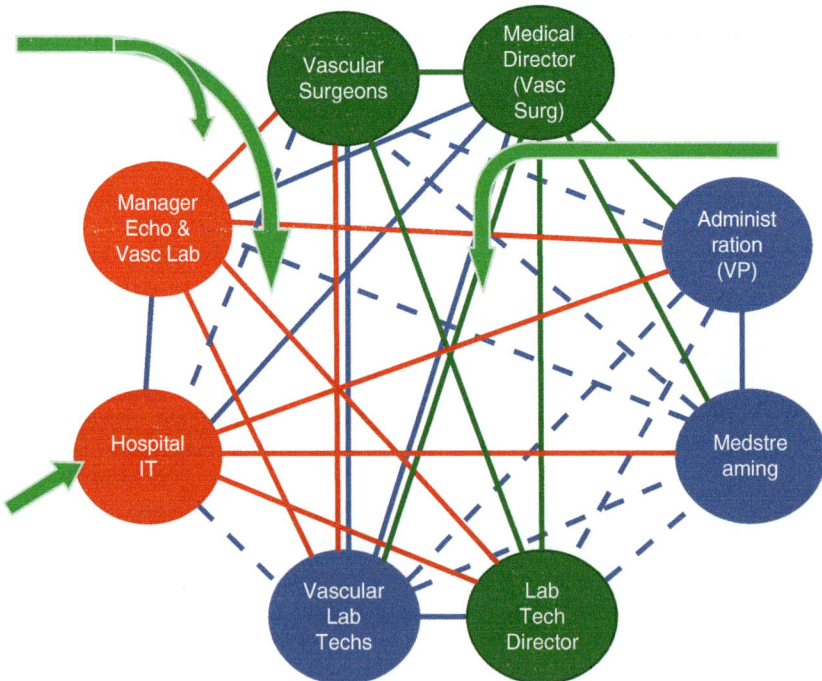

Fig. 16.1 Relational coordination schematic showing project team, process and evolution

The relational coordination analysis highlights the importance of involving boundary spanners in the process [4]. Boundary spanners possess a knowledge of multiple (specialty areas) and are able to build effective interpersonal bridges between those working in those areas. They communicate and translate important issues from people working in one realm to those working in another.

Results

We hoped and expected that implementation of the project would achieve several specific goals and have a positive impact on all stakeholders. At its core and most importantly, we expected to improve operational efficiency and reduce costs. We expected to improve stakeholder satisfaction across the health system including among reading physicians, lab technicians, referring physicians, patients, ancillary staff, the Emergency Department, and hospital administration. We fully anticipated vast improvements in image accessibility (currently paper only) and review. We hoped to improve data storage and management in addition to facilitating research and quality improvement (QI) projects. Finally, NewLab would allow for the posting of preliminary reports and facilitate tracking and reporting of studies read for training purposes by our residents and fellows.

There were several project specific challenges including the upfront cost of system purchase in resource constrained environment. The creation and maintenance of a large change team, that spanned many different departments was essential. The ongoing organizational expansion limits resources including those of capital and IT. The best solution may have warranted some degree of IT outsourcing, which the organization has traditionally preferred to avoid. Less importantly was the implementation of a new workflow after purchase.

The project gained traction and momentum through several major activities including stakeholders' meetings in which aspects of the program were reviewed. The need, ROI, and cost structure were discussed with administration, while integration, hardware and hosting strategies were discussed with IT. Meetings with clinical and technical staff that reviewed implementation, workflow, and report structure helped gather momentum at the user level.

Major accomplishments early in the articulation of the project included recognition of need and ultimately support from all stakeholders. Importantly, agreement that project can be remotely hosted on Amazon servers, a first for the medical center and a major cost savings, facilitated agreement and financial support from institution.

Ultimately, the team did well implementing the project and became increasingly cohesive over the course of the project. Review of the relational coordination diagram (Fig. 16.1) highlighted two salient points.

First, the relational coordination within groups improved significantly over the course of the project. In reality, this reflects alignment that was achieved within these groups as a result of open, ongoing and honest communication. This was most obviously manifested in the IT group, perhaps the largest and most diverse group by nature of the project requirements. Early considerations around project feasibility, labor required to build the necessary infrastructure, and the important question of whether remote hosting would ever be an option were resolved through open and frequent communication and a willingness to explore options outside of the institution's current operational strategies.

Second, the relational coordination between groups was equally improved. The most notable areas were between the IT Department and the Administration, who were able to reach consensus on the issues mentioned above and others, and between the Echo/Vascular Lab manager and the Vascular Surgeons as well as the Lab Technicians and Technical Director. Through constant dialogue everyone gained appreciation for the mutual and potential benefits of the proposed system and the importance of their coordinated efforts in moving the project forward.

While the process took longer than anticipated, there were times where we felt the project might be jeopardy of being placed "on hold". There were several breakthroughs along the way including an agreement to host the system remotely, the first at out institution. This agreement alone has a major impact for the project and the institution, as other projects may benefit from this strategy.

Discussion

Perhaps the most important lesson learned, or perhaps reinforced, was that projects of this scope require both grit and flexibility to see them through to completion [5]. The ability to invent and explore novel options with the team was essential. The project also highlighted the importance of leveraging relationships. In such an undertaking, which is both needed and justifiable on the merits, and which is nonetheless a big "ask", it was very helpful to be recognized at the outset as a group that does not ask for resources irresponsibly. Having established credibility by demonstrating institutional citizenship was helpful in consideration of the project, but was not, enough to complete it. Another important component that was highlighted was the importance of managing in all directions, with the many managers and administrators whose involvement was critical. I also came to appreciate the benefits of possessing a greater facility with finances and financing. In an era with so many competing priorities it was essential to be able to navigate the issues surrounding expense, cost structure, revenue generation, and financing options.

I was also reminded that what might seem obvious to those of us bringing the project forward, may not be so obvious to everyone else. It was important not to make assumptions, to lay out the project needs and goals clearly, and present relevant and factual data to support the project. Even so, presenting comprehensive data may not be enough to fuel the desire for change. "Show and tell" with pictures and/or visits to the site that highlights the current state can be very effective tools. It was important to pitch the idea thoughtfully and thoroughly, beginning with the concise and building to the comprehensive. One must understand the current local environment and culture they are operating within. This knowledge will allow one to be sensitive to the pressures on the larger organization and to understand its goals and

Table 16.12 Metrics and impact assessment

Metrics	Measures used	Baseline	Impact assessment
Efficiency	• Average study time • Turnaround time (TAT) for final reports	• Current study times • Current TAT	• Look to reduce study time by 20% • Reduce TAT 20%
Cost savings	• Overall costs • Eliminate use of paper	• Current DL costs • Current DM costs	• See TDABC and NPV analysis
Study quality	• Number of reports amended • Number of QI projects undertaken	• Current # amended reports • QI reviews past year	• Reduce amended reports and QI cases by 20%
Stakeholder satisfaction	• Satisfaction of physicians, technicians, referring physicians, and patients	• Current dissatisfaction • Improved recruitment and retention	• Improved satisfaction for all stakeholders • Improved lab recruitment/retention
Data availability, storage and retrieval	• Presence of images in PACS for interpreting physicians and referring providers • Availability of preliminary reports • Data stored on server	• Printed images only available • Preliminary reports not available on line • Data backed up on local computer	• All images on line • Images available to all clinical staff • Preliminary reports on line • Data stored and backed up on servers

drivers. A delineation of metrics and impact assessment helps define the parameters by which the ongoing success of the project will be measured (Table 16.12).

This scope of this project required an incorporation of key learnings from almost every aspect of our MBA program. Some concepts were more directly referable to the project than others including the following. Operations Management elaborated concepts that were essential for evaluating workflow and process. The team was thus able to formulate a solid understanding of the current and desired state and translate this to all project stakeholders. Managerial Accounting provided the basis and crux of the project, at least in terms of the anticipated cost savings. While many of us could see the waste in the system quantifying the potential gains in a granular way made the case clear. Relational Coordination provided the foundation for team building and maintaining high level functioning during the course of the project without disruption. Leadership and Organizational Behavior was essential for leading the change. Understanding the leader's role, fair process, and "going to the gemba" were the foundation and building blocks of the project. Taking on such a project also requires an understanding of the organization's culture in order to work effectively within it [6]. Healthcare Economics taught that the healthcare business is a network of several businesses each with their own model and structure. Understanding the interrelations between these businesses and their impact on each other are key elements of large-scale projects. Strategic Management brought forth concepts important for considering not only strategies for implementation, but also how this new resource will be incorporated into the comprehensive strategic plan.

Entrepreneurship taught concepts that were pivotal in "pitching the concept". While not necessarily an entrepreneurial project the lessons learned were applicable to the synthesis and presentation of the concept throughout the various phases and to all stakeholders [7]. Marketing course work helped our presentation to be more comprehensive than it might otherwise have been. Systems Thinking allowed us to demonstrate to others and ourselves the broader impact of a poorly functioning system beyond the direct touch points that seemed immediately obvious.

Conclusions

This project, while simple and narrowly defined in its objective, demonstrated the importance of applying a broad swath of business principles and practice in the process of achieving that objective. An appreciation of all aspects of business education including finance, leadership, operations, health care system, legal, relational coordination, etc. in addition to a detailed understanding of the clinical material was essential to understanding, incorporating and driving forward the positions of all stakeholders and making a case for such a large scale and important project. The ability to act as a boundary spanner, utilizing the principles highlighted above, facilitated this project and I expect will do so for many other projects that my classmates and I will undertake going forward.

Acknowledgements The author wishes to acknowledge the thoughtful and insightful contributions of Guy Nuki and Amir Taghinia in developing this project. I would also like to express my gratitude to my classmates, Professor Chilingerian and the entire faculty and staff of the Heller EMBA program for their inspiration and guidance during the entire program and beyond.

References

1. Kaplan RS, Anderson SR. Time-driven activity-based costing. Harvard Business Review, November 2004. https://hbr.org/search?N=4294923990&Ntt=time+directed+activity+based+costing#
2. Becker's Healthcare Financial Management enewsletter. What is the Financial Impact of Loising 5 ED Patients Per Day? May 22, 2012. http://www.beckershospitalreview.com/finance/what-is-the-financial-impact-of-losing-5-ed-patients-per-day.html.
3. Gittell JH. High performance healthcare: using the power of relationships to achieve quality, efficiency and resilience. United States: McGraw-Hill Education; 2009.
4. Gittell JH, Seidner R, Wimbush J. Relational model of how high-performance work systems work organization science. 2009;21(2):490–506. https://doi.org/10.1287/orsc.1090.0446.
5. Duckworth AL, Peterson C, Matthews MD, Kelly DR. Grit: perseverance and passion for long-term goals. J Pers Soc Psychol. 2007;92(6):1087–101. https://doi.org/10.1037/0022-3514.92.6.1087.
6. Chilingerian J. The discipline of strategic thinking in healthcare. In: Managing and leading in the allied health professions. In: Jones R, Jenkins F, editors. Routledge/Taylor and Francis, 2006/ebook 2021. https://heller.brandeis.edu/executive-education/pdfs/DisciplineofStrat.pdf
7. Applegate LM, Carlson C. Entrepreneurship reading: developing business plans and pitching opportunities. Harvard Business Publishing Education; 2014. https://hbsp.harvard.edu/product/8062-PDF-ENG

Use of Operations Management Tools to Improve Efficiency for Ambulatory Surgery Procedures

17

Mark Savarise and Ben Kragen

Key Learning Points

- Understand cost accounting in surgery, including actual costs of materials and per-minute costs of operating room time; and how this information can be used to determine lower cost alternatives to existing routines for surgical procedures.
- Understand how modern electronic medical records and other accounting tools can be used to obtain data necessary to accurately assess the true cost of surgical procedures.
- Understand the other determinants of value for surgical procedures beyond cost, including OR usage, patient satisfaction, and opportunity cost.
- Understand the other influences beyond cost that are drivers for preferential performance of ambulatory surgical procedures, and that other factors have a greater determination than cost on the decision to perform surgery at an ambulatory surgery center.

Executive Summary

Operating room cost accounting tools (ORCA) make it possible to break down the cost of operations into supply costs and OR time costs. This chapter looks at the use of ORCA to determine costs associated with four procedures: laparoscopic cholecystectomy, inguinal hernia repair, varicocelectomy, and artificial urinary sphincter. In an attempt to inspire efficiency, surgeons at a hospital system based in Utah were

---

M. Savarise (✉)
Department of Surgery, University of Utah South Jordan Health Center, South Jordan, UT, USA
e-mail: mark.savarise@hsc.utah.edu

B. Kragen
Heller School for Social Policy and Management, Brandeis University, Waltham, MA, USA

provided with ORCA data about the cost of their operations as compared to costs incurred by colleagues for the same operations. Results indicate that surgeries were often less expensive when procedures were performed at satellite ambulatory clinics compared to the main campus. This observation inspired a change management initiative where surgeries were redirected from the main campus to satellite clinics.

Introduction

University of Utah Healthcare (U of U Health) is an integrated academic health care provider in Salt Lake City that serves the larger population of Utah, southern Idaho, western Colorado, eastern Nevada, Montana and western Wyoming. U of U Health provides a full range of services, from primary care to quaternary referral care at its main campus in Salt Lake City. For thirty years, U of U Health has had primary care facilities outside the main campus in the Salt Lake region. In 2012, the organization completed construction on its first multi-specialty ambulatory care facility in South Jordan, Utah. South Jordan Health Center (SJHC) is larger and more comprehensive in scope than any of the other satellites, providing 24-hour emergency services, advanced imaging, and specialty care including ambulatory surgery. For the years from 2012–2015, South Jordan was among the fastest growing towns in the country [1]. SJHC is the first instance of U of U Health providing comprehensive specialty care away from its main campus. In 2015, surgical care included ENT, plastic surgery, urology, and general surgery. Surgeons and anesthesiologists were faculty members at the University who travelled to SJHC for outpatient clinics and procedures.

U of U Health measures its quality using several standardized methods. U of U Health is a member of the Vizient consortium for quality improvement (previously the University Health Care Consortium), and has consistently ranked among the top academic medical centers for quality in the Vizient annual rankings. In addition, U of U Health participates in Press-Ganey patient ranking. With a strong emphasis on Press-Ganey performance from senior administration, approximately half of U of U providers rank in the top 10% of Press-Ganey Exceptional Patient Experience (EPE) scoring every year.

U of U Health has been nationally recognized as a pioneer in the area of cost transparency, with its former Chief Executive Officer appearing in national media to endorse the concept [2]. This is in part due to our rollout of a new online tool in 2015 which gave physicians access to actual operating room supply costs, with physician-specific case information. The Operating Room Cost Accounting (ORCA) tool uses actual supply costs from hospital contracts for disposable instruments, supplies, sutures, drapes and other equipment pulled for a procedure, based upon surgeon preference cards. It also shows the actual cost of supplies opened and used during specific operative cases based upon nursing documentation in the Electronic Medical Record (EMR). Interestingly, physicians have access to their own data, as well as that of their peers, which is a decision that the hospital administration hopes will encourage cost reduction by adding context and friendly competition to their utilization. As an incentive, U of U Health supports "UP Projects", a policy whereby half of any cost savings from a project instituted by any U of U physician is passed on to the physician's department for a period up to 3 years.

ORCA is one of a series of Value Driven Outcomes (VDO) tools available in our institution. VDO tools were developed by the University of Utah Health Sciences center to measure costs against project objectives [3]. VDO tools are used to determine operating room costs on a per-minute basis, as well as similar costs-per-minute for our Same Day Surgery (SDS) unit and our Post Anesthesia Care Unit (PACU). Combined with traditional accounting data, such as case volume and procedure start and stop times, VDO tools make it possible to examine absolute and relative costs of care for similar operative procedures done at different sites or by different surgeons and anesthesiologists. This study compared cost at ambulatory centers against the main hospital campus.

Time-driven activity-based cost accounting for operating rooms has proven to be a transformative break from traditional accounting techniques in hospitals, allowing organizations to better weigh supply versus time cost, and further identify areas where underutilized staff represent opportunity cost [4, 5]. The cost of wages accounts for the majority of variable cost in surgeries, which is often several times the cost of supplies. Childers and Maggard-Gibbons [6] found that a minute spent in the OR cost roughly $37.45 for inpatient surgeries, and $36.14 for ambulatory surgeries. Direct expenses accounted for $20–21 of the total cost. The remaining variable cost was made up of $13–14 in wages and benefits and $2.50–3.50 in surgical supplies across California hospitals.

Prior findings demonstrated additional cost savings when surgeries were performed at ambulatory clinics compared to similar operations in main hospitals. In a multi-site study Fabricant et al. [7] demonstrated cost savings between 17% and 43% when orthopedic surgeries were performed at the ambulatory clinics. In line with a surgery examined for this paper, Rosen et al. [8] demonstrated that laparoscopic cholecystectomies performed at ambulatory clinics both decreased cost of surgery, and increased patient value in the areas of speedier recovery, reduced pain, and earlier return to work. Koenig [9] argues that growth of ambulatory surgical centers is likely to reduce Medicare spending because they bill at a lower rate than main hospitals for outpatient procedures. This study examines both the difference in cost between main hospitals and ambulatory centers, as well as some of the challenges that come with moving work from the main hospital to the outlying centers.

The Hospital System

By fiscal year 2015–2016, SJHC had been in operation for 3 years, and clinical volumes were expected to be reaching maturity. The population within 5 miles of the center had grown more than 5% per year. In addition, the University of Utah was preparing to open a second full service ambulatory center in Farmington, 22 miles north of the University campus. However, growth was not as rapid as expected. Operating room use remained below 50% of capacity at SJHC. Meanwhile, overcrowded block schedules and delays in operating room (OR) starts were commonplace at the main campus OR. Surgeons were reluctant to change practice habits by moving some of their elective outpatient surgical procedures out of the main hospital to one of the ambulatory centers. Both SJHC and the new ambulatory center in Farmington (FHC) were 30–60 min driving time from the main center, in areas of the Wasatch Front, Utah, that were unfamiliar to the University surgeons and anesthesiologists. This project was born out of an effort to incentivize use of these ambulatory centers. In this project, cost data was analyzed to measure real and potential savings. This information was used to drive policies and procedures with the aim of increasing patient volumes at the two ambulatory centers SJHC and FHC.

Methods

The research team examined cost drivers for frequently performed surgeries in the two specialties of general surgery and urology at SJHC, FHC, and the main campus. For general surgery, the team examined laparoscopic cholecystectomy (with or without intraoperative cholangiogram) and open inguinal hernia repair. For urology the team examined the cost for varicocelectomy and artificial urinary sphincter (AUS). These procedures were performed on outpatients at the two ambulatory clinics of SJHC and FHC, as well as at the main hospital, which acted as a natural comparison group for the two ambulatory clinics. The sample was limited to outpatient surgeries, and did not include emergency surgeries. Patients included in the sample had American Society of Anesthesiologists (ASA) scores of 3 or lower, and a BMI of less than or equal to 50 kg/m^2, which together made them eligible for outpatient surgery at the ambulatory centers. The team collected ORCA data for the procedures over the course of 2 years from electronic medical records.

Several operational differences existed between materials at the main clinic and SJHC. For open inguinal hernia repair, the three surgeons at SJHC agreed to standardize open inguinal hernia repairs to a single mesh choice. They agreed to three sizes of mesh to cover all general surgery procedures. SJHC was able to negotiate a very low cost for the simplest available mesh: uncoated mid-weight Parietene polypropylene, costing under $20 per individual item. The two larger sizes stocked at SJHC cost slightly more. In comparison, the main campus stocked a variety of specialty mesh products and surgeons were able to choose their preferred material. Cost variation in the selection at the main campus was large, with some synthetic mesh products costing nearly ten times the standard SJHC cost. This access to premium equipment at the main campus led us to suspect that supply costs would be lower at SJHC than at the main campus prior to the collection of ORCA data.

The team collected data on skin-to-skin operative times using medical records for the four procedures. This cost was then added to the supply costs using a standard rate cost-per-minute for the operating room assigned for analysis to all University of Utah facilities, creating an average total cost per OR case. The cost-per-minute data also accounted for anesthesia. The team did not account for the difference in cost-per-minute rate across facilities resulting from variation in overhead costs.

Lastly, the team looked at patient times in same day surgery both before and after surgery and post-anesthesia care unit (PACU) for our four index operations. A standard cost-per-minute rate was applied to each of these services and added to the total cost per operation. The same rate was applied to all facilities. The team did not look at differences in cost of pre-operative work-up of patients at the different facilities (for instance if patients were more likely to incur costs for electrocardiogram (EKG) or lab studies pre-op at one facility).

Results

Author's note: This data was collected and analyzed by hospital administrators as part of quality improvement efforts. Actual cost data in dollars are proprietary to University of Utah Healthcare. All data and figures in this chapter have been scrubbed of individual cost data; however, the relative cost comparisons and overall savings data are real and accurate.

Data demonstrated substantial cost savings for three of the four procedures at the ambulatory centers SJHC and FHC as compared to similar procedures on the main campus. All four procedures had savings from shorter OR times. This was not unexpected, as there was an apparent faster pace of OR cases at SJHC and FHC compared to the main campus.

One procedure, artificial urinary sphincter (AUS), had both increased supply costs and increased peri-operative costs at the ambulatory center. This finding prompted two members of the team to examine the factors that caused the higher costs. They determined that AUS was often performed on elderly men with frequent comorbidities, and that a number of patients required overnight observation stays (either anticipated or unanticipated). At the ambulatory sites, this was done in the same day surgery unit. The analysis showed that, overall, this was not cost effective, and the urology group has subsequently stopped doing this procedure at the ambulatory centers. For the other three procedures, cost savings were substantial; the largest coming from laparoscopic cholecystectomy, as displayed in Fig. 17.1.

Case	OR Cost Savings	Supply Cost Savings	Peri-op Cost Savings	Total Cost Savings
Laparoscopic Cholecystectomy	$367	$175	$175	$717
Repair Inguinal Hernia	$288	$95	$113	$496
Varicocelectomy	$331	$134	$5	$470
Artificial Urinary Sphincter	$224	($102)	($408)	($286)

Fig. 17.1 Cost savings by procedure

For all three procedures, there were savings in every phase of care over hospital outpatient surgery costs. In the perioperative phase of care, reduced cost was often due to the fact that we were spending less time getting patients ready. In the operative phase we spent less money because we were using fewer supplies and had faster procedures.

We also found that we spent less time inducing and awakening patients. We believe that this can be explained by the development of efficient practices by the anesthesia group assigned to outpatient surgery. Some of the observed efficiencies include (1) preoperative screening routines to sort out inappropriate patients for ambulatory surgery centers prior to the day of surgery; (2) an anesthesia team approach, where the anesthesiologist performed the preoperative assessment and managed PACU issues, while supervising 2–3 CRNA's performing the intra-operative anesthesia management; and (3) familiarity with total intravenous anesthesia techniques (TIVA) that were employed liberally, minimizing time of induction and awakening, while providing adequate levels of anesthesia for relatively short duration operations.

The largest variable cost noted in the data came from the mesh implant, which was found to have greater than three-fold variation in costs depending on the surgeon who did the procedure, as depicted in red in Fig. 17.2. This explains the significant difference in supply costs for inguinal hernia across locations. As previously discussed, a large amount of variation was explained by the choice of hernia mesh, which was the result of a prior LEAN project to obtain a supply of hernia mesh at the lowest possible cost.

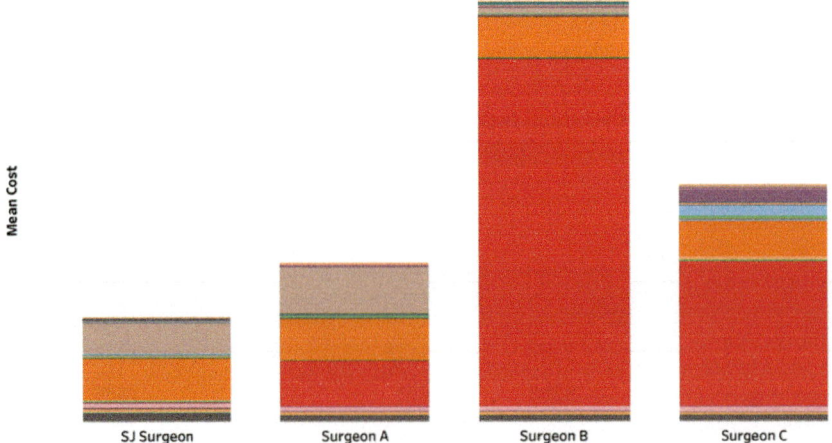

Fig. 17.2 Variation in open inguinal hernia repair supply cost by surgeon

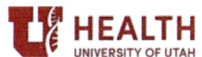

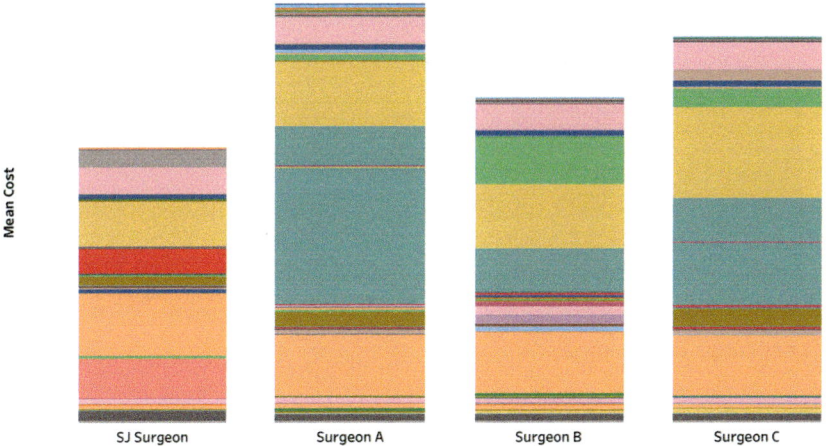

Fig. 17.3 Variation in OR supply costs for laparoscopic cholecystectomy

Figure 17.3 shows the OR supply costs for laparoscopic cholecystectomy, with or without cholangiogram. Here, the data shows even greater variability than for hernia repair. Again, standard items such as prep kits and drapes were included in the analysis. However, variation among surgeons is apparent in the use of disposable instruments and trocars. For example, some surgeons routinely employed disposable suction-irrigation devices, while others did so selectively. Others still chose to use a reusable suction device from the instrument tray. Because the data shows mean costs over all operative cases for surgeons, those who selectively used a disposable instrument showed lower per-case costs in the ORCA data than those whose preference card instructed staff to routinely open the instrument. Of note, not all surgeons in our institution employed routine cholangiography; both surgeons at SJHC in this analysis routinely did cholangiography, so the additional cost of the catheter, tubing, contrast and syringe were included in those surgeons' data. However, the difference in cost was substantial enough, even in consideration of this fact, that all cholecystectomies were included in the analysis.

The cost of materials used at SJHC was found to be substantially lower than at the main campus (other sites), as summarized in Fig. 17.4. We performed the same analysis for varicocelectomy and artificial urinary sphincter (data not shown). Cost savings for the ambulatory centers was seen in the urology data as well.

The duration of procedures was also found to be substantially lower at SJHC compared to the main campus (other sites). Figure 17.5 shows that procedure duration was on average more than 40 min greater at the main campus compared to SJHC for both Laproscopic Cholecystectomy and Open Inguinal Hernia. A

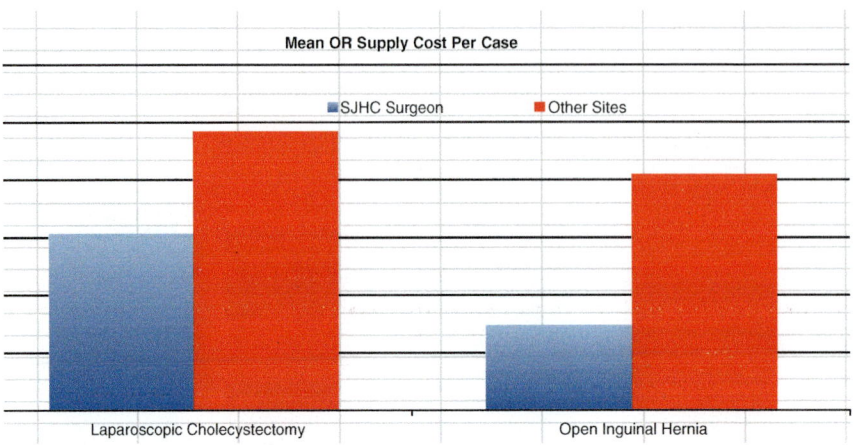

Fig. 17.4 OR supply cost per case

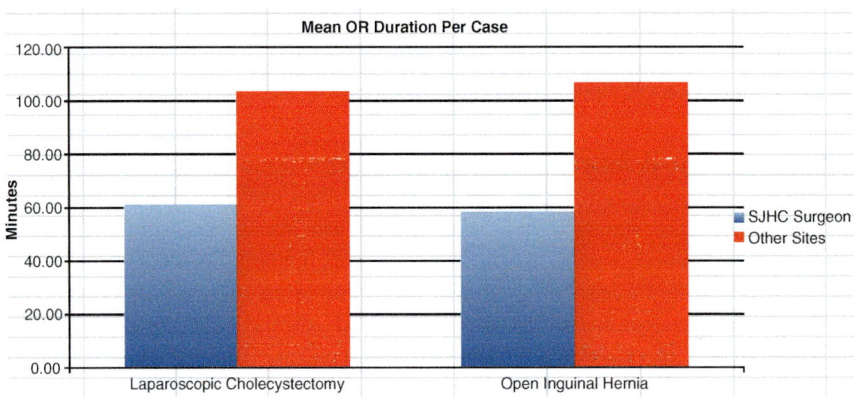

Fig. 17.5 OR duration per case

reduction in labor cost and other variable costs associated with using the operating room was a second contributing factor in the reduction of total cost per procedure at SJHC.

Supply Costs Vs. OR Time Cost

The analysis controlled for both supply and time costs in each procedure, which allowed us to understand the contribution of each factor to the average total cost per case.

In many cases there was a trade-off, where more expensive equipment reduced the procedure times. For instance, in the case of a laparoscopic inguinal hernia repair, certain types of formed or "self-gripping" mesh cost significantly more; but reduced operative time by eliminating the need for fixation with sutures or tacks. Balloon dissecting trocars also saved time in the initial dissection but came at a higher cost than standard trocars. To illustrate the cost-comparison for these devices, we analyzed laparoscopic hernia repair data to understand what combinations of equipment minimized the total cost and time spent on a procedure. At SJHC, the hernia surgeon used a balloon dissector, but a standard mesh with tacking device. At FHC, the hernia surgeon did not use a balloon dissector or tacking device; but used self-gripping mesh. The hernia surgeons on the main campus used standard trocars, standard mesh, and a tacking device.

We found that OR supply cost for laparoscopic hernia repair was 20% higher at SJHC and 4% higher at FHC than mean supply cost at the main campus. However, operative times were 29% lower at SJHC and 25% lower at FHC than at the main campus.

Total costs for laparoscopic hernia repair, shown in Fig. 17.6, were found to be lower at SJHC and FHC than on the main campus (other). This was a result of substantially shorter OR times which offset the cost of the equipment.

The lowest cost was obtained by the surgeon at FHC, whose supply choices resulted in the best combination of supply costs and OR time costs. This led to an overall cost-saving of 15% compared to surgeons at the main campus and 5% compared to the surgeon at SJHC.

Other surgeons in our institution have applied these methods to the use of advanced energy devices, for example Ligasure (Medtronic, Boston, MA) or the

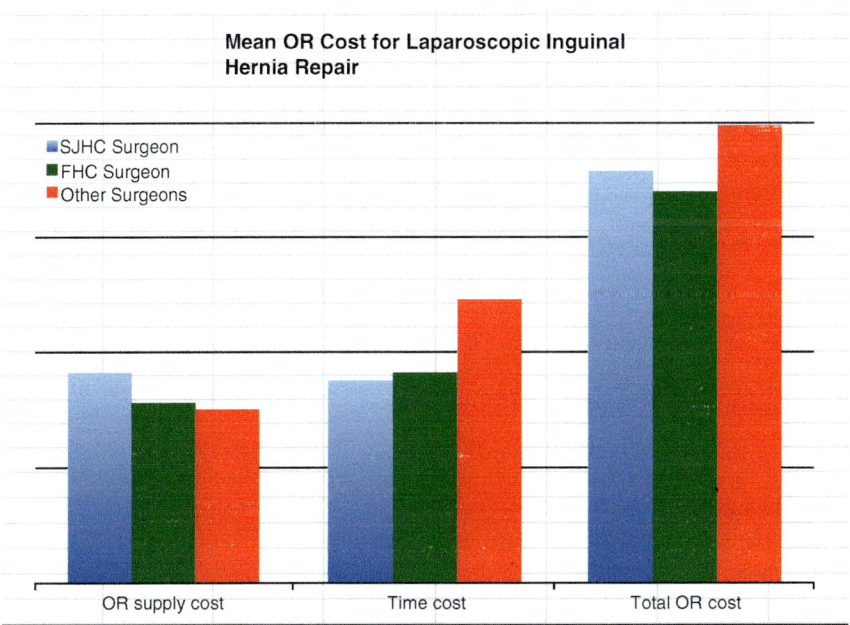

Fig. 17.6 OR cost for laparoscopic inguinal hernia repair by hospital

Harmonic Scalpel (Ethicon, Cincinnati, OH) and have found that cost savings from shorter OR times did not offset the additional cost of the devices for operations such as laparoscopic appendectomy or hemorrhoidectomy (Data not shown).

Discussion

Identifying areas for cost savings at the main campus and ambulatory centers was a good first step to lower overall expenses for the health system. We believed that the key to using this knowledge to implement change was to transfer cases from the main campus to the outlying ambulatory clinics.

The general surgery division had 30 faculty members, most of whom performed inguinal hernia repair and cholecystectomy. The urology division had 15 faculty, though only a few performed varicocelectomy or AUS placement regularly. As mentioned, the two ambulatory centers were remote from the main campus, requiring about an hour commute each direction. Most U of U surgeons had offices and/or research labs on the main campus. Convincing these surgeons to reschedule their elective outpatient operations at a remote ambulatory center proved to be a difficult task.

Upon the opening of SJHC, the Dean of the School of Medicine and Senior Vice President for Health Sciences had directed each Department Chair to tell clinical faculty to use the new facility for part of their practices. The response was not robust, and most specialties demonstrated poor rates of OR block utilization.

The notable exception was otolaryngology—head and neck surgery. Two otolaryngology surgeons established their primary clinical practices at SJHC when it opened and were able to build successful practices and fill OR block schedules. Eventually, other surgical divisions followed suit: general surgery, plastic surgery, ophthalmology, and urology hired surgeons with a specific focus on establishing clinical practices at SJHC (including the team participating in the study). Beyond the surgeons practicing primarily at FHC and SJHC, there was little interest among surgery faculty in scheduling their elective outpatient operations away from the hospital.

Influence of Schedulers

Scheduling of new patients was done primarily through a centralized process. UofU health employed schedulers at their Care Navigation Center. Schedulers were equipped with algorithms for patient referrals that vary for every department, and even for specialty sections in a department. For general surgery, the first step for a scheduler was to determine if a subspecialty (such as colon and rectal surgery or bariatric surgery) is appropriate. If a patient remained in the general surgery queue, then the scheduler referred the consult request to individual schedulers for each surgeon, based on a rotation. The exception to this process occurred when a referring provider made a specific request for a surgeon. A similar process occurred in urology.

Our group understood that enticing University-based surgeons to change their practice patterns would have limited success. Our approach, instead, was to address patient scheduling at the referral level. We instituted a policy that directed a higher percentage of appropriate patients to the surgical clinics at the ambulatory centers rather than at the hospital.

We began a process of hiring to meet the anticipated need for additional surgeons at the clinics. General surgery already had three surgeons working primarily at SJHC and hired a fourth to work primarily at FHC as this project started. Urology was able to add a third surgeon primarily at SJHC, who would also be the new executive medical director. Urology also simultaneously hired one of their finishing chief residents to work primarily at FHC.

In addition to changing the algorithms that ran the referral queue we focused on building direct contact between primary care staff and the surgical teams at FHC and SJHC. This began by establishing a dedicated boundary spanner role that was one administrative assistant who took charge of the patient referrals from internal UofU Health primary care clinics. General surgeons also met with referring providers, and over a few months, developed a routine of direct referral. This change was made easier by the fact that the clinics were largely under-burdened, which resulted in flexible schedules and short new-patient wait times. A second facilitating factor was that most of the patients seen by the primary care providers in U of U Community Clinics lived in closer proximity to the ambulatory centers than to the hospital main campus.

We came up with a scheme to assign patients to the outlying clinics based on geography of the region. We picked several roads that acted as geographic boundaries for the zone of the main campus and assigned patients to the main campus or the ambulatory clinics based on their position relative to these boundaries. A single addition to the referral algorithm at the Care Navigation Center accounted for the patient's home address. In practice this meant that any patient living west of I-15 in Salt Lake City, or outside the I-215 belt that encircled the city would be closer to SJHC or FHC than to the main campus and would be given the option of attending one of the two ambulatory centers.

Approval of this change required the buy-in of leaders and administrators of the affected departments, as well as the OR Executive Committee at the University Hospital. This constituted a second and formidable challenge, considering that the change to referral patterns would pull business from the main campus.

Building Buy-in

We began by reaching out to leadership teams that we believed would be in favor of growth at the ambulatory centers. First, we presented our data to the OR Executive Committee at SJHC, then to the Outpatient Surgery Leadership Team at the University. Before going any further at the University, we decided we needed a better case to make the necessary changes that would disrupt daily routine for some of the well-established senior surgeons.

Attending meetings of the OR block committee revealed that newly onboarded surgeons frequently had difficulty booking OR block time. Additionally, the census showed that the main hospital was often at capacity, which meant that elective operations were delayed until nursing supervisors could confirm bed availability. While these problems generally pertained to inpatient operations, the result was that some post-operative patients were housed for hours in the PACU awaiting beds. The congestion of PACU space also affected the ability to perform elective outpatient surgeries. This information led us to believe that the hospital was accruing significant opportunity cost by scheduling elective outpatient operations at the main campus.

We proposed that moving some of the patients would result in reduced delays for elective outpatient surgeries. In addition to increasing capacity, this approach would decrease patient wait times, which would further affect our scores for patient satisfaction. Our team went back over the previous year and identified the open inguinal hernia repairs, laparoscopic cholecystectomies, artificial urinary sphincter placements and varicocelectomies that could have been appropriately done at the ambulatory centers. We identified 374 operative cases, which accounted for 604 h of time in the main hospital OR's, or the equivalent of 12.2 h per week of operative time (Fig. 17.7).

Our group felt that a reasonable compromise would be to propose that half of the eligible patients be redirected to the ambulatory clinics. Based on the data we had accumulated, this hypothetical scenario would result in overall cost savings of $107,000 per year.

Furthermore, this would open six additional OR hours per week, which would appeal to the OR executive committee and Department Chairs. We applied the average value for our OR's per-hour revenue to the additional available OR blocks. If the 6 h of block time were filled it would result in over $200,000 per year in new revenue opportunities.

Our first presentation was to the Surgery Value Council. This council was made up of the Chief Value Officers (CVO's) of the surgical specialties, and was chaired by the Department CVO, a general surgeon who would be personally affected by any changes. The Value Council strongly endorsed the findings of our project.

Case	# of cases done 7/15-6/16	OR Hours	OR Hours/week	OR blocks/week
Inguinal hernia repair	204	326	6.5	0.81
Laparoscopic cholecystectomy	148	225	4.5	0.56
Artificial Urinary Sphincter	18	45	1	0.13
Varicocelectomy	4	8	0.2	0.03
Total	**374**	**604**	**12.2**	**1.53**

Fig. 17.7 Operative cases and hours

The next meeting was with the Chief of the Division of General Surgery and his senior administrative staff. With the endorsement of the CVO, we were able to secure approval for the geographic modification of the referral queue.

Riding high on these two wins, we approached the Chair of the Department of Surgery. Initially, the Chair was skeptical about the data and our extrapolations. However, he expressed his support for the concept and agreed that the information could be shown to the OR Executive Committee.

The OR Executive Committee included all of the Department Chairs and senior administrators with a stake in surgery at the institution. The Chief Medical Officer of Ambulatory Health made the presentation. The additional argument for opportunity cost put our argument over the top and the OR Executive Committee gave their official endorsement for redirecting ambulatory surgical procedures to the outlying clinics.

Retrospective

Two years after completing the ORCA analysis, we have made some progress and have experienced some setbacks. Patient volumes in surgical clinics at the outpatient facilities have grown over the years, as shown in Fig. 17.8. The surgeons at SJHC and FHC continue to perform at lower cost and maintain higher patient satisfaction scores than our colleagues at the main campus, and our ambulatory surgery facilities continue to have higher ratios of net operating margin to revenue than the surgery facilities at the main campus. The Surgery Department Chairman, who was

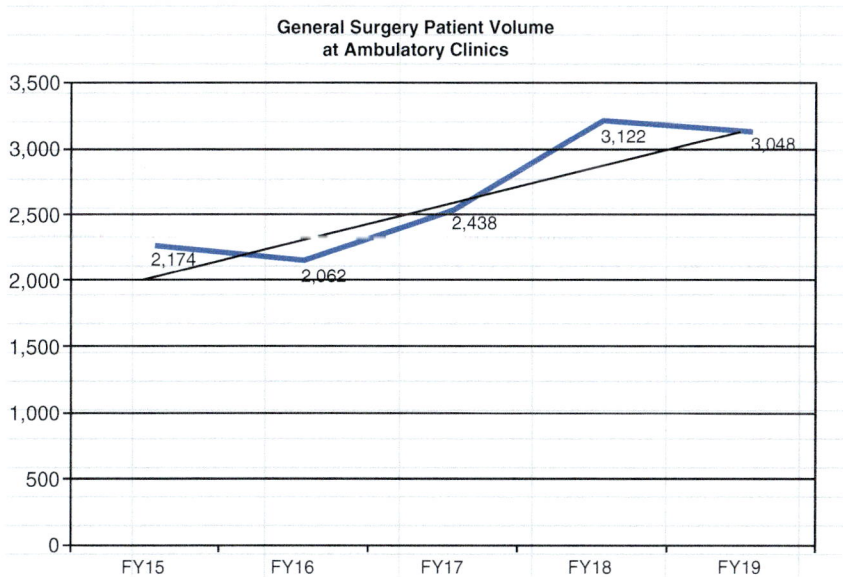

Fig. 17.8 General surgery patient volume at ambulatory clinics

skeptical at first, added an OR block at an ambulatory center to his schedule, and now drives from the main campus to do his ambulatory surgery procedures.

However, OR block utilization remains far below capacity at both centers and near capacity at the main campus. The culprit appears to be staff turnover. One of the three general surgeons at SJHC developed a serious illness that forced his retirement in 2017. Two of the three urologists at SJHC left the practice and only one has been replaced. The anesthesia lead for our project left for a private practice opportunity. We are currently working hard to not fall prey to staff turnover.

Conclusion

Cost accounting software is a powerful tool for driving change in behavior of surgeons, anesthesiologists and OR personnel. We found this tool to be critical to understanding the relative costs of equipment and OR time when developing strategies to minimize overall costs for common ambulatory operations. Data suggested that shifting operations to satellite clinics would decrease overall cost. However, cost-benefit analysis alone was not enough to institute change. We strategically sought backing from leadership, which was ultimately what gave us the social capital needed to translate cost accounting data into strategic action.

References

1. U.S. Census Bureau. U.S. Census Bureau QuickFacts: South Jordan city, Utah. 2020. https://www.census.gov/quickfacts/fact/table/southjordancityutah/INC110218. Accessed 2020 Feb 9.
2. Winchester S. CMS Administrator Seema Verma Commends University of Utah Health for its Commitment to Price Transparency. 2019. https://healthcare.utah.edu/publicaffairs/news/2019/01/price-transparency.php. Accessed 2020 Jun 28.
3. Kawamoto K, Martin CJ, Williams K, Tu M-C, Park CG, Hunter C, et al. Value Driven Outcomes (VDO): a pragmatic, modular, and extensible software framework for understanding and improving health care costs and outcomes. J Am Med Inform Assoc. 2015;22(1):223–35.
4. Akhavan S, Ward L, Bozic KJ. Time-driven activity-based costing more accurately reflects costs in arthroplasty surgery. Clin Orthop Relat Res. 2016;474(1):8–15.
5. Balakrishnan K, Goico B, Arjmand EM. Applying cost accounting to operating room staffing in otolaryngology: time-driven activity-based costing and outpatient adenotonsillectomy. Otolaryngol Head Neck Surg. 2015;152(4):684–90.
6. Childers CP, Maggard-Gibbons M. Understanding costs of care in the operating room. JAMA Surg. 2018;153(4):e176233.
7. Fabricant PD, Seeley MA, Rozell JC, Fieldston E, Flynn JM, Wells LM, et al. Cost savings from utilization of an ambulatory surgery center for orthopaedic day surgery. J Am Acad Orthop Surg. 2016;24(12):865–71.
8. Rosen MJ, Malm JA, Tarnoff M, Zuccala K, Ponsky JL. Cost-effectiveness of ambulatory laparoscopic cholecystectomy. Surg Laparosc Endosc Percutan Tech. 2001 Jun;11(3):182–4.
9. Koenig L, Gu Q. Growth of ambulatory surgical centers, surgery volume, and savings to medicare. Am J Gastroenterol. 2013;108(1):10–5.

Physician Engagement in Population Health: A Case Study in Project Selection and Practice Variation

18

Kim D. Ariyabuddhiphongs and Ben Kragen

Key Learning Points
- Small projects have a high likelihood of success.
- Focused projects that produce quantifiable results garner support.
- Projects should be influenced by alignment with organizational priorities, resource availability, time constraints, and competing priorities.
- Physician education is one of the most impactful strategies to reduce low-value care.
- Practice pattern variation can occur at the national, regional, state, local, and practice level leading to variations in outcomes and cost.
- Claims and EHR/clinical data allow for expansive study of data.
- Analytic projects need to be selective and focused in scope.
- Accountability and follow-through are key success factors in any initiative.
- Physicians are receptive to change.

Executive Summary

Physician practice pattern variation is a driver of unnecessary health care costs. We set out to reduce practice variation using Continuous Quality Improvement methods including stakeholder alignment and the Plan-Do-Study-Act framework. This informed the selection of a low risk intervention of educating providers about lab test ordering.

K. D. Ariyabuddhiphongs (✉)
Beth Israel Lahey Health Performance Network, Westwood, MA, USA
e-mail: kariyabu@bidmc.harvard.edu

B. Kragen
Heller School for Social Policy and Management, Brandeis University, Waltham, MA, USA

After performing a baseline analysis of the cost of labs, we created education materials, presented information at physician meetings, and performed trend analysis with 2018 and 2019 data. Data was presented and discussed at primary care physician (PCP) leadership meetings and select groups underwent intense follow-up with physician level analysis and more frequent follow-up meetings.

At the outset of this project each lab studied cost $20–60/test. Baseline analysis showed up to 15× variation in practice patterns by physician group in lab ordering for Chemistry 10, Lipid panel, Vitamin D, and TSH. Trend analysis showed groups with high intensity performance monitoring and follow-up had more favorable results and decreased the frequency of lab testing.

Although lab testing is a low contributor to total costs by percentage of total health care costs, this model informs strategies to introduce further cost-savings interventions to physicians through data, un-blinding, and frequent discussion. Future projects can be selected and designed with key learning from this project.

Physician leadership and engagement in cost reduction while improving patient care is necessary to bend the cost curve. Our program in low value care demonstrates that a combination of analytics and provider engagement approach is effective in decreasing lab frequency. This intervention has also informed current approaches to the physician role in decreasing health care costs in our system.

Background

The Case for Decreasing Health Care Costs

Meet the Weber family. Mr. Weber is 45 years old and installs fences for a living. Mrs. Weber is a teacher. They have two children. Their family moves to a new community and Mr. Weber sees a physician for symptoms of cough and weight loss. Unable to obtain records from a previous work-up, the physician orders labs and imaging. The Webers have a high-deductible health plan (HDHP) for health insurance coverage. Their high deductible of $2000 is high for their family. It will mean the difference between taking a family vacation or forgoing other purchases that year. Mr. Weber undergoes the lab and imaging, creating unnecessary duplication of tests and hitting his deductible for the year. The repetition of work-up is normal but the Webers are left with high health care costs that year.

The Webers' story is echoed nationally as health care costs rise and individuals and families take on more health care costs out of their own pockets [1]. A predictable portion of health care services is of low-value to patients' overall health [2, 3]. Physicians can take an active leadership role in reining in skyrocketing health care costs considering their position as the leader of the health care team and because of their direct role in defining health care costs [4]. Physicians are well positioned to directly impact health care costs given their familiarity with clinical guidelines and their role in making recommendations to patients.

Health Policy Focuses on Cost

The 2010 Affordable Care Act (ACA) initiated several cost-control mechanisms and health care delivery reform nationally [5]. Although the ACA primarily focused on increasing access to health care by decreasing the uninsured population, it funded and spurred several programs that have led to the creation and expansion of Accountable Care Organizations (ACOs) throughout the country. ACOs are networks of physicians and hospitals that come together and agree to take on financial risk to care for a population of individuals [6]. ACOs are financially incentivized to improve the experience of care, improve population outcomes, and keep per capita spending down, health care's Triple Aim [7]. As early as 2003, health care systems had already started moving in the direction of 'Population Health,' broadly defined as improving the health outcomes of a population of individuals, while decreasing costs [8].

Successful ACO's early savings were realized with nurse care management and decrease in post-acute care costs, neither of which required significant change in physician behavior or practice. Lack of attention to evidence-based medicine, or the use of scientific evidence to support medical practice, contributes to variation in outcomes [9]. Variation has been detected in screening, diagnostic testing and procedures, treatment, and management, which lead to regional and local variation in clinical practice as well as cost [10].

In recent years there has been increased attention to unnecessary care and waste in the health care system, including "low value care". Low value care is care that is provided to patients but does not improve outcomes [2]. Several of these areas include frequently ordered labs, radiology, and procedures. While these areas represent lower percentages of the total cost of care compared to the high-cost areas of inpatient medical and surgical admissions, they represent the intersection of unnecessary care, strong clinical guidelines, and collectively account for significant cost savings despite having low per unit costs. These represent focus areas of evidence-based medicine and clear guidance from medical societies with clinical guidelines. Several past initiatives have addressed these target areas, including the Choosing Wisely campaign from the American Board of Internal Medicine which publishes recommendations from specialty organizations to reduce unnecessary care by engaging physicians to follow clinical guidelines [11].

Physician Engagement

Physicians' decisions, practice patterns, and actions directly impact patient outcomes as well as the total cost of care. Physician engagement is central to quality improvement efforts in health care organizations [12]. Physician champions who can effectively share knowledge, facilitate reflective practice, and create a supportive environment can drive cost-conscious care [13]. While the majority of practicing physicians have not been trained to recognize the costs of health care, recent literature suggests that this practice can increase the value of care [13]. A systematic literature review found that physician education and clinical decision support through EHR were the two most successful interventions to reduce low-value care [14]. In the context of a heterogeneous mix of practices, a combination of stakeholder analysis and physician education were found to be effective to mitigate overuse [15].

Context of the Organization

Our organization in Eastern Massachusetts (MA) was one of the Medicare Pioneer ACOs in the state and achieved cost savings and higher performance on quality performance in the early years of the program. This was accomplished by examining and decreasing unnecessary costs in post-hospitalization care, also known as post-acute care. Additional savings had been more challenging to generate in subsequent years. However, quality measure performance continued to be strong and the management team evaluated ways to continue to decrease cost while continuing to provide excellent clinical care within the network. We turned to physician engagement and leadership as a way to contain costs moving forward.

The organization has more than 500 primary care physicians in a combination of employed groups and independent practices. The physicians are structured in large employed groups (>100 PCPs) and span a variety of sizes down to solo practitioners. With this variety of settings come a variety of Population Health infrastructure supports such as nurse care management and quality improvement or population health specialist roles. Physicians were also on different Electronic Health Record (EHR) platforms with different workflows in place. This means that there is a heterogeneous mix of decision support in EHRs, population health quality leads, nurse care management, and EHR registry support across the network.

In early 2019, our health system was on the cusp of merging with another health system in the second largest health system merger in Massachusetts. This induced feelings of optimism and creativity across the legacy organizations but also created uncertainty. The impact on investment in new projects was significant before the transaction, during the transition period, and continued well after the merger.

In the year preceding the merger there were constraints on resources in order to prepare for the upcoming structural changes. Understanding these constraints, we looked for a project that was focused and aligned with organizational goals, was feasible within our resource constraints, and was relevant to our goals of improving quality or decreasing cost. We also selected a project that could be completed in the same year a major merger was occurring. The factors that contributed to us picking a data management and physician engagement project stemmed from both the desired deliverables but also the environment within which the project was set: the financial, policy, state, cultural, economic, and organizational structures that impacted our health system.

Choosing the Project: Stakeholder Alignment, CQI

Generally, when thinking about the likelihood of success of a given project, the external, internal, and local environments are critical to understand because they greatly influence interest and appetite to invest resources [14]. Aligning stakeholder interests is a critical step in developing mutually satisfying reciprocal relationships with adjacent efforts. Building in the goals of adjacent efforts is a strategic move to reinforce the success of a given project [16]. This is an easy way to develop investment of physicians and leadership that are not directly involved in the project. Mapping the distribution of benefits and costs onto the different stakeholders that are tangentially involved in the intervention can help to illuminate strategies to shape the project to be more politically feasible [17].

Given the multiple competing priorities facing our organization, a "good change" required a relatively small manageable project that required low resources and had defined deliverables that aligned with organizational goals and quality measures [18]. While the selection of a smaller goal is absolutely critical in resource constrained primary care settings like the ones described in this paper, the strategy is generalizable to all organizations as part of a strategy for continuous quality improvement (CQI).

CQI is a strategy that builds on Imai's Kaizen principles of "good change", which advocates for small improvements to fine tune a system [19]. O'Donnell and Gupta (2020) suggest choosing projects that have specific, quantifiable operational or patient care outcomes [20]. Several methods have been proposed to implement CQI [20]. This project employs the Plan-Do-Study-Act cycle, which is discussed in the methods section.

It's worth noting that CQI extends beyond any project, and is instead part of a larger management style. While each project is important and can help to achieve specific goals, it is important to nest the project in the larger theme of change in the organization. CQI thrives when an organization has developed a culture of implementing frequent small changes that together amount to large but gradual shifts in the organization [18].

Methods

Continuous Quality Improvement: Plan Do Study Act

Continuous quality improvement (CQI) was implemented in this study using the Plan-Do-Study-Act (PDSA) method [20].

"Plan"

The planning stage involved defining the problem, the field of study, and objectives for the study. Guided by the principles of CQI, as discussed in the background, we selected a small quantifiable project that aligned with the larger goals of the health care organization and health care environment broadly.

Our team considered the health systems population health goals, the fact that our health system was merging, the need for physician engagement, and the resources required for a focused project when making our decision about which low-value care category to focus on. Lab tests were selected as an area that was understood to be an opportunity to reduce costs and align with clinical guidelines by management in several departments, as well as at the organizational level. It further aligned with the appetite to reduce low-value work. A last benefit was that lab work was quantified in the organization, allowing for a measure of success. This can be helpful in stimulating interest in future quality improvement projects.

To demonstrate pre/post intervention variation, our project required looking at labs that had high enough physician ordering frequency and allowed for sufficient data collection to smooth over outliers and other biasing effects. This both helped us to get a sense of appropriate variation; and was convincing to physicians who otherwise might have questioned the generalizability of our findings to their practice. We looked at the variety of labs that were ordered and selected the labs that were most often ordered redundantly. We identified lab orders assessing Vitamin D, cholesterol, thyroid stimulating hormone (TSH) and Chemistry 10/Comprehensive Metabolic Panel (CMP) as the best opportunities to decrease low value care. Our network spends more than $3 million on these four lab tests per year.

With this information in hand, we convened a small nimble team of physician leaders, a project manager, and data analysis specialists to determine the suitable intervention to address lab ordering. We were guided by the literature to consider either a physician education initiative or a clinician decision support initiative. Considering the disparate and noncommunicating EHR platforms employed by our different provider groups, we decided to rule out a clinician decision support initiative and move forward with a physician education and data un-blinding project.

"Do"

We talked to physicians about the incentives to reduce additional lab work. We were careful to align incentives by explaining to our physicians that reducing low value care would benefit their practice by reducing overall work and align with clinical guidelines. We explained that eliminating extraneous procedures would help the ACO to meet financial goals, which will increase shared savings. In this way we framed the project as one that reduces work rather than requires extra work, something that is often associated with quality improvement projects.

We talked with physicians about the different types of low value care, including radiological imaging, lab ordering, and decreasing the use of antibiotics in viral infections. Through consensus, lab ordering was identified as the area of focus.

Once we secured buy-in from physicians we designed a program to address unnecessary lab ordering. We used practice pattern variation analysis to produce unblinded data. We used an educational approach by sharing unblinded data, reviewing clinical guidelines, discussing potential cost savings, and identifying top 25 physician utilizers across the network. All physicians received a broad education intervention and select groups received more intense education and regular monitoring through more frequent follow-up meetings compared to their peers.

Primary care physicians and their practices were organized into 22 separate groups within the larger network based on geography. Each group represents approximately 25 physicians (Actual group numbers have been de-identified). We analyzed baseline lab utilization by group for the time period Jan-September 2018 (first three quarters of the calendar year). Results were not risk-adjusted.

Physician leaders received baseline analysis of their group and review of low-value care literature. We obtained PCP leadership engagement and support of the initiative, and together held frequent and well-attended physician meeting forums to review clinical guidelines and data. After subsequent analysis, three groups received higher intensity intervention compared to their peers. These groups were selected based on their engagement and higher baseline lab ordering frequency. Group 14 received monthly group level analysis on lab frequency whereas the other two groups received quarterly reminders through a less intense intervention.

"Study"

We studied the impact of intervention on lab and radiology exam ordering using retrospective data analysis. We used a combination of claims data and EHR/clinical data to capture both the patient and provider interactions, as well as the services billed for each patient. Baseline data from 2018 and follow up data from 2019 was used to do an analysis of lab and radiology exams ordering. Our variables were generated from ICD-10 codes and Current Procedural Terminology (CPT) codes incorporated into the written code for the baseline and follow-up analysis.

"Act"

We are currently in the final "act" stage. If the project was unsuccessful, we would repeat the PDSA cycle and incorporate the insight gained in the first cycle. However, in the case of this study the intervention was successful in achieving the goal of changing lab ordering patterns. When a project is successful like this, O'Donnell and Gupta suggest regular check-ins to insure continued compliance [20]. It is also possible to maintain momentum and scale the intervention to address additional low-value lab and radiology ordering.

Results

Continuous Quality Improvement

The change initiative was adopted in the organization by both managers and providers. Overall, we found that physicians were accustomed to quality measurement, practice pattern variation analyses, and the logic behind the ACO model that incentivized waste reduction. Rollout of the provider education intervention was successful and met little resistance from providers. The three most engaged roles in this project were (1) physician champion, (2) project manager, and (3) data analyst.

Baseline Analysis Reveals Wide Variation in Practice Patterns

Baseline data revealed wide variation for all four lab tests. On the heat map shown in Fig. 18.1 green represents lower frequency of testing and red represents higher frequency of testing. Measurement was performed in tests per 1000 patient member months (or mm, defined as 1 patient enrolled in the ACO for 1 month). The largest variation in ordering practices was found for the

Lab Testing Frequency/1000 patients				
GROUP	CMP	Lipid Panel	Vitamin D*	TSH
1	62.8	353.7	88.0	433.0
2	167.5	542.9	111.8	435.2
3	208.1	549.4	63.1	425.6
4	61.0	470.3	82.5	427.3
5	264.0	519.8	113.8	398.4
6	236.3	488.1	100.3	326.7
7	103.3	447.8	111.2	386.7
8	49.4	217.5	54.1	158.7
9	253.4	297.0	44.7	193.1
10	42.2	357.5	110.3	257.4
11	76.7	249.9	71.1	204.0
12	396.8	354.9	69.7	167.9
13	394.5	668.7	226.8	298.3
14	339.6	454.6	163.7	312.6
15	658.3	733.3	124.7	235.7
16	79.4	391.7	75.1	411.7
17	486.2	514.3	131.9	310.7
18	406.7	635.9	170.2	281.2
19	325.8	504.1	165.9	196.5
20	108.3	201.1	63.8	129.4
21	588.9	646.6	118.4	288.1
22	346.7	540.4	145.5	235.7
TOTAL	229.1	437.6	104.6	296.4
Cost per test	$33.20	$21.54	$61.09	$39.69

Fig. 18.1 Jan–Sept 2018 Baseline Lab frequency/1000 patient member months by group. *: Vitamin D testing measured as testing without documented indications consistent with clinical guidelines. All other lab testing is observed frequency

Comprehensive Metabolic Panel (CMP), which ranged from 42 tests per 1000 mm ordered by group 10, to 658 tests per 1000 mm ordered by group 15. Orders placed for Vitamin D tests had the smallest variation, ranging from 45 tests per 1000 mm to 227 tests per 1000 mm. Several groups (groups 8–11, group 20) showed lower frequency of testing for all four tests studied. Groups 13, 15, 18, and 21 generally ordered more tests on the whole. The majority of groups demonstrated variation both in the frequency of test types that they ordered within their group, as well as variation with the frequency of specific tests ordered by their group as compared to other groups. Figure 18.1 shows the baseline analysis.

Monthly Provider Education Was Associated with Decrease in Lab Ordering

Table 18.1 shows the change in lab ordering for Groups 14, 17 and 18 compared to the entire network total (the benchmark) from baseline in 2018–2019, approximately 1 year after the bundled intervention. Group 14 received the most intense intervention with regular engagement with physicians, reminders at monthly meetings, and performance tracking over time. This group of physicians had the biggest change in lab frequency compared to the benchmark. Groups 17 and 18, who did not receive regular follow-up, had mixed results.

Trend analysis showed Group 14, the group that received the highest intensity performance monitoring and follow-up, demonstrated a favorable decrease in lab ordering frequency across all four tests from 2018 to 2019 compared to the trends exhibited by the total PCP network (Fig. 18.2).

Table 18.1 2018 and 2019 trends for three Higher Intensity Intervention Groups compared to overall lab frequency trends

2019 Group	2019	CMP	LIPID	VIT D	TSH
14	Test Count	1216	1897	480	1253
	Util/1000	305.3	474.1	132.6	313.9
	Trend 2018–2019	−10.1%	4.3%	−19.0%	1.1%
17	Test Count	2831	2852	533	1393
	Util/1000	558.8	562.9	106.9	279.6
	Trend 2018–2019	14.9%	9.4%	−19.0%	−10.0%
18	Test Count	1249	2121	542	962
	Util/1000	405.4	680.3	173.2	309.6
	Trend 2018–2019	−0.3%	7.0%	1.8%	10.1%
Total	Test Count	23,712	47,413	9485	29,042
	Util/1000	255.5	472.1	105.2	311.0
	Trend 2018–2019	11.5%	7.9%	0.5%	4.9%

Util/1000 Trend refers to lab frequency per 1000 patients

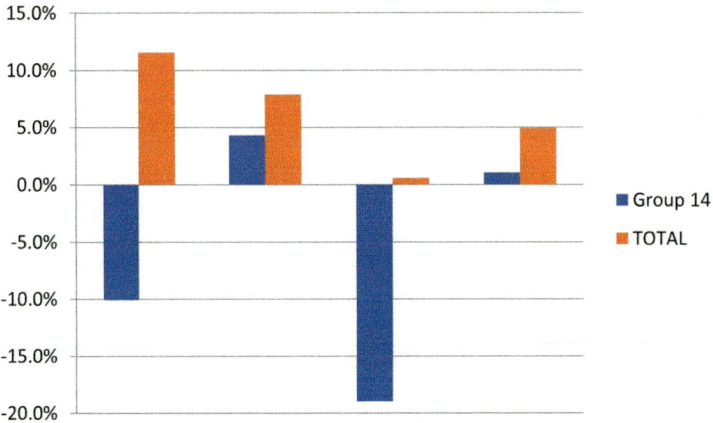

Fig. 18.2 Group 14 2018–2019 lab frequency trends compared to overall network

Discussion

Our analysis revealed large variation in lab ordering across a large physician network. Results indicate that for our treatment group, group 14, that the combination of a focused initiative, engaged PCP leadership, the use of various data sources, review of clinical guidelines, and regular discussion at physician meetings was associated with a decrease in lab ordering frequency. Similar interventions have been shown to impact physician behavior in other settings [21].

Given the multiple areas of opportunity, we observed that it is tempting for physician leaders to have expansive goals at the outset of identifying population health initiatives. We found success in choosing a project that is narrowly scoped, quantifiable, and required low financial investment. We also noted that shifting priorities, as observed during the merger, have the potential to put projects at risk. Notable was the fact that external pressures and internal constraints threatened the success of the project. Our choice to focus on a discrete low-value care project was ultimately appropriate for an organization that was in flux because it did not require significant future commitment and served as a pilot for other more involved quality improvement projects. In this way the project had three successful outcomes; (1) it was associated with a reduction in low-value lab ordering, and (2) it informed future quality improvement initiatives, and (3) it helped to validate a strategy of continuous quality improvement.

Conclusion

This project demonstrates the ability of a small team to produce change in a large organization. In this case we were able to roll out provider education about lab test ordering which impacted provider results. In lieu of workflow changes or decision support in EHRs at the point of ordering, regular engagement meetings with physicians, performance tracking at the group level, and widely accepted clinical guidelines were key to achieving outcomes. We found additional success in having a benchmark for comparison between peers.

The Triple Aim remains relevant today with goals of improving patient experience, improving the quality of care, and decreasing cost. Throughout the era of health care delivery reform, physician engagement remains a core principle necessary for success in improving Population Health while decreasing cost.

Acknowledgement We would like to acknowledge Elizabeth Kelleher and Julianne Hunn for their contributions to this project.

References

1. Berwick DM, Hackbarth AD. Eliminating waste in US health care. JAMA. 2012;307(14):1513–6. https://doi.org/10.1001/jama.2012.362.
2. Schwartz AL, Landon BE, Elshaug AG, Chernew ME, McWilliams JM. Measuring low-value care in Medicare. JAMA Intern Med. 2014;174(7):1067–76. https://doi.org/10.1001/jamainternmed.2014.1541.
3. O'Sullivan JW, Stevens S, Oke J, Hobbs FDR, Salisbury C, Little P, et al. Practice variation in the use of tests in UK primary care: a retrospective analysis of 16 million tests performed over 3.3 million patient years in 2015/16. BMC Med. 2018;16(1):229. https://doi.org/10.1186/s12916-018-1217-1.
4. Lee TH, Cosgrove T. Six tests for physicians and their leaders for the decade ahead. NEJM Catal Innov Care Deliv. 2020;1(4) https://doi-org.ezp-prod1.hul.harvard.edu/10.1056/CAT.19.1045
5. Strokoff SL, Grossman EG. Office of the Legislative Counsel. 2010. p. 974.
6. Gold J. Accountable care organizations, explained. Kaiser Health News. 2015, Sept 14. https://khn.org/news/aco-accountable-care-organization-faq/
7. Berwick DM, Nolan TW, Whittington J. The triple aim: care, health, and cost. Health Aff. 2008;27(3):759–69.
8. Kindig D, Stoddart G. What is population health? Am J Public Health. 2003;93(3):380–3. https://doi.org/10.2105/ajph.93.3.380.
9. Hisham R, Ng CJ, Liew SM, Hamzah N, Ho GJ. Why is there variation in the practice of evidence-based medicine in primary care? A qualitative study. BMJ Open. 2016;6(3):e010565. https://doi.org/10.1136/bmjopen-2015-010565.
10. Eddy DM. Practice: the role of uncertainty. Health Aff. 1984;3(2) https://doi.org/10.1377/hlthaff.3.2.74.
11. Choosing Wisely. An initiative of the American board of internal medicine. Available from https://www.choosingwisely.org/
12. McGonigal M, Bauer M, Post C. Physician engagement: a key concept in the journey for quality improvement. JAMA. 2015;314(22):2384–400. https://doi.org/10.1001/jama.2015.16353.
13. Stanmen LA, Stalmeijer RE, Peternotte E, Pool AO, Driessen EW, Scheele F, et al. Training physicians to provide high-value, cost-conscious care: a systematic review. JAMA. 2015;314(22):2384–400. https://doi.org/10.1001/jama.2015.16353.
14. Scanlon D, Beich J, Leitzell B, Shaw B, Alexander J, Christianson J, et al. The aligning forces for quality initiative: background and evolution from 2005 to 2015. Am J Manag Care. 2016;22(12 Suppl):s346–59.
15. Colla CH, Mainor AJ, Hargreaves C, Sequist T, Morden N. Interventions aimed at reducing use of low-value health services: a systematic review. Med Care Res Rev. 2017;74(5):507–50.

16. Miles JA. Stakeholder theory. In: Management and organization theory: a Jossey-Bass reader. The Jossey-Bass business & management reader series. 1st. ed. San Francisco, CA: Jossey-Bass; 2012. p. 305–11.
17. Langley A, Denis J-L. Beyond evidence: the micropolitics of improvement. BMJ Qual Saf. 2011;20(Suppl_1):i43–6.
18. Knechtges P, Decker MC. Application of kaizen methodology to foster departmental engagement in quality improvement. J Am Coll Radiol. 2014;11(12 Pt A):1126–30.
19. Singh J, Singh H. 5 1 kaizen philosophy: a review of literature kaizen philosophy: a review of literature. IUP J Oper Manag. 2009;8:51–72.
20. O'Donnell B, Gupta V. Continuous quality improvement. In: StatPearls. Treasure Island, FL: StatPearls Publishing; 2020 [cited 2021 Jan 27]. Available from: http://www.ncbi.nlm.nih.gov/books/NBK559239/
21. Cammisa C, Partridge G, Ardans C, Buehrer K, Chapman B, Beckman H. Engaging physicians in change: results of a safety net quality improvement program to reduce overuse. Am J Med Qual. 2011;26(1):26–33.

Late Surgical Cancellations in a Pediatric Surgical Practice

19

Vivek Singh, Usha E. A. Beijnen, and Amir H. Taghinia

Key Learning Points
- Most preventable cases can be attributable to patient factors, with illness accounting for almost half of all canceled cases.
- Health care facilities may seek to establish a dedicated line of provider-patient communication on weekends to avoid a buildup of canceled appointments on Mondays.
- When patient illness is suspected ahead of a surgery, it may be advantageous to schedule the patient for an end-of-day procedure to avoid disrupting workflow in the event of a cancellation.
- Procedures such as nevi excisions and other non-urgent skin excisions are more prone to patient cancellation and thus should be scheduled toward the end of the day if possible.
- Patient non-adherence to preoperative guidelines is a substantial source of same-day cancellations, indicating a need to clarify preoperative instructions.
- Office staff should confirm patient insurance status prior to surgery.
- Patient phone numbers should be verified upon each visit.

Executive Summary

Surgical cancellations within 1 day of the procedure (late-cancellations) impact the ability of the OR to function efficiently. A study was designed to identify the factors associated with these cancellations in a pediatric surgical practice [1]. The medical records of patients treated by plastic and oral surgery services at our institution from 2010 to 2015 were queried, and a total of 10,730 scheduled operating room cases

---

V. Singh · U. E. A. Beijnen · A. H. Taghinia (✉)
Department of Plastic and Oral Surgery, Boston Children's Hospital, Boston, MA, USA
e-mail: amir.taghinia@childrens.harvard.edu

were included. Our analysis indicated that most late surgical cancellations were preventable or possibly preventable. Additionally, the timing of the cancellation was critical because those occurring near the scheduled procedure time disrupted redistribution of operating room resources and personnel. Addressing cancellations deemed preventable or possibly preventable will improve efficiency and ensure timely patient access to surgical procedures.

Introduction

Fixed costs of the operating room compose approximately 60% of the total cost of surgery with an approximate cost of over $15 per minute excluding professional fees [2–4]. These costs are primarily personnel costs, but also include equipment, real estate, and utilities. An unused operating room incurs significant costs during a normal workday as it generates a mismatch between demand (another patient who cannot get care) and supply (resources to provide care) and can worsen existing supply constraints. Thus, late surgical cancellation can result in substantial financial cost to healthcare facilities due to wasted resources, reduced internal efficiency, and underutilization of personnel. During the time between cases, physicians and other staff must take an extended break, losing valuable momentum while waiting for the next procedure. Surgeries that are rescheduled may also incur increased costs for each episode of care, often requiring repeat appointments and additional out of pocket costs [5]. In the pediatric setting, these issues are compounded since at least one parent is required to be present for the duration of procedures. This may generate stress by requiring parents to take time off from work and coordinate care for other children.

By contrast, cancellations with ample lead time allow hospital staff to reschedule cases such that there are minimal losses to operating room utilization. Hospitals are increasingly striving to reduce inefficiencies to improve patient care while minimizing the cost of each encounter. Thus, understanding the reasons for late surgical cancellations may prevent downstream untoward consequences.

Methods

The study employed a retrospective chart review of cases cancelled within 24 h of scheduled procedure time. Data were obtained from the Boston Children's Hospital Department of Plastic and Oral Surgery. Inpatient cases, late scheduled cases, and cases in which the primary surgeon was part of a different department were excluded from the analysis. In total, 444 cases met inclusion criteria and were further analyzed for time of and reason for cancellation. Patient age, gender, diagnosis, and procedure type were also tabulated and analyzed.

Cancellations were categorized based on whether they could be addressed with interventions such as new guidelines or fail-safes. Four groups of cases were generated: preventable, possibly preventable, unpreventable, and undocumented.

Preventable cancellations included those in which there was either inadequate preprocedural preparation or system inefficiency. This included cases with missing preoperative laboratory testing or clinical consultations, cases in which patients did not adhere to preoperative instructions, as well as cases that were cancelled due to scheduling errors. Possible preventable cancellations included those in which illness in either patients or hospital staff prevented surgical procedures from taking place. It was postulated that some illnesses may present with early signs or symptoms, which—if reported early enough—could signal the need to reschedule a procedure. Unpreventable cancellations included those in which there was inclement weather, death, or emergent procedures by the health care team.

Results

Table 19.1 shows the reasons for surgical procedure cancellation as well as the category of cancellation. In sum, 10,730 surgical cases were analyzed and 584 cases were cancelled, of which 444 met criteria for inclusion in the study. One hundred and forty-seven cases were cancelled after 1 PM the day before the procedure and 297 were cancelled the day of the procedure. In all, 42% of all cancellations were categorized as preventable, 45.3% as possibly preventable, and 2.5% as unpreventable. Three hundred and thirty-four (75.3%) preventable and possible preventable

Table 19.1 Reasons for cancellations [1]

Category of cancellation	Reason for cancellation	Number of cancellations	Percent of total cancellations (%)
Preventable (41.7%)	Patient not fasted	39	8.8
	Cancelled by parent	29	6.5
	Cancelled by office	27	6.1
	Operation/procedure not necessary	19	4.3
	Patient failed to attend/or late	18	4.1
	Patient needed more work up	12	2.7
	Insurance denied	12	2.7
	Other	29	6.5
Unpreventable (2.5%)	Inclement weather	8	1.8
	Emergency case	2	0.5
	Death in family	1	0.2
Possibly preventable (45.3%)	Patient illness	197	44.4
	Surgeon illness	4	0.9
Undocumented (10.6%)		47	10.6

Reprinted from Beijnen UEA, Noonan Caillouette C, Flath-Sporn SJ, Maclellan RA, Sanchez K, Labow BI, Meara JG, Taghinia AH. Factors Associated With Late Surgical Cancellations in Pediatric Plastic and Oral Surgery, Annals of Plastic Surgery, https://journals.lww.com/annalsplasticsurgery/Abstract/2018/04000/Factors_Associated_With_Late_Surgical.21.aspx, 2018 Apr;80(4):412–415, with permission from Wolters Kluwer Health, Inc.

cancellations could be attributed to the patient and 52 (11.7%) cancellations could be attributed to the surgical team. Patient illness accounted for 44.4% of all cancelled cases and was the most commonly cited reason for cancellation.

Table 19.2 shows the prevalence of cancellation by case type. The highest percentages of cancellations were skin surgeries (36%), dentoalveolar procedures (14%), and palatoplasties (12%).

Figure 19.1 shows the frequency of cancellation by month, with the highest cancellation rates occurring during cold and flu season in the months of December and January. Figure 19.2 shows the frequency of cancellation by day of the week normalized for case volume and shows the highest of rates occurring on Mondays.

Table 19.2 Prevalence of cancellation by case type [1]

Case type	OR cases per year (%)	OR cancellations (%)
Skin	21	36
Cleft	17	12
Dentoalveolar	9	14
Maxillofacial	7	5
Breast	5	2
Hand	5	10
Vascular Anomalies	5	5
Ear	4	6
Craniofacial	3	1
Other	24	9

Reprinted from Beijnen UEA, Noonan Caillouette C, Flath-Sporn SJ, Maclellan RA, Sanchez K, Labow BI, Meara JG, Taghinia AH. Factors Associated With Late Surgical Cancellations in Pediatric Plastic and Oral Surgery, Annals of Plastic Surgery, https://journals.lww.com/annalsplasticsurgery/Abstract/2018/04000/Factors_Associated_With_Late_Surgical.21.aspx, 2018 Apr;80(4):412–415, with permission from Wolters Kluwer Health, Inc.

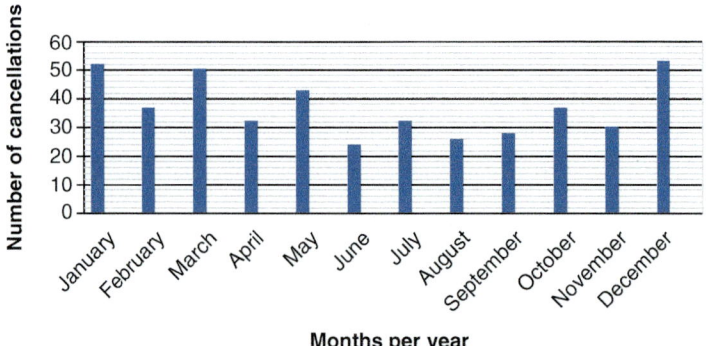

Fig. 19.1 Frequency of cancellations by month [1]. Reprinted from Beijnen UEA, Noonan Caillouette C, Flath-Sporn SJ, Maclellan RA, Sanchez K, Labow BI, Meara JG, Taghinia AH. Factors Associated With Late Surgical Cancellations in Pediatric Plastic and Oral Surgery, Annals of Plastic Surgery, https://journals.lww.com/annalsplasticsurgery/Abstract/2018/04000/Factors_Associated_With_Late_Surgical.21.aspx, 2018 Apr;80(4):412–415, with permission from Wolters Kluwer Health, Inc.

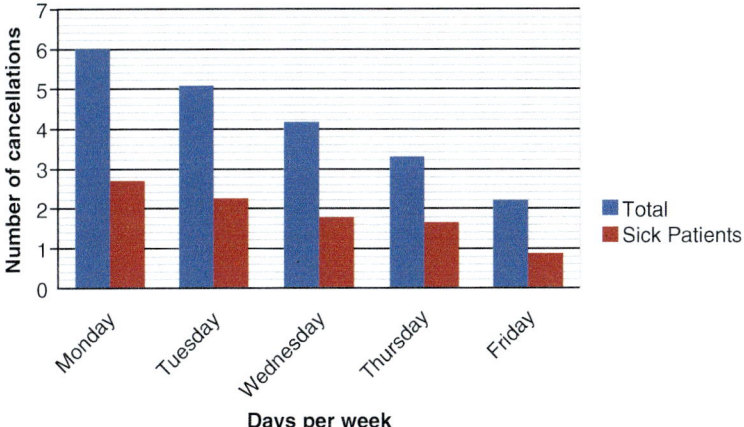

Fig. 19.2 Cancellation numbers normalized for case volume by weekday [1]. Reprinted from Beijnen UEA, Noonan Caillouette C, Flath-Sporn SJ, Maclellan RA, Sanchez K, Labow BI, Meara JG, Taghinia AH. Factors Associated With Late Surgical Cancellations in Pediatric Plastic and Oral Surgery, Annals of Plastic Surgery, https://journals.lww.com/annalsplasticsurgery/Abstract/2018/04000/Factors_Associated_With_Late_Surgical.21.aspx, 2018 Apr;80(4):412–415, with permission from Wolters Kluwer Health, Inc.

Discussion

Results of the study showed that rates of preventable and possibly preventable cancellations were high, which suggests a potential area of improvement. Though the Plastic and Oral Surgery Department at Boston Children's Hospital has a below-average rate of surgical visit cancellation compared with literature values, interventions informed by the results of this study could aid in lowering these rates further [6]. From 2010 to 2015, 444 cases (4.1%) were cancelled, with notable increases in cancellation rate occurring in the months of January and December. The most common reason for cancellation was patient illness, which may have increased the cancellation rate in the winter months when upper respiratory infections are more common [7]. Cancellation was most common on Mondays. Since offices are generally closed on the weekends, communication between patients and administrators can be challenging, which may lead to increases in cancellation at the start of each week.

These results demonstrate the importance of communicating patient illness status to reduce late cancellations. Implementing a 48-h fever free rule could achieve this by allowing patients and their families to reach hospital administrators ahead of the scheduled procedure day and time. Likewise, establishing a dedicated call center accessible during the weekends could allow patients to readily communicate on non-business days and reduce cancellation rates earlier in the week. During preoperative counseling, families should be informed to contact the surgical scheduling team if their child develops a fever or cold symptoms. Families should also be advised on how to avoid or prevent illness, especially during the winter months. Because bouts of illness vary in severity, it may be possible to reschedule a case of non-severe or questionable illness to the end of the daily surgical schedule to allow time for preoperative evaluation. If the case gets cancelled, resources could be diverted to another more urgent or add-on case rather than waiting for the case to follow.

Interestingly, there was a significant number of cancellations coded 'operation/procedure not necessary.' These cancellations were all cyst excision cases where the cyst had self-resolved between the time of scheduling and time of surgery. In these instances, families could be informed about the growth and potential involution of these lesions during the initial consult and during preoperative scheduling. Since it would be unlikely for cysts to resolve the day before surgery, families may report self-resolution of cysts early enough for the scheduling team to reschedule cases for that day.

It is also important to note that most late OR cancellations were for skin excisions. Since these procedures are small and non-urgent, parents may be under the impression that last-minute cancellations are not problematic for the hospital. Patient counseling is critical for patients to understand that late cancellations have much broader effects on the system than the last-minute cancellation of a simple clinic visit. Another category of late cancellations was patient nonadherence to nil per os (NPO) guidelines ($n = 39$). In these cases, compliance could be improved by better communicating guidelines and simplifying information presented on handouts. Cancellations due to issues with insurance were also identified ($n = 12$). This possibility should be communicated to patient families by the surgeon's administrative office pre-procedurally so these cases may be rescheduled in the event of insurance denial.

Another possible target for improving cancellation rates was phone communication with patients during the pre-operative period. Though messages may appear to be delivered to patients and their families via voicemail or the like, it is not certain these communications are actually received. Likewise, during attempts to contact patients, administrative offices may discover that patient phone numbers are inaccurate, voicemail inboxes are full, or patients or their families are not inclined to return calls. It is imperative that offices ensure a perioperative line of communication. Patient phone numbers should be verified at each visit and at the last visit prior to procedure date. They must also be informed that they will be called by the hospital and that they must return calls in a timely manner (Fig. 19.3).

Previous studies have shown how addressing the common causes of cancellations through organizational change can improve OR efficiency, cut costs, and enhance patient access to surgical care [8]. Potential strategies have included protocols for preoperative phone calls as well as new-employee orientations of OR guidelines. Overall, these changes resulted in the cancellation rate reducing from 15.0 to 5.9% in 2014. It should be mentioned that while organizational changes to surgical

> - Dedicated phone line for issues over the weekend
> - 48-hour fever free rule
> - Possible sick patient moved to the end of the day
> - Simplifying handouts for NPO guidelines
> - Verifying contact information of patients/guardians

Fig. 19.3 Recommendations to prevent late surgical cancellations [1]. Reprinted from Beijnen UEA, Noonan Caillouette C, Flath-Sporn SJ, Maclellan RA, Sanchez K, Labow BI, Meara JG, Taghinia AH. Factors Associated With Late Surgical Cancellations in Pediatric Plastic and Oral Surgery, Annals of Plastic Surgery, https://journals.lww.com/annalsplasticsurgery/Abstract/2018/04000/Factors_Associated_With_Late_Surgical.21.aspx, 2018 Apr;80(4):412–415, with permission from Wolters Kluwer Health, Inc.

schedules, provider-patient administrative communication, and preoperative compliance could be difficult to implement in an existing medical facility, the expected returns in efficiency would be substantial. This efficiency could, in turn, translate to improved patient care and provider morale.

Conclusion

Late surgical cancellations are a barrier to maximizing hospital resource use in the pediatric care setting. By better utilizing personnel and operating room space, more procedures can be performed. Thus, more patients can access surgical care. Our findings show that although patient illness was the most frequently reported cause of late cancellation, a large portion of cancellations were preventable or possible preventable. If these illness cases were reported earlier, it may be possible to redistribute the hospital resources that would have been wasted in the event of late cancellation. Likewise, interventions such as improved evaluation of patient illness, education of patient families, and adherence to preoperative requirements may reduce the rates of late cancellation.

It may be argued that the interventions proposed here are cost-ineffective and that the relatively low cancellation rate at the study center could not be reduced further without incurring diminishing returns. While this concern is legitimate, the potential benefits of small, incremental changes to hospital procedure could dramatically reduce inefficiency in the long term. If best-practice guidelines were implemented and sequentially studied, costs could be controlled, and interventions could be tested without significant burden of cost. The implementation of these changes could thus provide a low-cost, low-risk approach to maximizing operating room utilization. Nevertheless, additional prospective studies are needed to further interrogate the aforementioned interventions and assess their efficacy and cost-savings.

References

1. Beijnen UEA, Noonan Caillouette C, Flath-Sporn SJ, Maclellan RA, Sanchez K, Labow BI, Meara JG, Taghinia AH. Factors associated with late surgical cancellations in pediatric plastic and oral surgery. Ann Plast Surg. 2018;80(4):412–5.
2. Macario A, Vitez T, Dunn B, McDonald T. Where are the costs in perioperative care? Analysis of hospital costs and charges for inpatient surgical care. Anesthesiology. 1995;83(6):1138–44.
3. Stoutzenberger TL. Using lean strategies to improve operating room efficiency. OR Manager. 2014;30(1):18–20.
4. Cima RR, Brown MJ, Hebl JR, Moore R, Rogers JC, Kollengode A, et al. Use of lean and six sigma methodology to improve operating room efficiency in a high-volume tertiary-care academic medical center. J Am Coll Surg. 2011;213(1):83–92.
5. Tait AR, Voepel-Lewis T, Munro HM, Gutstein HB, Reynolds PI. Cancellation of pediatric outpatient surgery: economic and emotional implications for patients and their families. J Clin Anesth. 1997;9(3):213–9.
6. Boudreau SA, Gibson MJ. Surgical cancellations: a review of elective surgery cancellations in a tertiary care pediatric institution. J Perianesth Nurs. 2011;26(5):315–22.
7. Eccles R. An explanation for the seasonality of acute upper respiratory tract viral infections. Acta Otolaryngol. 2002;122(2):183–91.
8. Kaye AD, McDowell JL, Diaz JH, Buras JA, Young AE, Urman RD. Effective strategies in improving operating room case delays and cancellations at an academic medical center. J Med Pract Manag. 2015;30(6 Spec No):24–9.

Routine Post-reduction Radiographs After Closed Reduction of Pediatric Wrist and Forearm Fractures Is Unnecessary: Effecting Process Change and Eliminating Waste in the Pediatric Emergency Department

Aristides I. Cruz Jr

Key Learning Points
- Pediatric forearm and wrist fractures are one of the most common pediatric fractures evaluated in Emergency Departments.
- Formal post-reduction plain radiographs used in pediatric wrist and forearm fractures increases radiation exposure, cost, and time spent in the ED.
- The use of digital fluoroscopy provides real-time, point of care images that can be used instead of post-reduction plain radiographs.
- Fluoroscopy is reliable in assessing fracture reduction, eliminating the use of routine post-reduction radiographs following treatment of pediatric upper extremity fractures.
- The time spent during each encounter between the end of the fracture reduction procedure and postreduction radiographs that could potentially be eliminated from a process change represents an annual opportunity cost that institutions can use to meet additional ED patients.

Executive Summary

Initiating process change in healthcare is an important aspect of streamlining the delivery of care. Safely increasing operational efficiency can benefit multiple stakeholders including healthcare systems, providers of care, and patients. When

A. I. Cruz Jr (✉)
Department of Orthopaedic Surgery, Hasbro Children's Hospital, Warren Alpert Medical School, Brown University, Providence, RI, USA
e-mail: aristides_cruz@brown.edu

considering a change, no process is too small or modest to be deemed worthwhile and in fact, small, incremental change is often preferred. Small changes in processes can be rapidly deployed, studied, and altered as needed with the goal of cementing process change for the benefit of all involved. The Plan-Do-Study-Act (PDSA) paradigm is a useful tool for evaluating and testing a proposed change in process.

Introduction

Pediatric forearm and wrist fractures account for approximately 25–50% of pediatric fractures and are one of the most common causes of acute Emergency Department evaluation [1–4] (Fig. 20.1). The rate of distal radius and forearm fractures among children and adolescents has increased over time [5] and it is estimated that the cost of treatment for these injuries is upwards of $2 billion annually [6]. Without proper treatment of these injuries, permanent loss of forearm or wrist motion and limitation in arm movement can result.

With the changing landscape of healthcare costs and the drive towards value-based decisions, certain aspects of care must be reexamined for methods to improve efficiency of care (decreased patient and provider time spent, increased patient throughput), quality of care (increased safety, decreased radiation exposure), and decreased cost [both direct costs (e.g. costs of radiographs) and indirect costs (e.g. opportunity costs of unnecessary care)]. The evaluation and treatment of pediatric wrist and forearm fractures in the Emergency Department (ED) commonly involves closed reduction [wherein the fractured extremity is manually manipulated to realign the bone(s)] and cast application. This procedure is frequently performed under sedation and with fluoroscopy (i.e., live, real-time, point-of-care X-ray), which is followed by formal post-reduction plain radiographs to confirm adequate fracture reduction (i.e. realignment) (Fig. 20.1).

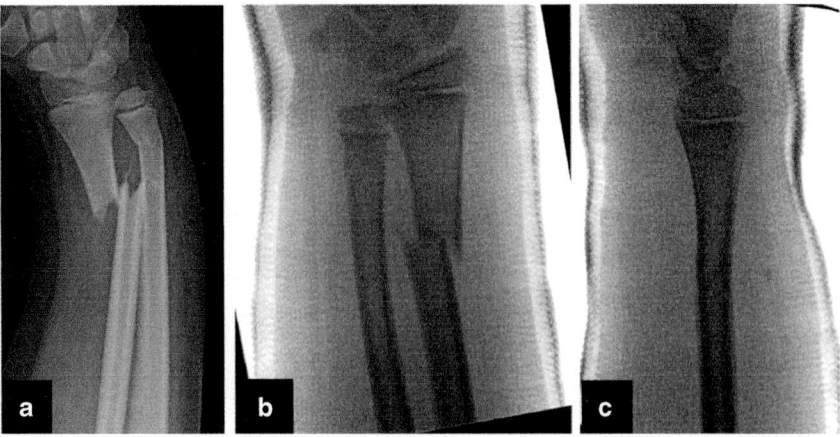

Fig. 20.1 Injury (Panel **a**) and post-reduction (Panels **b** and **c**) radiographs of a pediatric patient with a wrist (distal radius and distal ulna) fracture

Obtaining these additional radiographs after closed reduction is not without their drawbacks, however. This additional step increases radiation exposure, cost, and time spent in the ED [7]. As patient safety, satisfaction, and organizational efficiency become progressively more important in the current healthcare environment, it is critical to evaluate each aspect of patient care.

Ostensibly, the benefit of the post-reduction radiograph is to more carefully evaluate post-manipulation fracture reduction and may potentially demonstrate a need for a repeat intervention. However, given the proliferation of digital fluoroscopy, with high-quality, real-time, point of care images that can be saved to the medical record, this final step may be unnecessary. Past literature has shown that the use of fluoroscopy has been shown to improve quality of reduction, decrease the need for operative treatment, decrease radiation exposure, and allow for a shorter consultation time [1, 8–10]. In this chapter, I describe two separate but related projects regarding the elimination of the routine use of post-reduction radiographs in the pediatric emergency department at our institution. I first discuss and present the results of the initial project where my team initiated process change in the ED in order to streamline patient care, decrease cost and radiation exposure, and improve operational efficiency. I then discuss the second project which involved the follow-up study examining the process change we had initiated and the results from the follow-up study.

Methodology

Initial Study

My team and I first collected baseline data evaluating the current state of operations within a large, urban, tertiary care pediatric emergency department. We sought to quantify the time and costs associated with performing closed reduction in pediatric patients with wrist and forearm fractures as well as the rate of repeat closed reduction following primary, fluoroscopy-guided closed reduction. Our hypothesis during the first project was that obtaining routine post-reduction radiographs for isolated pediatric wrist and forearm fractures does not change management. By implication, patients who receive routine post-reduction radiographs are faced with unnecessarily increased time in the ED, radiation exposure, and cost, without commensurate benefit. We postulated that eliminating the routine use of post-reduction radiographs would benefit patients, providers, and the institution by making care delivery more efficient without affecting quality.

Following Institutional Review Board approval, a retrospective chart review was performed for all patients with fractures of the wrist [distal radius and/or distal ulna (DR/DU) and forearm (FA)] presenting to the Emergency Department at an urban Level I pediatric trauma center over a 6-month period (April 1, 2015—September 20, 2015). Patients were excluded if the fracture was open, not isolated, did not require sedated reduction, or if the information contained within the electronic medical record was incomplete.

All patients were treated with the same standard protocol, which included pre-reduction radiographs, evaluation by the on-call orthopaedic resident, and discussion with family (and patient, as appropriate). If reduction was deemed necessary (i.e., angulation or rotation that was beyond acceptable radiographic parameters [11]), the ED provider provided procedural sedation to the patient to allow for reduction and casting/splinting with mini C-arm fluoroscopy guidance. Per our department's policy, post-reduction radiographs were routinely obtained after all fracture reductions to evaluate adequacy of reduction. Medical record time stamp data was recorded and different time intervals were calculated, including ED length of stay, total sedation time, and time between end of sedation and end of post-reduction radiographs (Fig. 20.2).

Each record was reviewed to determine if the patient required re-reduction in the ED, or if subsequent surgery was performed at our institution. These variables served as our primary outcomes when determining the utility of obtaining routine post-reduction radiographs.

Direct and variable indirect cost and charge data was obtained for each patient's encounter from the corporate financial database at our institution. Costs for the post-reduction time period was calculated by multiplying the entire encounter cost by the fraction of encounter time between the end of sedation and post-reduction radiographs. Cost-to-charge ratio was calculated for all patients available in total, and the direct cost of the post-reduction radiograph itself was calculated by multiplying the X-ray charge by this cost-to-charge ratio.

We expressed the opportunity cost of routine post-reduction radiographs in terms of potential extra ED patient throughput. The average number of ED patients seen over the previous 9-year period was used as an estimate of annual patient volume. This was translated to minutes spent per patient by dividing the average patient volume by minutes in a year. Because the patients in our sample only represented a portion of the year, we prorated this number to estimate the annual number of patients who required a post-reduction radiograph after a DR/DU or FA fracture. This number was then used to estimate annual time savings which was subsequently translated to potential extra ED patient throughout per year.

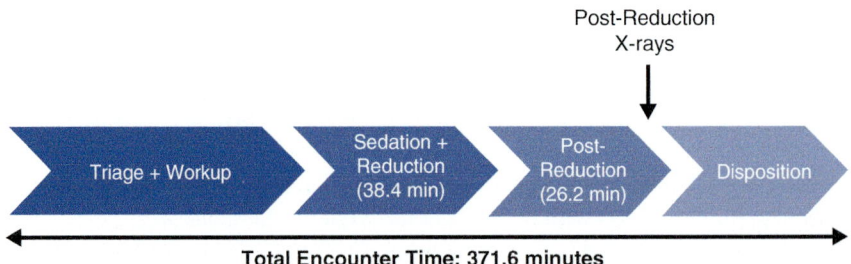

Fig. 20.2 Patient flow through the Emergency Department. Time data shown are part of baseline data collection project. Reprinted from Goodman AD, Zonfrillo MR, Chiou D, Eberson CP, Cruz AI; The cost and utility of postreduction radiographs after closed reduction of pediatric wrist and forearm fractures; Journal of Pediatric Orthopaedics; 2019 Jan;39(1):e8–e11; https://journals.lww.com/pedorthopaedics/Citation/2019/01000/The_Cost_and_Utility_of_Postreduction_Radiographs.4.aspx; with permission from Wolters Kluwer Health, Inc. [7]

Standard descriptive statistics were used. Chi-squared tests were used to evaluate categorical variables, and paired Student's t-tests were used to analyze for statistical significance of time differences. Significance was set to $p < 0.05$ *a priori*.

Results

Initial Study

The initial search included 210 patients, of whom 91 were excluded. Of the 119 patients included, 80 (67.2%) had DR/DU fractures, while 39 (32.8%) had FA fractures. Among the 119 patients, zero patients required fracture re-reduction. Three patients (3.8%) in the DR/DU group and eight patients (20.5%) in the FA group went on to surgery at our institution ($p = 0.012$). Post-reduction radiographs were completed after a mean of 26.2 min after sedation end (SD 19.2 min, range 0–99 min, 7.3% of ED time), which was similar between the two groups ($p = 0.740$, Table 20.1).

The marginal time cost of the post-reduction radiographs was a mean of 7.3% of the total encounter cost (median: 5.6%, standard deviation: 5.3%); these were similar between both the DR/DU and FA groups ($p = 0.400$). For all included patients, the direct X-ray cost was a mean of 2.6% of the total encounter cost.

Opportunity Costs

With a mean of 26 min for each encounter between the end of sedation and post-reduction radiographs that could potentially be eliminated from an estimated 255 similar encounters per year, the estimated annual opportunity cost was 111.5 h. Over the past 9 years, our institution had an average of 51,500 annual ED visits, or 10.2 min per patient. Our annual opportunity cost was therefore calculated to be 656 emergency department patients seen (Table 20.2).

Table 20.1 Interventions and time course through the Emergency Department [7]

Intervention	DR/DU	FA	Overall	Significance
# Re-reductions	0	0	0	$p = 1$
# Surgery	3 (3.8%)	8 (20.5%)	11 (9.2%)	[a]($p = 0.012$)
Timing				
Total ER time (min)	379 ± 64	357 ± 67	372 ± 98	$p = 0.006$
Sedation time (min)	38 ± 3	39 ± 4	38 ± 15	$p = 0.627$
Sedation-XR time (min)	26 ± 27	27 ± 14	26 ± 19	$p = 0.099$
Sedation as % of total	*5.5%*	*7.0%*	*5.9%*	$p = 0.003$

[a] Fisher exact test

Reprinted from Goodman AD, Zonfrillo MR, Chiou D, Eberson CP, Cruz AI; The cost and utility of postreduction radiographs after closed reduction of pediatric wrist and forearm fractures; Journal of Pediatric Orthopaedics; 2019 Jan;39(1):e8–e11; https://journals.lww.com/pedorthopaedics/Citation/2019/01000/The_Cost_and_Utility_of_Postreduction_Radiographs.4.aspx; with permission from Wolters Kluwer Health, Inc. [7]

Table 20.2 Opportunity cost calculations [7]

Row	Variable	Quantity	Notes
1	Mean annual patient volume	51,532	(Range 49,233–53,060; SD 1259)
2	Minutes per year	525,600	
3	Avg. patients seen per minute	0.098	Row 1 ÷ Row 2
4	Patients in sample	119	
5	Days in sample	170	
6	% year in sample	46.6%	Row 5 ÷ 365 days
7	Prorated patients seen per year	255	Row 4 ÷ Row 6
8	Potential times savings (min) per patient	26.2	
9	Potential time savings (min) per year	6691	Row 7 × Row 8
10	Potential extra patients seen per year	656	Row 3 × Row 9

Reprinted from Goodman AD, Zonfrillo MR, Chiou D, Eberson CP, Cruz AI; The cost and utility of postreduction radiographs after closed reduction of pediatric wrist and forearm fractures; Journal of Pediatric Orthopaedics; 2019 Jan;39(1):e8–e11; https://journals.lww.com/pedorthopaedics/Citation/2019/01000/The_Cost_and_Utility_of_Postreduction_Radiographs.4.aspx; with permission from Wolters Kluwer Health, Inc. [7]

Methods

Follow-Up Study

The follow-up study was an important part of the "Plan, Do, Study, Act" cycle of process change and continuous improvement [12]. Our institution changed the ED pediatric forearm and wrist fracture management protocol in 2017 to reflect the findings above. We no longer mandated formal radiographs after fluoroscopy-assisted reductions, leaving the choice of obtaining post-reduction imaging up to the responsible orthopedic provider on a case-by-case basis. If the provider felt that the mini C-arm fluoroscopy was sufficient, then that became the definitive imaging; otherwise, a formal radiograph was obtained. In this follow-up study we sought to evaluate this change in protocol—specifically, its safety, efficacy, and effect on ED visit time and cost. We hypothesized that the new protocol of fluoroscopy as definitive post-reduction imaging would not change total encounter time and cost, or incidence of re-reduction or surgery, compared with obtaining formal radiographs.

Change in Protocol

A retrospective chart review was performed for all patients with isolated, closed wrist or forearm fractures that required sedation and reduction (under mini C-arm fluoroscopy) presenting to our institution both before and after this policy change was instituted in June 2017. The "before" period was from April 1, 2015—September 20, 2015, while the "after" period was from July 31, 2017—November 30, 2017.

All patients were managed with a standardized protocol as described above. If the fracture had angulation or rotation that was unacceptable, the fracture was reduced using mini C-arm fluoroscopy under procedural sedation given by emergency medicine providers. After reduction, a cast or splint was applied, and alignment assessed again with anteroposterior (AP), lateral, and oblique views on the mini C-arm fluoroscopy unit to ensure adequacy of reduction. These final images were saved in electronic format to the patient's health record [Picture Archiving and Communication System (PACS), made available through collaboration with the Information Technology department] and reviewed at the daily orthopedic departmental fracture conference.

Prior to this change in departmental policy, all patients had formal post-reduction radiographs in the Radiology Department after the patient recovered from sedation, or nearly so (as they remained under close observation). After the change, the decision to obtain these was left to the provider (most often the on-call resident, although this was discussed with the attending surgeon if any questions remained). If they deemed the mini C-arm fluoroscopy to be insufficient to gauge length, rotation, or alignment of the fracture reduction, a formal radiograph was ordered and was performed once the patient had recovered from sedation. If re-reduction was deemed necessary based on the post-reduction fracture alignment, a second sedation (and reduction) would be performed. Patients were followed for up to 6 months from the index injury.

Data Collection

After Institutional Review Board approval, codes from the International Classification of Diseases, Ninth/Tenth edition (ICD-9/10) were chosen to capture all patients with closed forearm and wrist injuries. Demographic information was collected, and fractures were classified as distal radius and/or distal ulna (DR/DU), or forearm (FA). Timestamp data was collected from the Epic electronic health record (Epic Systems Corporation, Madison, WI) and different intervals were determined, including total sedation time, total ED length of stay, and time between sedation end and discharge.

Each chart was further reviewed to determine subsequent re-reduction or surgery (safety outcomes). The need for surgery was a joint decision based on reduction quality, deformity, stability, or patient/parent preference, and was made with the patient, family, and pediatric orthopedic surgeon. Charge data in United States dollars were collected from the corporate financial database at our institution.

Analysis

Our primary endpoint was the total ED encounter time, while our secondary endpoints were the rate of re-reduction and surgery, as well as total encounter charge. In addition to standard descriptive statistics, between-group differences were analyzed with Student's t-test and Chi-square test. Multivariable linear and logistic regression was used to determine risk factors (including fluoroscopy-as-definitive-imaging) for additional time spent in the ED, as well as need for surgery, and cost. Statistical significance was set at $p < 0.05$ *a priori*; analysis was performed with Microsoft Excel 2016 (Redmond, WA).

Results

Follow-Up Study

Two hundred and forty-three patients were included (119 before the protocol change, and 124 after). Of these, 165 patients sustained DR/DU fractures, and 78 sustained FA fractures (Table 20.3). Demographic data were broadly similar between the before and after groups. After the protocol change, 80/85 (94.1%) of the DR/DU fractures had fluoroscopy as definitive imaging, compared with 7/78 FA fractures (9.0%).

Post protocol implementation, sedation times were longer by 17 min and 13 min for DR/DU and FA fractures, respectively, while the total ED time and the time from sedation beginning to discharge were similar (Table 20.4).

Table 20.3 Demographic data for patients undergoing sedation and reduction of a closed, isolated wrist or forearm fracture [13]

	DR/DU only			BBFA only		
	Before	After	p-value[a]	Before	After	p-value[a]
# Patients	80	85		39	39	
Mean age (years)	8.6	9.3	0.186	7.5	8.8	0.127
# Male (%)	63 (78.8%)	59 (69.4%)	0.214	17 (43.6%)	22 (56.4%)	0.365
Mean weight (kg)	35.4	43.7	0.012	31.3	36.6	0.177
Mean weight percentile for age	62.7%	69.1%	0.279	60.9%	58.2%	0.400

DR/DU distal radius/distal ulna fracture, *BBFA* both bone forearm fracture
[a]Student's t-test for continues data; Chi-square test for categorical data
Reprinted from Goodman AD, Walsh DF, Zonfrillo MR, Eberson CP, Cruz AI Jr.; Fluoroscopy as Definitive Postreduction Imaging of Pediatric Wrist and Forearm Fractures is Safe and Saves Time; Journal of Pediatric Orthopedics; 2020 Jan;40(1):e14–e18; https://journals.lww.com/pedorthopaedics/Abstract/2020/01000/Fluoroscopy_as_Definitive_Postreduction_Imaging_of.4.aspx; with permission from Wolters Kluwer Health, Inc. [13]

Table 20.4 Time outcomes before and after protocol change [13]

	DR/DU only			BBFA only		
	Before	After	p value[a]	Before	After	p value[a]
Sedation (min)[b]	**39**	**56**	**<0.001**	**38**	**51**	**0.003**
Sedation begin → Discharge (min)[b]	128	125	0.599	**130**	**149**	**0.043**
Total ED time (min)[b]	379	353	0.098	357	351	0.787
Surgery	3 (3.8%)	6 (7.1%)	0.497	7 (17.9%)	10 (25.6%)	0.410

[a]Student's t-test for continuous data; Chi-square test for categorical data. Values in bold denote statistical significance
[b]Values expressed as means
Reprinted from Goodman AD, Walsh DF, Zonfrillo MR, Eberson CP, Cruz AI Jr.; Fluoroscopy as Definitive Postreduction Imaging of Pediatric Wrist and Forearm Fractures is Safe and Saves Time; Journal of Pediatric Orthopedics; 2020 Jan;40(1):e14–e18; https://journals.lww.com/pedorthopaedics/Abstract/2020/01000/Fluoroscopy_as_Definitive_Postreduction_Imaging_of.4.aspx; with permission from Wolters Kluwer Health, Inc. [13]

After multivariable regression analysis for all patients combined, "fluoroscopy-as-definitive-imaging" was the main variable that was an independent determinant of the various time intervals, compared to using post-reduction formal radiography. Using fluoroscopy as the final imaging modality was associated with a length of sedation that was 13.8 min longer (95% CI 7.9–19.7, p < 0.001), while the interval from sedation beginning to discharge was 15.8 min shorter (95% CI −27.4 to −4.3, p = 0.007), and total ED time was 33.0 min shorter (95% CI −60.2 to −5.8, p = 0.018).

Charges increased significantly between the before and after groups; for the total encounter for DR/DU fractures, the charge increased from $5127 to $5523 (7.7% increase, p < 0.0001), while charges for FA fractures increased from $5069 to $5787 (14.2% increase, p = 0.011). The charges for most individual items (for medications, staff time, and other resources) increased between 2 and 15% over the same timeframe. The charges for formal radiographs ($141 per series, stable between groups) were not applied to those patients who had fluoroscopy as definitive imaging. On multivariable regression, being in the after group did increase charges by $533 (p = 0.004). However, using fluoroscopy as definitive imaging did not increase charges (p = 0.657). These increased charges may be due to annual medical inflation [14].

Discussion

Pediatric wrist and forearm fractures are among the most common injuries evaluated in the ED. Many of these injuries can be successfully treated with closed reduction and casting. Radiographs are needed to assess the adequacy of reduction, however, with the advent of "point-of-care" radiography in the form of mini C-arm fluoroscopy, the routine use of post-reduction radiographs may be unnecessary. While the literature is mixed on whether radiation exposure to the patient is decreased with the use of mini C-arm fluoroscopy [8, 9, 15–17], this method of fracture assessment after closed reduction has been found to be reliable. Our findings corroborate this, with no patients needing a re-reduction after using this method of radiographic evaluation.

In addition to the potential for time savings in the ED, the use of mini C-arm fluoroscopy has also been shown in the literature to increase efficiency and throughput in the outpatient setting [10]. In line with this finding, we demonstrated that the time between end of sedation and completion of x-rays comprised 7.3% of the total encounter time. Because mini C-arm fluoroscopy is reliable in assessing fracture reduction, eliminating the use of routine post-reduction radiographs following treatment of pediatric upper extremity fractures has the potential to result in significant time and cost savings, increased practice efficiency and throughput, and possibly improved patient experience. We calculated the opportunity cost of post-reduction radiographs in terms of additional patient throughput in the ED. Although the cost of extra imaging is relatively modest, the additional time (and cost thereof) spent to obtain them is significant. Because of this, the opportunity cost is also quite large, amounting to more than 110 h of clinical time each year at our institution. This time could either be used to increase patient throughput or potentially decrease staffing costs. This improved efficiency not only improves institutional metrics but can also improve patients' and families experience during these emergency department visits. In addition to decreasing time spent in the emergency department, mini C-arm fluoroscopy use has the potential to decrease radiation exposure, which may be a valued safety measure for families.

Lessons Learned/Principles

The most important lesson learned from implementing these two projects is that process change is difficult, even for a modest and focused change such as eliminating routine use of X-rays for a specific set of injuries seen in a pediatric emergency department. However, just because a project is small or modest, does not mean that it is unimportant. This is an important lesson for those looking to implement change in their organization. Lean management principles emphasize small, rapid-fire projects in order to garner small, tangible wins. The first project described above was relatively small in scope but provided actionable data that was used to implement change (i.e. no patient required re-reduction and therefore this step can be eliminated). Lean principles also emphasize streamlining processes which was accomplished as a result of the first project. Utilizing "Plan, Do, Study, Act" (PDSA) principles (Fig. 20.3), the knowledge gained from the initial project was used to implement process change in the emergency department. This change was also

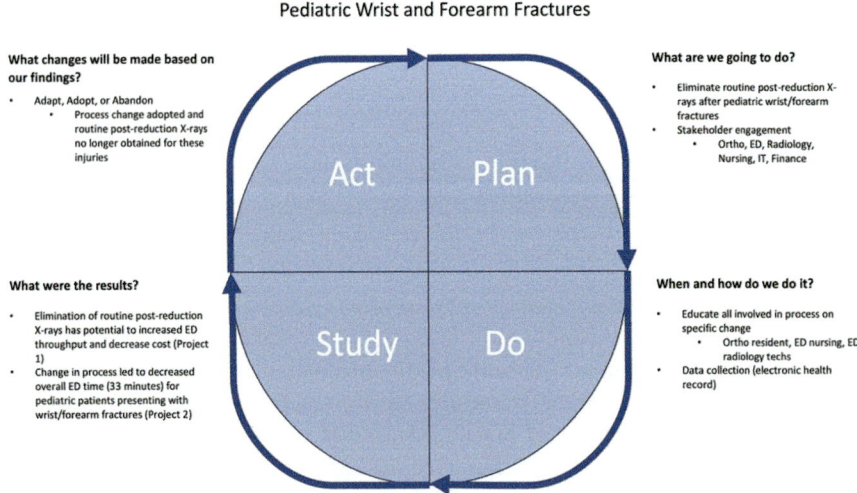

Fig. 20.3 Example schematic of PDSA principles utilized in described projects

studied and confirmed that it was not detrimental to care and was beneficial for reducing time spent in the emergency department after these injuries. This process change resulted in benefits for multiple stakeholders including the emergency department, radiology department, orthopedic department, nursing, and most importantly, patients and families [14].

Another important lesson is to engage more parties earlier in the process [18]. A major delay in the initial project was obtaining financial data from hospital administration. Part of the initial strategy was to first collect the pertinent clinical data to present to the hospital administration in order to justify obtaining the financial data. In retrospect, it would have been beneficial to have engaged the hospital administration sooner and made them a part of the initial planning of the project. This would have saved time and may have possibly added another dimension to our data collection methods. Another party to engage earlier in the process was the hospital's IT department. While it may be dependent on one's specific institution, implementing a change into our institution's electronic health record (specifically, the ability to electronically upload mini C-arm fluoroscopy unit images directly into the electronic health record) was a time-consuming and often frustrating task. Something as simple as generating a new order in the electronic health records system took more than 6 weeks. We then had to spend a significant amount of time troubleshooting the electronic workflow of changing this process. IT experts should have been involved sooner in the planning of the initial project in anticipation of this obstacle.

Conclusions

With increased pressure to demonstrate value in healthcare delivery, minimizing unnecessary services is important. The projects described above support others in the literature that showed value in the use of mini C-arm imaging in the emergency department for assessment of pediatric wrist and forearm fractures. With the addition of small changes (such as the ability to electronically upload images from the mini C-arm into the electronic health record) and empowering providers to determine the necessity of formal imaging, the process change described is a widely generalizable method for helping to control costs while maintaining quality of care of pediatric upper extremity fractures. These projects can serve as examples on how to effect process change within healthcare organizations particularly within the context of the Plan-Do-Study-Act paradigm.

References

1. Lee MC, Stone NE, Ritting AW, Silverstein EA, Pierz KA, Johnson DA, et al. Mini-C-arm fluoroscopy for emergency-department reduction of pediatric forearm fractures. J Bone Joint Surg Am. 2011;93(15):1442–7. Available from: https://journals.lww.com/jbjsjournal/Abstract/2011/08030/Mini_C_Arm_Fluoroscopy_for_Emergency_Department.9.aspx. https://doi.org/10.2106/JBJS.J.01052.

2. De Putter CE, Van Beeck EF, Looman CWN, Toet H, Hovius SER, Selles RW. Trends in wrist fractures in children and adolescents, 1997–2009. J Hand Surg Am. 2011;36(11):1810–1815. e2. https://doi.org/10.1016/j.jhsa.2011.08.006.
3. Khosla S, Melton LJ III, Dekutoski MB, Achenbach SJ, Oberg AL, Riggs BL. Incidence of childhood distal forearm fractures over 30 years. JAMA. 2003;290(11):1479. Available from: http://jama.jamanetwork.com/article.aspx? https://doi.org/10.1001/jama.290.11.1479.
4. Naranje SM, Erali RA, Warner WC, Sawyer JR, Kelly DM. Epidemiology of pediatric fractures presenting to emergency departments in the United States. J Pediatr Orthop. 2016;36(4):e45–8. https://doi.org/10.1097/BPO.0000000000000595.
5. Cruz AI, Kleiner JE, DeFroda SF, Gil JA, Daniels AH, Eberson CP. Increasing rates of surgical treatment for paediatric diaphyseal forearm fractures: a national database study from 2000 to 2012. J Child Orthop. 2017;11(3):201–9. https://doi.org/10.1302/1863-2548.11.170017.
6. Nellans KW, Kowalski E, Chung K. The epidemiology of distal radius fractures. Hand Clin. 2012;28(2):113–25. Available from: https://www.hand.theclinics.com/article/S0749-0712(12)00002-9/fulltext
7. Goodman AD, Zonfrillo MR, Chiou D, Eberson CP, Cruz AI. The cost and utility of postreduction radiographs after closed reduction of pediatric wrist and forearm fractures. J Pediatr Orthop. 2019;39(1):e8–e11. https://doi.org/10.1097/BPO.0000000000001081.
8. Gendelberg D, Hennrikus W, Slough J, Armstrong D, King S. A radiation safety training program results in reduced radiation exposure for orthopaedic residents using the mini C-arm. Clin Orthop Relat Res. 2016;474(2):580–4. https://doi.org/10.1007/s11999-015-4631-0.
9. Sharieff GQ, Kanegaye J, Wallace CD, McCaslin RI, Harley JR. Can portable bedside fluoroscopy replace standard, postreduction radiographs in the management of pediatric fractures? Pediatr Emerg Care. 1999;15(4):249–51.
10. Fanelli MG, Hennrikus WL, Slough Hill JM, Armstrong DG, King SH. The mini C-arm adds quality and efficiency to the pediatric orthopedic outpatient clinic. Orthopedics. 2016;39(6):e1097–9. https://doi.org/10.3928/01477447-20160808-01.
11. Noonan KJ, Price CT. Forearm and distal radius fractures in children. J Am Acad Orthop Surg. 1998;6(3):146–56. Available from: https://journals.lww.com/jaaos/Abstract/1998/05000/Forearm_and_Distal_Radius_Fractures_in_Children.2.aspx with authorized username and password
12. IHI Resources. Plan/Do/Study/Act (PDSA) Worksheet. Institute for Healthcare Improvement. 2020. Available from: http://www.ihi.org/resources/Pages/Tools/PlanDoStudyActWorksheet.aspx
13. Goodman AD, Walsh DF, Zonfrillo MR, Eberson CP, Cruz AI J Jr. Fluoroscopy as definitive postreduction imaging of pediatric wrist and forearm fractures is safe and saves time. Pediatr Orthop. 2020;40(1):e14–8. https://doi.org/10.1097/BPO.0000000000001388.
14. US Bureau of Labor and Statistics. Measuring Price Change in the CPI: Medical Care. 2020 Mar 20 [cited 2019 Sep 12]. Available from: https://www.bls.gov/cpi/factsheets/medical-care.htm
15. Athwal GS, Bueno RA Jr, Wolfe SW. Radiation exposure in hand surgery: mini versus standard C-arm. J Hand Surg Am. 2005;30(6):1310–6. https://doi.org/10.1016/j.jhsa.2005.06.023.
16. Singer G, Herron B, Herron D. Exposure from the large C-arm versus the mini C-arm using hand/wrist and elbow phantoms. J Hand Surg Am. 2011;36(4):628–31. https://doi.org/10.1016/j.jhsa.2011.01.010.
17. Sumko MJ, Hennrikus W, Slough J, Jensen K, Armstrong D, King S, Urish K. Measurement of radiation exposure when using the mini C-arm to reduce pediatric upper extremity fractures. J Pediatr Orthop. 2016;36:122–5.
18. Brandeis/The Heller School for Social Policy and Management. Relational Coordination Research Collaborative. [Internet] [cited 2019 Sep 12]. Available from: https://heller.brandeis.edu/relational-coordination/

Index

A
Absorptive capacity, 15
Academic emergency department, 240
Academic excellence, 267–268
Accountability, 141
Accountable Care Organizations (ACOs), 333
Administrative protocols, 231
Affordable Care Act (ACA) 2010, 17, 333
American Society of Anesthesiologists (ASA), 320
Application programming interfaces (APIs), 231
Arteriovenous malformations (AVM), 262
Artificial urinary sphincter (AUS), 317, 320, 321, 323

B
Baseline analysis, 338–339
BlueWater Emergency Partners (BWEP), 96
  engagement, 97, 98
  internal changes, 100–102
  overview, 96, 97
Boundary spanner, 136
Buprenorphine/medication-assisted treatment (MAT) programs, 215

C
Cardiac resuscitation teams (CRTs), 6
C-arm fluoroscopy, 357, 359
Center of Excellence (COE)
  academic excellence, 267–268
  acoustic neuromas, 262
  business proposition, 268–269
  cavernous malformations, 262
  clinical interdependency, 265–267
  craniofacial neoplasms, 262
  leadership framework, 268–271
  management structure for, 263
  monetary support, 268
  neurosurgical COE, 262–263
  pituitary adenomas, 262
  referral system, 264–265
  skull base meningiomas, 262
  skull base surgery, 262
  strategic location of, 264, 265
  trigeminal neuralgias, 262
Cerebrospinal fluid (CSF) leaks, 262
Change management
  ACS Children's Verification of Surgery program, 176
  authority, 178
  Beaumont Children's Hospital (BCH), 166–168
  buy-in, 177
  cultural issues, 179
  decision-making, 177
  HPS
    analysis, 173
    goals and timing, 170, 171
    indications, 169
    nurses and surgical residents, 171
    nursing and resident education, 171, 172
    policy team, 172, 173
    pre- and post-intervention, 171
    results, 173, 174
    structured vs. ad libitum feeding, 171
  implementation, 180
  informal networks, 175, 176
  institutional history, 179
  laparoscopic pyloromyotomies, 175
  leadership, 178

Change management (*cont.*)
  LOS
    analysis, 173
    ERAS protocols, 172
    goals and timing, 170, 171
    nonprocedural care, 169
    nurses and surgical residents, 171
    nursing and resident education, 171, 172
    policy team, 172, 173
    pre- and post-intervention, 171
    results, 173, 174
    structured *vs.* ad libitum feeding, 171
  proxy wars, 178
  pyloric pager, 176
  quality improvement project, 168, 169
  relational coordination framework, 175
  service line/program, 175
  social capital, 175, 179
  stakeholder perspective, 164–166
  strategic plan, 175
Chiari malformations, 262
Chief Executive Officer (CEO), 187
Chief Medical Information Officer (CMIO), 191
Chief Medical Officer (CMO)
  academic children's hospital, 191
  challenges for, 184
  collective problem-solving, 194
  cultural and institutional changes, 193
  100-day plan, 193
  healthcare executive administration, 185
  initial visit, 189
  institutional capacity and patient flow, 193
  national rankings, 188
  operational excellence, 191
  reinforce relationships, 194
  relational barriers and distinctions, 192
  relationship and communication, 190–191
  reporting structure, 187
  robust market analyses, 193
  role of, 186
  Vizient rankings, 188
Chief Nursing Officer (CNO), 191
Chief Operating Officer (COO), 186
Chief Quality Officer (CQO), 183, 191
Chief Value Officers (CVO), 328
Cholangiography, 323
Chronic care management protocols, 217
Communication, 208
Community-based information, 231
Community-based prevention program, 214, 215
Comprehensive metabolic panel (CMP), 339
Congenital heart disease (CHD)
  additional factors, 256
  congenital heart malformations, 252
  fetal echocardiogram database, 253, 255, 257
  maternal fetal medicine, 257
  prenatal consultation, 257
  prenatal diagnosis of, 252
  survey questions, 254
Congenital heart surgery (CHS), fast track strategy
  change management, 159
  complications/survival, 151
  cost analysis, 153–155
  demographics, 151
  early versus late extubation/determinants of failure, 151–153
  limitations, 156
  organization or clinical practice, 156–158
  overview, 148
  procedural details, 151
  project's organizational format/participants, 150
  quality improvement, 146
  statistical analysis, 149, 150
  team performance and leadership, 158, 159
  variables, 148, 149
Continuous quality improvement (CQI), 335–339
Cost variation, 320
COVID-19 pandemic, 212
Critical Access Hospitals (CAH), 95
Critical CHD (CCHD), 252
Culture change, 137, 143
Current Procedural Terminology (CPT), 337

D

Decision aid (DA), 241
Delphi exercise, 241

E

Electrocardiogram (EKG), 321
Electronic health record (EHR) platforms, 334
Electronic medical record (EMR), 295, 296, 318
Emergency department (ED), 237, 352
  ED-based PS, 238
Emergency Medical Services (EMS), 212
Emergency medicine (EM), 238
Emergency physicians (EPs), 238
Enhanced Recovery After Surgery (ERAS) protocols, 131, 172, 180

Index

Epic electronic health record, 357
Etomidate, 238
Evidence-based care, 263
Evidence-based medicine, 333

F
Fixed costs, 300, 344
Fluoroscopy-as-definitive-imaging, 359

G
Glenn's school project, 258

H
Health care costs, 332
Health care delivery system, 215
Health information exchanges (HIEs), 231
Hepatitis C, 220
High-deductible health plan (HDHP), 332
High-value health care, 3–4
Hospital system, 319–320
Hypertrophic pyloric stenosis (HPS)
    analysis, 173
    goals and timing, 170, 171
    indications, 169
    nurses and surgical residents, 171
    nursing and resident education, 171, 172
    policy team, 172, 173
    pre- and post-intervention, 171
    results, 173, 174
    structured *vs.* ad libitum feeding, 171

I
Imai's Kaizen principles, 335
Inguinal hernia repair, 317
In-hospital cardiac arrest (IHCA), 14, 15
Inova Health System ("IHS"), 113, 114
Intermountain Healthcare (IHC), 16, 17

K
Ketamine, 238

L
Laparoscopic cholecystectomy, 317, 319, 321, 323
Late surgical cancellations
    frequency of cancellations, 346
    late surgical cancellations, 349
    OR cancellations, 348
    patient illness, 347
    phone communication with patients, 348
    possible preventable cancellations, 345
    pre-operative counseling, 347
    preventable cancellations, 345
    reasons for, 345
    reduced internal efficiency, 344
    surgical procedure cancellation, 345
    underutilization of personnel, 344
    unpreventable cancellations, 345
Leadership, 206–208, 269–271
Leadership alignment, 208
Lean management system, 15
    principles, 360
Length of stay (LOS)
    analysis, 173
    ERAS protocols, 172
    goals and timing, 170, 171
    nonprocedural care, 169
    nurses and surgical residents, 171
    nursing and resident education, 171, 172
    policy team, 172, 173
    pre- and post-intervention, 171
    reduction, 275
    results, 173, 174
    structured *vs.* ad libitum feeding, 171
Licensed practical nurses (LPN), 227
LSU Health Shreveport, 262

M
Medical assistants (MA), 227
Medication-assisted treatment (MAT), 215
Minimally invasive cardiac surgery (MICS), 11, 12
Minimally invasive surgery, 274
Multi-specialty health system, 232

N
Naloxone, 213, 215
National surgical quality improvement program (NSQIP)
    change management, 203–204
    data collection and assessment goals, 201
    documentation, 204
    hospital's performance, 200
    hypothesized benefits, 202
    innovation and excellence, 200
    leadership, 206–208
    outlier analysis, 202, 203
    poor patient outcomes, 202
    ratings, 204–206
    surgical quality measurement, 200

Nemours Children's Health System (NCHS), 253
Net present value (NPV), 304, 306, 308, 309
Neuro-ophthalmology, 266
Neurosurgery, 262, 264
Non-incremental cash outflows, 300

O

Open inguinal hernia, 323
Operating room cost accounting tools (ORCA)
    ambulatory clinics, 329
    ambulatory surgery procedures, 330
    artificial urinary sphincter, 317
    building buy-in, 327–329
    cost savings, 321
    duration per case, 324
    head and neck surgery, 326
    hospital system, 319–320
    influence of schedulers, 326–327
    inguinal hernia repair, 317
    laparoscopic cholecystectomy, 317, 323
    laparoscopic inguinal hernia repair, 325
    LEAN project, 322
    open inguinal hernia repair, 322
    operational differences, 320
    operative cases and hours, 328
    SJHC and FHC, 320
    supply cost per case, 324
    supply costs *vs.* OR time cost, 324–326
    varicocelectomy, 317
    VDO tools, 319
Operating room efficiency
    billing, 132
    block utilization, 326
    challenges, 131, 132
    communication and relationship patterns, 113
    data gathering
        neutral interaction, 120
        on-time surgical start time, 124, 128
        operating room nurses/leadership, 120
        participants, 120
        pre-op nurses/leadership, 120
        relational coordination, 123–127
        relational coordination domains, 120, 121
        surgical process, 122, 123
        working relationship, 120
    definition, 114
    IHS, 113, 114
    improvement opportunities, 131
    issues, 131
    preliminary hypothesis, 114
    project planning
        process improvement tools, 115–117
        project initiation, 117–120
    results, 129–131
    Six Sigma, 112, 113
Operational excellence, 191, 192, 194
Opioid abuse, 212
Opioid epidemic, 214
Opioid overdose, 212
Opioid use disorders (OUD)
    community-based prevention program, 214, 215
    community-based primary care practices, 214
    pain management model, 216–217
    reducing barriers to care, 217–219
    substance use disorder, 220
    synthetic opioids, 214
    team-based primary care, 219
    treatment of chronic pain, 219
    U.S. overdose deaths, 212
Opportunity costs, 355–356
Oral and maxillofacial surgery (OMFS), 266
Organizational alignment, 280
Organizational leadership, 215
Organizational learning, 11, 12
Organizational structure analysis, 140, 141
Outlier analysis, 202, 203

P

Patient care, 268
Patient decision aid (DA) tool, 244
Pediatric EM fellowships, 238
Pediatric wrist and forearm fractures
    change in protocol, 356–357
    data collection, 357
    follow-up study, 356, 358–359
    on-call orthopaedic resident, 353
    opportunity costs, 355–356
    post protocol implementation, 358
    post-reduction radiographs, 353, 355
    post-reduction time period, 354
    value-based decisions, 352
Physician assistant (PA), 258
Physician engagement, 333, 334
    biomedical sciences, 5–8
    leadership on performance, 9, 10

management training, 4
  in quality improvement, 2, 3
  technical organizations, 8, 9
  transitioning from clinical staff member to manager, 10, 11
  value revolution, 3, 4
Physician leadership, 337
  and engagement, 332
Physician-led team-based care, 227
Picture archiving and communication system (PACS), 357
Plan-Do-Study-Act cycle, 335
Plan-Do-Study-Act (PDSA) method, 335
  framework, 331
  principles, 360
"Point-of-care" radiography, 359
Possible preventable cancellations, 345
Post-acute care, 334
Post anesthesia care unit (PACU), 319, 321
Prenatal pediatric cardiology, 255
Prescription monitoring programs (PMPs), 217
Primary care physician (PCP), 332
Primary Cares Initiative, 227
Problem-solving, 194
Procedural sedation (PS), 237
  adverse event, 241
  decision aid, 241
  evidence-based medicine, 244
  evidence-based risks, 238
  federal reimbursement rules, 239
  graphical representations of, 242
  incidence of adverse events, 243
  informed consent process, 242
  learning and new awareness, 240
  multidisciplinary work, 244
  providers and patient feedback, 245
  relational coordination, 245
  risk communication, 244
  SAEs, 242, 244
  sedative medications, 238
  short-acting sedative agents, 238
  use of short-acting analgesics, 238
  verbal affirmation for minors, 240
Process cycle efficiency (PCE), 116
Project management, 207
Propofol, 238

Q
Quadruple performance problem, 4
Quality control, 58, 59
Quality improvement, 340

R
RedCap, 269
Registered nurses (RN), 227
Reimbursement models, 227
Relational coordination (RC) theory, 116, 136, 175, 312
Risk-standardized mortality, 13, 14
Robotic surgery (RS) program
  accreditation of, 274
  benefits of, 274
  competitive advantage, 279
  current status of, 275
  environment, 274–275
  executive change team, 277
  growth, 285
  key success factors, 279
  leadership reflections, 287–288
  metrics, 284
  operating environment, 282
  organizational alignment, 280
  outcomes, 285–287
  project deliverables, 283–284
  project plan, 278
  reason for accreditation, 276
  relational coordination, 279
  resources needed, 278
  sizing up external environment, 282
  stakeholders, 277
  unexpected obstacles, 278
Rural hospitals
  BWEP, 96–98
  CAH, 95
  challenges, 107
  emergency department (ED)
    BWEP, 100–102
    quality patient care, 98
    quality work, 99
    relational/cultural/political, 99, 100
    staffing and finance, 98, 99
  financial performance, 106
  leadership, 106
  patients arrival, 107, 108
  results, 102–106
  sign-out meeting, 107
  team members, 107

S
Same day surgery (SDS), 319
Sedation costs, 239
Serious adverse events (SAEs), 239, 240, 244
Seven S factor analysis, 280, 281
Shared decision making, 242

Shouldice Hospital, 87–90
    ambulation, 27
    archival data analysis, observation and interviews, 33
    backstage at, 40, 41, 48, 49
    caregivers, 65, 66
    care program, 37, 38
    challenges, 71–73
    chronic post-operative pain and complications, 69, 70
    clinical activity, 41
    conscious sedation, 38, 39
    continuous ambulation, 39, 40
    cross-functional relationships, 36
    customization, 78
    effectiveness, 31
    evolutionary history of hernia surgery, 29, 30
    focused factory, 32, 33
    follow-up interviews, 34
    frontstage, 40
    general anesthesia, 36
    hernia recurrence, 68, 69
    high-volume clinic, 40
    high volume of cases, 40
    immediate ambulation, 39, 40
    integrating culture, 83
    laparoscopic and mesh repairs, 25, 26
    leveraging value to patients, 77, 78
    Lichtenstein mesh technique, 31
    lifetime value, 82, 83
    local anesthesia, 36
    nonmesh repair, 30, 31
    open mesh, 31
    operating room
        motivating environment, 56–58
        post-operative length-of-stay, 55, 56
        service process flow, 53–55
        working as team, 52, 53
    operating strategy, 24, 52
    organizational culture, 24
    patient demand
        for hernia repairs, 73
        management, 78–81
    patient flow, 78–81
    patient-caregiver co-production, 81, 82
    patient-centered accountability, 58, 59
    patient-centered culture, 85
    patient-centered focus, 83–85
    patient value proposition, 25, 47, 48
    positioning, 76, 77
    pre-admission and investigation, 41–47
    preoperative to postoperative care, 36
    quadruple performance problem, 27, 28
    quality of care, 25
    results and performance, 31, 62, 66–68
    service concept, 51, 52
    service delivery system
        human resource investment in training, 61, 62
        organization structure and people management, 59, 60
        patient-centered facility, 62–65
        people and job design, 60, 61
    staff echoes and voices, 65, 66
    standardization, 78
    structured and unstructured interviews, 33
    supply-side competitive forces, 34–36
    surgery complexities, 31
    surgical training program, 31
    targeted patient segments, 49–51
    team-based culture, 85
    tier one patients, 74
    tier three patients, 75
    tier two patients, 75
    tier zero patients, 74
    value creation, 70, 71
    value innovation, 85, 86
Skull base surgery, 262, 269
Skyrocketing health care costs, 332
Stakeholder alignment, 335
Substance use disorder, 220
Surgical culture
    accountability, 141
    anesthesia group, 142
    care process, 142
    change management, 142, 143
    communication, 142
    front-line workers, 142
    informants, 139
    nurses as boundary spanners, 138
    organizational structures analysis, 140, 141
    physician of the day (POD), 137
    policy decisions, 138, 139
    qualitative interviews, 137
    Relational Coordination stakeholder map, 137
    relational mapping, 139, 140
    skill sets, 138
    stakeholder group, 137
Sweet spot analysis, 280
Synthetic opioids, 214

T
Team-based care
    chronic disease burden, 226
    co-location, 229

5-minute daily morning huddle, 229
four core principles, 228
four-stage office visit, 229–230
implementation, 231
medical assistants and nurses role, 230
patient experience, 234
pre-visit planning, 229
primary care delivery, 227
primary care setting, 226
provider and staff experience, 234
provider capacity, 232
role of good data, 227–228, 230–231
vs. traditional practice model, 233
Team-based models, 219
Team building, 258
Team performance, 287–288
Thyroid stimulating hormone (TSH), 336
Time driven activity-based costing (TDABC)
analysis, 301
accounting, 319
Total intravenous anesthesia techniques
(TIVA), 322
Traditional practice model, 233
Trend analysis, 339

U
Unpreventable cancellations, 345

V
Value-adding opportunity, 17
Value-based payment models, 227
Value driven outcomes (VDO) tools, 319
Value stream mapping (VSM), 116
Variable costs, 300
Varicocelectomy, 317, 320, 323

Vascular laboratory
cash inflows
cost of capital, 309
cost savings, 301–303
discounted cash flow analysis, 304–307
patient service revenue, 303, 304
patient volume, 306, 308
technician costs, 309
cash outflows, 300
direct labor time, 299
hospital acquisitions and affiliations, 295
image acquisition, management and
storage, 295, 296
incremental revenues/cost savings, 298
institution's financial status, 295
leadership, 297
metrics and impact assessment, 315
opportunity costs, 299
outpatient sites, 294
post study evaluation, 297
pre-study evaluation, 297
project team, process, and evolution,
312, 313
qualitative issues, 310, 311
results, 312–314
storage space, 299
storages discs, 299
sunk cost, 299
Vice President of Medical affairs
(VPMA), 183–184
Vizient annual rankings, 318

W
Webers' story, 332
Well-managed health care organization, *see*
Shouldice Hospital

Printed by Printforce, United Kingdom